CARDIOLOGY RESEARCH AND CLINICAL DEVELOPMENTS

MYOCARDIAL INFARCTIONS

RISK FACTORS, EMERGENCY MANAGEMENT AND LONG-TERM HEALTH OUTCOMES

CARDIOLOGY RESEARCH AND CLINICAL DEVELOPMENTS

Additional books in this series can be found on Nova's website under the Series tab.

Additional e-books in this series can be found on Nova's website under the e-book tab.

CARDIOLOGY RESEARCH AND CLINICAL DEVELOPMENTS

MYOCARDIAL INFARCTIONS

RISK FACTORS, EMERGENCY MANAGEMENT AND LONG-TERM HEALTH OUTCOMES

PATTIE WILKONSON
EDITOR

New York

Library of Congress Cataloging-in-Publication Data

ISBN: 978-1-63321-726-3

Library of Congress Control Number: 2014947412

Published by Nova Science Publishers, Inc. † New York

Contents

Preface

Acute myocardial infarction (AMI) is a major cause of morbidity and mortality. The almost exclusive cause of acute coronary syndromes (ACS), including unstable angina, AMI with or without ST-segment elevation, and sudden cardiac death is atherothrombosis. This book discusses risk factors, emergency management and long-term health outcomes of myocardial infarctions. Some of the topics discussed include MI and cardiogenic shock; risk of MI in the pathophysiology and treatment of prostatic diseases; albuminuria; essential roles of monocytes/macrophages in ACI; and management of unstable angina/non-ST segment MI.

Chapter 1 - Cardiogenic shock (CS) or acute systolic heart failure after myocardial infarction carries high mortality risk and remains a major medical challenge. Its incidence is about 10% in patients with ST-segment elevation myocardial infarction (STEMI) based on queries of almost 2 million patients from the 2003-2010 Nationwide Inpatient Sample databases. Compared with STEMI shock, NSTEMI shock was more likely in older and women patients; and in patients with diabetes mellitus, hypertension, previous heart failure, MI, or peripheral arterial disease; and who received coronary artery bypass grafting but less likely to have received percutaneous coronary intervention. The phosphaturic hormone fibroblast growth factor 23 (FGF-23) has been introduced as a novel biomarker for predictor for mortality in heart failure. In CS, a tremendous increase in FGF-23 occurs, and high levels of FGF-23 are associated with poor outcome. In patients with acute MI, new right bundle branch block on admission ECG is associated with the highest risk of CS development, frequent left main coronary artery affection, and unsuccessful revascularization. It is also an independent predictor of one-year mortality. The authors have witnessed evolution of modern therapy for acute MI and CS with heavy emphasis on early and aggressive revascularization therapy. For elderly population > 75 years-old, there was 50% reduction in hospital mortality (23% vs. 46%, $P < 0.001$) in the invasive strategy group, as reported by the Korea Acute Myocardial Infarction Registry. For patients who presented with acute right ventricular infarct and CS, without reperfusion therapy the in-hospital mortality was 80%, with thrombolytic therapy the mortality was 100%, and with primary percutaneous coronary intervention, the rate decreased to 44%. There was an increase in early mechanical revascularization (30.4% to 50.7%, $P <0.001$) and intra-aortic balloon pump (IABP) use (44.8% to 53.7%, $P<0.001$) in these patients over the 8-year period from 2003 to 2010. (2) However the large IABP-SHOCK II Trial did not demonstrate 30-day survival benefit in patients with acute MI who underwent PCI or coronary artery bypass surgery using with or without IABP support. IABP support did reduce 30-day mortality in the patients with shock due to ventricular septal rupture and acute mitral regurgitation complicating acute myocardial infarction. For patients in CS requiring emergent hemodynamic support, Percutaneous cardiac assist devices (pVAD) compared with surgical support (ECMO) alternative, pVAD therapy offers a less invasive alternative that can be deployed sooner, resulting in better outcomes, shorter LOS, lower costs and with no incremental cost, and a survival benefit. Early initiation of hemodynamic support prior to PCI with Impella 2.5 is associated with more complete revascularization and improved survival in the setting of refractory CS complicating an AMI. Finally, the mortality remains elevated in elderly patients (>75 year-old) with STEMI complicated by CS and treated by PCI at 30 days (39% vs 69%; P=.01) and 1 year (51% vs 79%; P<.001). compared with younger counterparts.

Chapter 2 - Optical coherence tomography (OCT) is a high-resolution intravascular imaging modality able to visualize the micro-environment of the atheromatic plaque and assess intracoronary stents in great detail. As a result, OCT is a valuable research tool for examining the role of morphological characteristics of atheromatic plaque in the progression of coronary artery disease and plaque destabilization, which lead to the clinical manifestation of acute coronary syndromes. Several OCT studies have focused on expanding the current understanding of the pathomechanisms of acute myocardial infarction. Moreover, as OCT is being increasingly used in clinical practice, potential clinical applications of OCT in myocardial infarction are emerging. Despite the lack of established indications for OCT imaging in myocardial infarction thus far, OCT could be potentially of assistance in interventional guidance in several clinical scenarios such as culprit lesion identification, assessment of the underlying mechanisms of stent thrombosis, and guidance of local and systematic antithrombotic therapy. The current chapter summarizes the pathophysiological insights obtained by OCT imaging in acute myocardial infarction, and critically reviews potential areas of clinical application of this imaging modality in myocardial infarction.

Chapter 3 - *Introduction:* according to the literature, psychosocial factors significantly contribute to both pathogenesis and expression of coronary artery disease (CAD). Depression, anxiety, anger and hostility, social isolation and stressful life-style represent the main contributing factors both to higher prevalence of unhealthy behaviors (poor diet, physical inactivity, alcohol use or smoking) and adverse pathophysiological mechanisms, such as neuroendocrine and platelet activation.

Material and method: over the past few decades, there has been an increasing interest in investigating the relationship between psychosocial risk factors and cardiovascular disease, leading to a growing pool of clinical and epidemiological data on the subject. Specifically, a large case–control trial, involving 52 countries, has identified nine potentially modifiable risk factors for CAD, among which psychosocial factors have been included and divided into two general categories: chronic stressors and emotional factors. These are believed to exacerbate the development of cardiovascular disease by two mechanisms: 1) encouraging unhealthy behaviors and increasing the non-compliance to treatments; and 2) eliciting physiological responses that may lead to insufficient oxygen delivery to the heart muscle, threatening heart rhythms, more vulnerable plaque, and the potential for blood clotting. Etiological controlled studies also confirmed this relationship.

In this work, the authors outline the psychosocial domains significantly considered associated with increased risk of cardiovascular morbidity and mortality. They also discuss critical pathophysiological mechanisms and pathways that, operating in a synergistic and integrative way, promote related clinical manifestations. Also, the impact of cardiac rehabilitation programs on psychological-related cardiovascular events is discussed.

Discussion: the importance of psychosocial variables in the development, clinical manifestations, and prognosis of patients with heart disease received increased attention in recent years. However, the influence of psychosocial risk factors in cardiovascular disease remains under-estimated when compared with the conventional ones. To recognize this relationship and to offers an important target for cardiovascular education, counseling and behavioral interventions, even after controlling for major risk factors. Cardiac rehabilitation programs considering a multidisciplinary approach are then widely recommended for the management of risk factors, nutritional, psychological, behavioral and social aspects potentially affecting patient outcomes.

Chapter 4 - Benign prostatic hyperplasia (BPH) and prostate cancer (PC) have shown an increased prevalence among elderly population in the last ten years leading to a significant deterioration in the quality of life and life span. BPH is a non-malignant adenofibromyomatous overgrowth of the periurethral portion of prostate gland that becomes clinically manifest through bladder outlet obstruction symptoms. PC is the most common malignancy in men and often shows an adenocarcinoma histology with symptoms such as hematuria and obstruct urine flow.

Pharmacological treatment of BPH includes α-adrenergic blockers and PDE-5 inhibitors though surgery is necessary if medical therapy fails or obstructive symptoms are impressive. Transurethral resection of the prostate (TURP) is the gold standard surgery for PBH; however open prostatectomy could also be considered as an option.

PC therapy is determined by PSA level, grade and stage of tumor, age and comorbidity. Generally, surgery or radiation therapy are preferred for localized cancer while hormonal therapy, radiation therapy or chemotherapy are utilized for symptomatic, advanced, and metastatic PC.

Particularly, in patients with a locally advanced tumor or metastases, androgen deprivation therapy (ADT) by bilateral orchiectomy or medical therapy with gonadotropin-releasing hormone (GnRH) agonists and antagonist are commonly utilized.

Recently, several studies exploring the relationship between cardiovascular (CV) risk and prostatic diseases have been published. In fact, there are some factors involved in the pathophysiology and treatment of prostatic diseases that may influence the establishment and progression of myocardial infarction (MI) in elderly patients with comorbidities.

First of all, perioperative and postoperative urological surgery are associated with cardiological complications as MI. Indeed, some studies showed an increase in MI-related mortality after TURP vs open prostatectomy. Furthermore, ADT (GnRH agonists and orchiectomy) induces a status of hypogonadism, which is related to adverse events as metabolic syndrome, diabetes and CV diseases. In fact, it has been demonstrated an increased risk of a CV events (coronary heart disease, MI and cardiac death) in PC patients treated with GnRH agonists. Besides, 6-months therapy with GnRH agonists is related to an earlier timing of fatal MI in elderly patients while GnRH antagonists administration decreases cardiac events (ischemic cerebrovascular diseases, MI, and other ischemic heart disease) in patients with preexisting CV disease during the first year of treatment compared to GnRH agonists.

Therefore, in this chapter the authors will analyze in detail the aforementioned data of the literature and they will discuss the CV, hormonal and metabolic factors involved in the development either of MI than prostatic disease. In particular, establishment of metabolic syndrome increases the estrogen-to-androgen ratio leading to sympathetic overactivity and influences the progression of BPH. Subsequently the authors will evaluate the surgical elements and the factors related to medical therapy for prostatic disease that are connected to myocardial damage.

Finally the authors will emphasize that in patients with prostatic disease is very important to evaluate pre-existing CV diseases and myocardial function and to strictly recommend a healthy lifestyle that includes a moderate and adequate exercise training associated to a balanced diet.

Chapter 5 - Background/Aims: Albuminuria is a marker of a cardiovascular morbimortality. The authors assessed the relationship between albuminuria, atrial fibrillation and mortality in a cohort of patients with acute myocardial infarction.

Methods: In the observational prospective study, the authors examined 636 consecutive patients with a diagnosis of acute myocardial infarction. Urine specimens were analyzed for albuminuria and were corrected with urinary creatinine to obtain a reliable estimate of Albumin/Creatinine rate. Albumin/Creatinine $\geq$30 mg/g^{-1} was considered abnormal. Association between Albumin/Creatinine, atrial fibrillation and mortality was assessed by multivariate analysis.

Results: The incidence of atrial fibrillation was 7.5% when Albumin/Creatinine was normal. When the albuminuria ranged from 30 to 300 mg.Cr^{-1}, the incidence of atrial fibrillation was 17.8%. Macroproteinuria (>300 mg.Cr^{-1}) was detected in 48 patients and the incidence of atrial fibrillation was 27%. In-hospital mortality was 42 (6.6%) and increased to 16.7% when macroalbuminuria was present. In a multivariate adjusted risk, Albumin/Creatinine $\geq$30 mg.Cr^{-1} (OR=1.8;1.1-2.9), previous coronary artery by-pass (OR=2;1.1-4) and chronic renal disease (OR=1.6;1-2.6) were independent prognostic factors for the incidence of atrial fibrillation. Albuminuria increased the model prediction (C-statistic analysis) for atrial fibrillation in 0.026. Neither albuminuria nor atrial fibrillation increased the model prediction for mortality. In a multivariate analysis for mortality, the most important prognostic factors were a Killip class>1 (OR=6;2.8-15) and initial or complicate Bundle Brunch Block (OR=3;1.5-6) on admission meanwhile a previous history of hypertension had a protective factor (OR=0.22; 011-0.45)(<0.001)

Conclusions: An early increase of albuminuria was associated with atrial instability but was not a marker for a poor in-hospital prognosis in patients with acute myocardial infarction.

Chapter 6 - Acute myocardial infarction (AMI) is one of the leading causes of death in the adult population. Myocardial ischemia/reperfusion (I/R) injury is an important complication of acute coronary arterial occlusion and subsequent recanalization, whether it is spontaneous or therapeutic. Following AMI, therapeutic coronary artery recanalization by thrombolytic therapy or percutaneous coronary intervention (PCI) is used to minimize infarct size. In most cases, the damaged structure can be repaired, and heart function can be restored to its basal level through reperfusion. However, in some instances, I/R exerts the opposite effect, not only failing to improve heart function but instead exacerbating cardiac function and worsening structural damage. Cellular damage after reperfusion of previously viable ischemic tissue is defined as I/R injury (IRI).

There is growing evidence that apoptosis plays a key role during myocardial I/R and much discussion has been undertaken to elucidate the detailed mechanisms, relevant gene expression, and signaling transduction pathways. Protection of cardiomyocytes from I/R induced cell death would in principle increase the viable myocardium, thus providing acute and chronic benefits after AMI. Therefore, cardiomyocyte apoptosis may be an excellent target for therapeutic modulation in the context of AMI and IRI. Drug pretreatment has been one of the main focus for ameliorating IRI.

Luteolin is a common flavonoid that exists in many types of plants, including fruits, vegetables and medicinal herbs. Preclinical studies have revealed the diverse beneficial effects of luteolin, such as cardiovascular protection, antioxidant, anti-inflammatory, antimicrobial, anticancer effects and other biological activities. Recent studies have suggested that administration of luteolin yields cardioprotective effects during I/R in rats. Pretreatment with luteolin can improve cardiomyocyte shortening amplitude, decrease the apoptosis rate, upregulate Bcl-2/Bax ratio under a simulated I/R condition. Moreover, luteolin pretreatment can activate multiple endogenous signaling pathways such as PI3K/Akt, JAK/STAT and MAPKs, which further protect the myocardium against IRI through different mechanisms. The aim of this chapter is to summarize luteolin's anti-apoptotic roles and mechanisms following I/R in rats, and luteolin may be a potential candidate for preventing and treating cardiovascular diseases.

Chapter 7 - Despite improvements in interventional and pharmacological therapy of acute coronary syndrome (ACS), it is still the leading cause of death.

Hence, there is a need for further development of effective therapeutic approaches. This requires better understanding of the molecular mechanisms and pathophysiology of the disease.

During the long-term process of initiation and progression of an atherosclerotic plaque, monocytes/macrophages plays a major role in this process. Macrophages, which are differentiated from circulating monocytes, give rise to foam cells by excessive accumulation of modified lipoproteins. Atherogenesis subsequently progress through necrotic core expansion associated with the death of macrophage, followed by the transition to vulnerable plaques.

The transition from stable atherosclerotic plaques to rupture of the atherosclerotic plaque, finally resulting in acute thrombus formation in ACS is the consequence of an inflammatory process. It is well recognized that plaque growth is not continuous and plaque rupture may suddenly occur during the acute inflammatory phase.

Here, the authors discuss the impact of monocytes/macrophages on both advanced plaque progression and onset of ACS, focusing on the potential targeting of inflammatory process in atherosclerosis.

Chapter 8 - Acute myocardial infarction (AMI) remains the leading cause of mortality in Western countries as well as in Asia. The remarkable progress achieved in the treatment of cardiovascular disease over the past few decades has resulted in decreased mortality worldwide. In particular, advances in intensive management in patients with AMI, such as the use of primary percutaneous coronary intervention (PCI) and development of coronary care units, have contributed to increases in in-hospital survival rates. However, increases in the rates of postinfarction morbidity and mortality are a growing problem, especially with respect to the frequency of admission for congestive heart failure.

AMI pathologically progresses in the coronary arteries in sequence from plaque formation to destabilization to rupture. A predisposition toward atherosclerosis and the effects of a hyperinflammatory state play important roles in the onset of AMI. In-hospital mortality due to AMI, particularly in cases of ST-segment elevation myocardial infarction, is primarily caused by arrhythmias, acute heart failure and/or cardiac rupture, whereas the severity of postinfarction complications depends on the magnitude of left ventricular remodeling, consequently resulting in a reduced left ventricular function.

In this chapter, the authors review the potentially predictive risk factors for long-term outcomes and suggest preventive measures at each stage: before a PCI-capable hospital, before primary PCI, during primary PCI, after primary PCI and before hospital discharge. Finally, they propose acute-phase strategies for improving long-term outcomes in patients with AMI.

Chapter 9 - Cardiogenic shock is a well-recognized leading cause of death in patients with an acute myocardial infarction even in the era of early prompt percutaneous coronary intervention (PCI). So far the intensive strategy such as an early use of mechanical circulatory support with PCI also failed to provide significant clinical benefits in those with a cardiogenic shock complicating acute myocardial infarction. As one of the main considerations, systemic mal-perfusion and also high incidence of failed myocardial tissue-level reperfusion may have a critical role in the fatal pathogenesis of a cardiogenic shock complicating acute myocardial infarction. Recently the authors found an association of exaggerated inflammation with systemic and myocardial tissue-level mal-perfusion in patients treated with PCI for a cardiogenic shock complicating acute myocardial infarction. Here they present an overview of critical issues and then think of the best challenges to provide better clinical outcomes in patients with a cardiogenic shock complicating acute myocardial infarction.

Chapter 10 - Unstable angina is a classification of acute coronary syndrome (ACS). Indeed, ACS spans the spectrum of unstable angina, non-ST segment myocardial infarction, and ST segment elevation myocardial infarction. Millions of Americans present to medical care professionals with unstable angina. While the disease process and treatment varies with ACS presentation and degree of injury, there are certain characteristics that are common to each clinical scenario. A through history and physical examination, diagnostics including electrocardiogram, and biochemical markers help to establish the diagnosis and degree of ACS. By determining the extent of injury to a patient, physicians are able to guide appropriate treatment goals based on risk/benefit ratio. Medical treatment includes anti-ischemic, antiplatelet, antianginal, and statin therapies. Finally, invasive measures including revascularization plays a prominent role in treating unstable angina. Beyond revascularization, cardiac rehabilitation is increasingly recognized in treating patients who present with unstable angina.

In: Myocardial Infarctions
Editor: Pattie Wilkonson

ISBN: 978-1-63321-726-3

Chapter 1

Myocardial Infarction and Cardiogenic Shock

Denise M. Zingrone, D.O., FACC and David H. Hsi*, MD, FACC, FASE
Deborah Heart and Lung Center, Browns Mills, New Jersey, US

Abstract

Cardiogenic shock (CS) or acute systolic heart failure after myocardial infarction carries high mortality risk and remains a major medical challenge. Its incidence is about 10% in patients with ST-segment elevation myocardial infarction (STEMI) based on queries of almost 2 million patients from the 2003-2010 Nationwide Inpatient Sample databases. [1] Compared with STEMI shock, NSTEMI shock was more likely in older and women patients; and in patients with diabetes mellitus, hypertension, previous heart failure, MI, or peripheral arterial disease; and who received coronary artery bypass grafting but less likely to have received percutaneous coronary intervention. [2] The phosphaturic hormone fibroblast growth factor 23 (FGF-23) has been introduced as a novel biomarker for predictor for mortality in heart failure. In CS, a tremendous increase in FGF-23 occurs, and high levels of FGF-23 are associated with poor outcome. [3] In patients with acute MI, new right bundle branch block on admission ECG is associated with the highest risk of CS development, frequent left main coronary artery affection, and unsuccessful revascularization. It is also an independent predictor of one-year mortality. [4] We have witnessed evolution of modern therapy for acute MI and CS with heavy emphasis on early and aggressive revascularization therapy. For elderly population > 75 years-old, there was 50% reduction in hospital mortality (23% vs. 46%, $P < 0.001$) in the invasive strategy group, as reported by the Korea Acute Myocardial Infarction Registry. [5] For patients who presented with acute right ventricular infarct and CS, without reperfusion therapy the in-hospital mortality was 80%, with thrombolytic therapy the mortality was 100%, and with primary percutaneous coronary intervention, the rate decreased to 44%. [6] There was an increase in early mechanical revascularization (30.4% to 50.7%, $P <0.001$) and intra-aortic balloon pump (IABP) use (44.8% to 53.7%,

* Corresponding Author: David H. Hsi, MD, FACC, FASE; Email: davidhsi.md@gmail.com.

P<0.001) in these patients over the 8-year period from 2003 to 2010. (2) However the large IABP-SHOCK II Trial did not demonstrate 30-day survival benefit in patients with acute MI who underwent PCI or coronary artery bypass surgery using with or without IABP support. [7] IABP support did reduce 30-day mortality in the patients with shock due to ventricular septal rupture and acute mitral regurgitation complicating acute myocardial infarction. [8] For patients in CS requiring emergent hemodynamic support, Percutaneous cardiac assist devices (pVAD) compared with surgical support (ECMO) alternative, pVAD therapy offers a less invasive alternative that can be deployed sooner, resulting in better outcomes, shorter LOS, lower costs and with no incremental cost, and a survival benefit [9] Early initiation of hemodynamic support prior to PCI with Impella 2.5 is associated with more complete revascularization and improved survival in the setting of refractory CS complicating an AMI. [10] Finally, the mortality remains elevated in elderly patients (>75 year-old) with STEMI complicated by CS and treated by PCI at 30 days (39% vs 69%; P=.01) and 1 year (51% vs 79%; P<.001). compared with younger counterparts. [11]

References

[1] Kolte D, Khera S, Aronow WSJ, et al: Trends in incidence, management, and outcomes of cardiogenic shock complicating ST-elevation myocardial infarction in the United States. *Am Heart Assoc.* 2014 Jan 13;3(1):e000590.

[2] Anderson ML, Peterson ED, Peng SA, et al: Differences in the profile, treatment, and prognosis of patients with cardiogenic shock by myocardial infarction classification: A report from NCDR. *Circ Cardiovasc Qual Outcomes.* 2013 Nov;6(6):708-15.

[3] Janine Pöss, Felix Mahfoud, Sarah Seiler, et al: FGF-23 is associated with increased disease severity and early mortality in cardiogenic shock. European Heart Journal: Acute Cardiovascular Care September 2013 2: 211-218,

[4] Jakl M, Stasek J, Kala P, et al: Acute myocardial infarction complicated by shock: outcome analysis based on initial electrocardiogram. *Scand Cardiovasc J.* 2014 Feb;48(1):13-9.

[5] Yoo YP and Korean Acute Myocardial Infarction Registry Investigators. *J Geriatr Cardiol.* 2013 Sep;10(3):235-41

[6] Lupi-Herrera E, González-Pacheco H, Juárez-Herrera U, et al: Primary reperfusion in acute right ventricular infarction: An observational study. *World J Cardiol.* 2014 Jan 26;6(1):14-22.

[7] Thiele H and the IABP-SHOCK II Trial Investigators: Intraaortic Balloon Support for Myocardial Infarction with Cardiogenic Shock *N Engl J Med* 2012; 367:1287-1296 October 4, 2012

[8] Kettner J, Sramko M, Holek M, Pirk J, Kautzner J. Utility of intra-aortic balloon pump support for ventricular septal rupture and acute mitral regurgitation complicating acute myocardial infarction. *Am J Cardiol.* 2013 Dec 1;112(11):1709-13.

[9] Maini B, Gregory D, Scotti DJ, Buyantseva L. Percutaneous cardiac assist devices compared with surgical hemodynamic support alternatives: cost-effectiveness in the emergent setting. *Catheter Cardiovasc Interv.* 2013 Oct 15.

[10] O'Neill WW, Schreiber T, Wohns DH, et al: The Current Use of Impella 2.5 in Acute Myocardial Infarction Complicated by Cardiogenic Shock: Results from the USpella Registry. *J Interv Cardiol.* 2014 Feb;27(1):1-11.

[11] De Felice F1, Guerra E, Fiorilli R, et al: One-year clinical outcome of elderly patients undergoing angioplasty for ST-elevation myocardial infarction complicated by cardiogenic shock: the importance of 3-vessel disease and final TIMI-3 flow grade. *J Invasive Cardiol.* 2014 Mar;26(3):114-8.

Cardiogenic shock is the leading cause of death among hospitalized patients after a myocardial infarction. Recent guidelines focus on timely recognition and initiation of rapid therapy. The cornerstone of treatment is early coronary revascularization to correct underling ischemia. This chapter focuses on cardiogenic shock as a complication of myocardial infarction and aims to review the recent updates and relevant data related to guideline recommendations.

Definition

Cardiogenic shock (CS) is a critical condition characterized by inadequate systemic perfusion resulting from decreased cardiac output. The most common etiology occurs in the setting of an acute myocardial infarction. Clinically, the patient presents with signs and symptoms of diminished cardiac output. The most notable features are poor mentation, oliguria, metabolic acidosis, and cold mottled extremities. Classically, CS is defined by persistent hypotension (<90mmHg) in the presence of adequate intravascular volume. Reduced cardiac index (<2.2 L/min/m2) will predispose to poor tissue perfusion and acidosis, and an elevated pulmonary capillary wedge pressure (>15 mmHg) will lead to pulmonary congestion and hypoxia.

Hemodynamic evaluation is not only paramount in aiding the rapid diagnosis of cardiogenic shock, but also serves as an objective means to guide and tailor therapeutics. Hemodynamic parameters obtained from either the insertion of a pulmonary artery (PA) catheter or from a carefully performed transthoracic echocardiography and Doppler can aid the clinicians in rapid diagnosis and management. PA catheters are able to be inserted at the bedside by a skilled physician. However, as with any invasive procedure there are well-documented risks associated with insertion. Also, if proper care is not taken in interpretation and maintenance, the information received may not be truly reflective of the hemodynamic profile. Doppler echocardiography is an alternative noninvasive means for gathering the hemodynamic assessments. A clinician trained in this modality is able to obtain an estimate of right atrial pressures, PA systolic, diastolic and mean pressures, and an assessment of cardiac output (CO), cardiac index (CI) and left ventricular end-diastolic pressure (LVEDP). Patient positioning and body habitus may impair the ability to image the necessary parameters.

Incidence

Cardiogenic shock or acute systolic failure after myocardial infarction portends a high mortality risk and remains a major medical challenge. According to the 2003-2010 Nationwide Inpatient Sample database, 7.9% of patients with STEMI were complicated by CS. [1] Interestingly, an increase in early revascularization and intra-aortic balloon pump counter-pulsation did not affect the numbers of those diagnosed. Despite increasing incidence over this eight year period, the database did report decreasing in-hospital mortality from 44.6% to 33.8% [1]. There was no appreciable difference in mortality rates when subgroups were compared, particularly in patients <75 years of age and >75 years of age, and between the opposite sexes.

Non-ST segment elevation myocardial infarction (NSTEMI) patients may also present with CS, although less likely than with ST segment elevation myocardial infarction (STEMI). Compared with their STEMI counterparts, NSTEMI patients with shock were more likely to be older and female. They are also more likely to have diabetes mellitus, hypertension, and prior history of MI, heart failure or evidence of peripheral arterial disease. One study comparing differences between STEMI and NSTEMI patients form 2007-2011 found that cardiogenic shock with NSTEMI carried a higher mortality (40.8% shock vs. 2.3% no shock) than with STEMI patients (33.1% shock vs. 2.0% no shock). [2] This may be attributed to the fact that NSTEMI patients with shock had longer delays to revascularization seen both with PCI as well as CABG.

While heightened awareness allows early and more accurate diagnosis, the true incidence and prevalence will always be difficult to accurately measure due to patients dying prior to hospital arrival. As recent guidelines and evidence based medicine continue to recommend and emphasize a more aggressive and early PCI based treatment strategy, the incidence of shock complicating myocardial infarction will hopefully improve.

Although the purpose of the chapter is to review and examine cardiogenic shock secondary to myocardial infarctions, it is important to note other etiologies may develop CS as well. It is important to consider and exclude other diagnoses if a patient presents with cardiogenic shock and an acute coronary syndrome has been ruled out. Table 1 presents the other etiologics of cardiogenic shock.

Table 1. Differential Diagnosis of Cardiogenic Shock

Myocarditis
Sepsis with Underlying Cardiomyopathy
Myocardial Contusion and Trauma
Prolonged Cardiopulmonary Bypass
Intractable Ventricular Dysrhythmias
Acute Mitral Regurgitation
Acute Aortic Regurgitation
Hypertrophic Obstructive Cardiomyopathy
Massive Pulmonary Embolism
Acute Aortic Dissection

Pathophysiology

Cardiogenic shock is characterized by both systolic and diastolic dysfunction. When the ejection fraction is depressed there are several compensatory reflexes activated. Neurohormonal activation results in tachycardia, vasoconstriction, and sodium and fluid retention. The end result is increased decreased ventricular compliance, increased oxygen demand, and ongoing ischemia. Figure 1 outlines the progressive spiral which occurs.

Evidence of a systemic inflammatory response (SIR) cascade is seen in many patients with cardiogenic shock similar to what is witnessed in sepsis or trauma. CS patients with the SIR syndrome often have low systemic vascular resistance. Overproduction of nitric oxide has been postulated to be the etiology for this response. Other markers of inflammation in CS include the cytokine interleukin-6 and tumor necrosis factor alpha. Both of these mediators may further reduce myocardial function. [3]

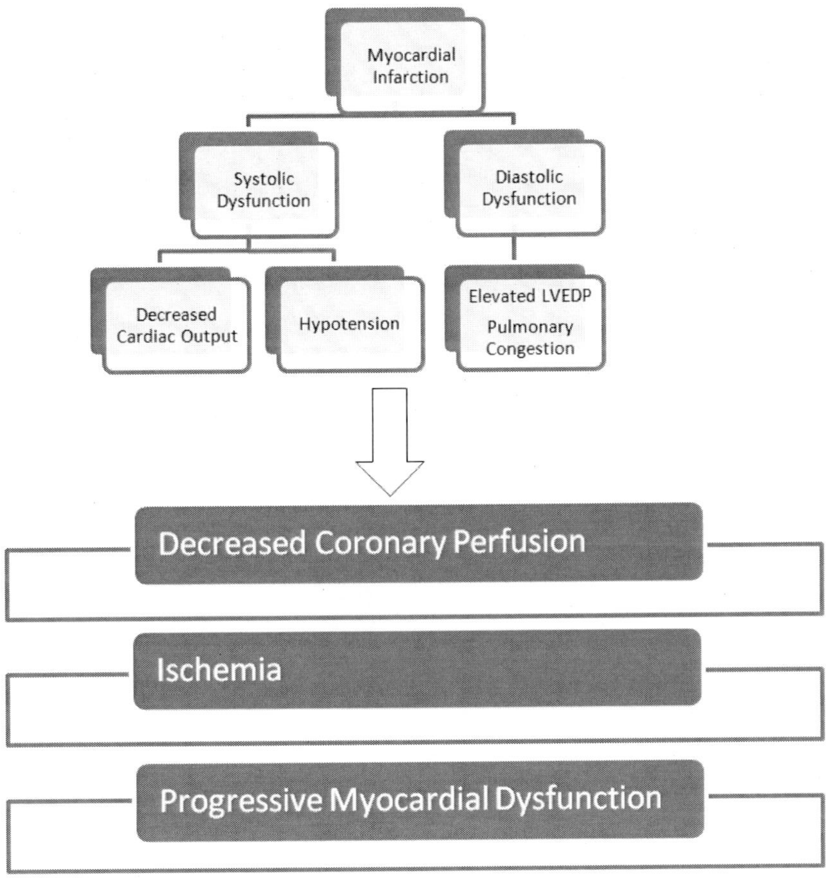

Figure 1. Pathophysiology of Cardiogenic Shock.

Risk Stratification

Mortality from cardiogenic shock remains high at approximately 50%. Therefore, it is imperative to stratify all patients presenting with an acute infarct to attempt to identify which individuals may deteriorate. Traditional risk factors which have been shown to predict increased mortality include advanced age, cerebral hypoxia, low left ventricular ejection fraction (LVEF), and delay of revascularization. With increasing delay between symptom onset and admission, the risk of development of cardiogenic shock increases. In the one German percutaneous coronary intervention (PCI) registry, patients presenting later than 6-12 hours after symptom onset had a 25% higher in-hospital mortality compared to patients who presented earlier. [4]

CS is a systemic condition associated with the release of a cascade of inflammatory markers. Novel biomarkers are under investigation not only as a potential line of therapeutics, but to also aid in risk stratification. One of the novel biomarkers currently under investigation is phosphaturic hormone fibroblast growth factor 23 (FGF-23). This recently has been introduced as a predictor of mortality in patients with chronic systolic heart failure. FGF-23 was measured in 51 patients with CS, 18 patients with uncomplicated MI, and 940 patients undergoing elective PCI for stable CAD. FGF-23 was found to be elevated in the patients with CS but not with uncomplicated MI or with stable CAD. Furthermore, the CS patients were categorized according to survival. CS patients who died had much higher levels than the CS patients who lived. [5]

The admission electrocardiogram (ECG) has not only diagnostic importance but also imparts prognostic information. Stasek et.al reported on the relationship between the initial ECG, presence of risk factors, angiography results and outcomes in patients with AMI and CS. Data from 5572 patients were analyzed over a three year period. Patients were divided into four groups based on presenting ECG: ST-segment elevation, bundle branch block (BBB), ST segment depression, and other ECG findings of acute MI. Cardiogenic shock developed most frequently among patients with BBB. The risk of CS progression was similar in individuals with (Left) LBBB and (Right) RBBB. However, the one year mortality was highest among patients with RBBB (66.7% vs. 48.6% with LBBB). Also, RBBB patients were associated with higher rates of left main coronary stenosis and unsuccessful revascularization. [6]

Etiology

The most common cause of cardiogenic shock is extensive myocardial infarction which compromises a critical mass of the left ventricle. In the SHOCK (Should we emergently revascularize Occluded Coronary arteries for Shock) trial registry, 55% of infarctions were anterior, 46% inferior, 21% were posterior, and 50% were in several locations. [7] While one usually associates a large infarct with the development of shock, it is important to emphasize that the presence of a relatively small infarct in a patient with a concominent cardiomyopathy may precipitate the systemic hypotension and end organ hypoperfusion.

Characteristics which increase the likelihood of developing cardiogenic shock in the setting of an infarct include advanced age, associated diabetes and hypertension, diminished ejection fraction, and the presence of new left bundle branch block. [8] Cardiogenic shock that has a delayed onset may result from infarct extension, occlusion of a previously patent artery, or development of left ventricular dysfunction form viable but hibernating myocardium.

Angiography most often demonstrates the presence of multi-vessel coronary disease. The SHOCK trial registry reports left main occlusion in 29 % of patients, triple vessel disease in 58%, two-vessel disease in 20%, and single vessel occlusion in 22% of afflicted individuals. [7] Theses angiographic findings demonstrate a key concept in the pathophysiology of shock. Compensatory hyperkinesis develops normally in myocardial segments not involved in an acute infarct. This serves to maintain the stroke volume and cardiac output of the left ventricle. Failure to promote this compensatory response due to multivessel disease is a key risk factor in developing CS.

Mechanical Complications of Myocardial Infarction

While MI with LV impairment is the most common predictor of developing cardiogenic shock, there are several other mechanical complications which may occur. Acute severe mitral regurgitation, interventricular septal rupture, and left ventricular free wall rupture all present dramatically and lead to fulminate cardiogenic shock and death if not quickly appreciated and treated. In the SHOCK registry the vast majority had predominately left ventricular failure. However, 8.3% had mitral regurgitation, 4.6% had VSR, 3.4% had isolated RV failure, and 1.7% had free wall rupture and tamponade[7].

The clinician must have a high index of suspicion and act rapidly to avoid the significant mortality associated with these complications. Echocardiography should be performed to confirm their presence. Ventricular septal rupture (VSR) carries the worst prognosis and highest mortality of 85%. VSR almost always occurs within days of the acute infarct and is more common in patients with hypertension. This condition presents abruptly with systemic hypotension. A new pansystolic murmur and thrill may be appreciated during physical exam. The classic finding is a "step-up" in oxygen saturation from the right atrium to the right ventricle as a result of the VSR.

Echocardiography is essential in confirming the diagnosis. Often on 2D imaging the exact rupture location is difficult to isolate as many VSRs present as a serpiginous tract rather than a discrete lesion. This is particularly true if an inferior infarction is associated with a VSR. Inferior wall infarcts may cause rupture of the basal inferior septum. These ruptures are particularly challenging for the surgeon as well as have a much worse prognosis than VSRs related to anterior wall infarcts. Anterior wall infarcts will cause rupture in the apical septum. Figure 2 and 3 depicts a VSR with left to right shunting.

Acute severe mitral regurgitation after inferior wall myocardial infarction may result from either transient ischemia or infarction of the papillary muscle. The posteromedial papillary muscle has a single blood supply from the posterior descending artery as opposed to the anterolateral papillary which has a dual supply from the left anterior descending and circumflex. Acute mitral regurgitation presents approximately four to seven days after infarct with acute pulmonary edema, hypotension and shock. Patients with this condition are unable to lay flay due to the increased in pulmonary capillary wedge pressure. A murmur may not be appreciated at the bedside and should not rule out the presence of significant regurgitation. There is rapid equalization of pressures in the left atrium and ventricle which accounts for a soft or absent murmur. A precordial thrill is not observed and is a useful diagnostic tool for distinguishing between VSR and acute MR.

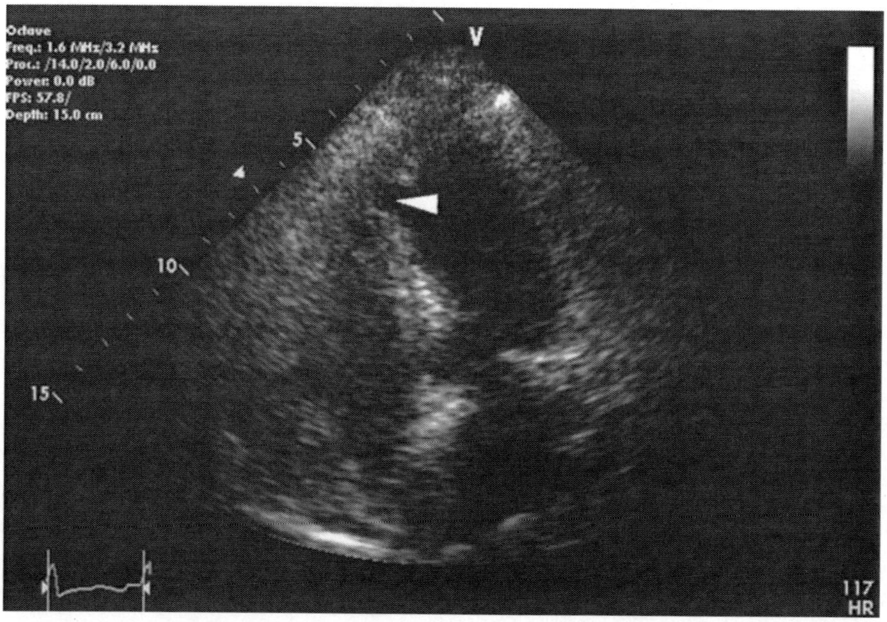

Figure 2. Ventricular Septal Rupture (arrowhead).

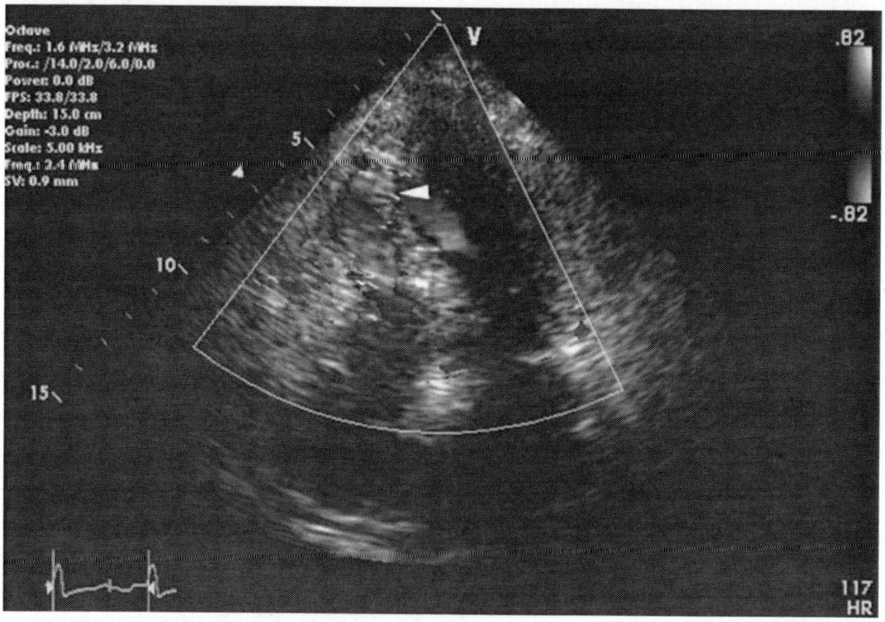

Figure 3. VSR with evidence of LV to RV shunting (arrowhead).

Transthoracic echo may also frequently miss acute severe MR due to the rapid pressure equalization. Therefore, if one considers acute severe MR as an etiology for CS, TEE is the preferred modality to assess the mitral valve in this setting. Figure 4 and 5 is a TEE of severe MR due to flail posterior leaflet.

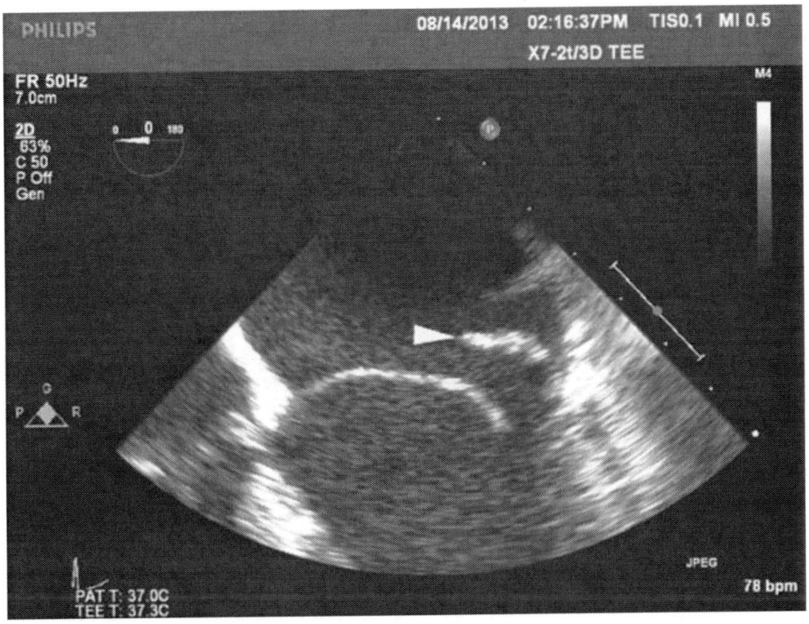

Figure 4. TEE with flail posterior leaflet (arrowhead).

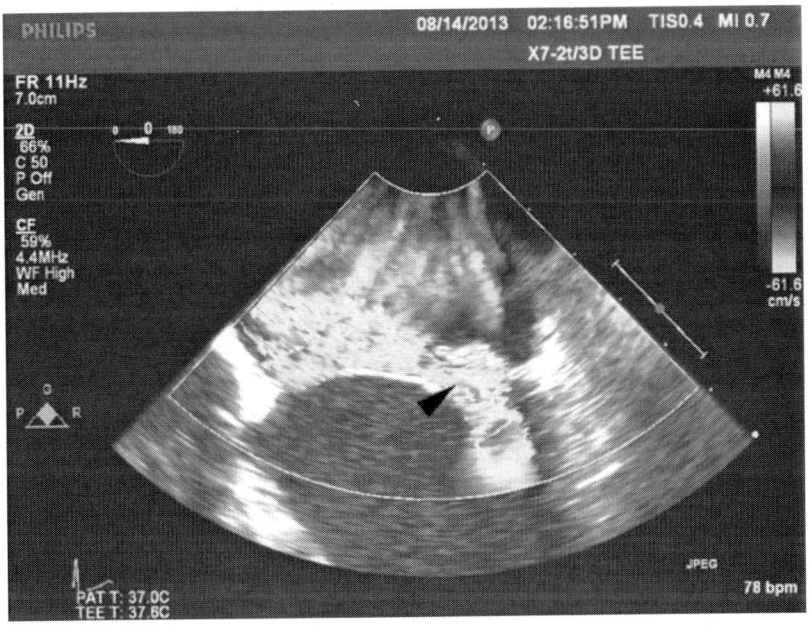

Figure 5. TEE of Severe MR (arrowhead).

Rupture of the myocardial free wall usually presents either with sudden death or with pericardial tamponade (Fig 6). The typical patient is elderly, female, and hypertensive. Other significant risk factors for this condition include the use of steroids, nonsteroidals, and anticoagulants.

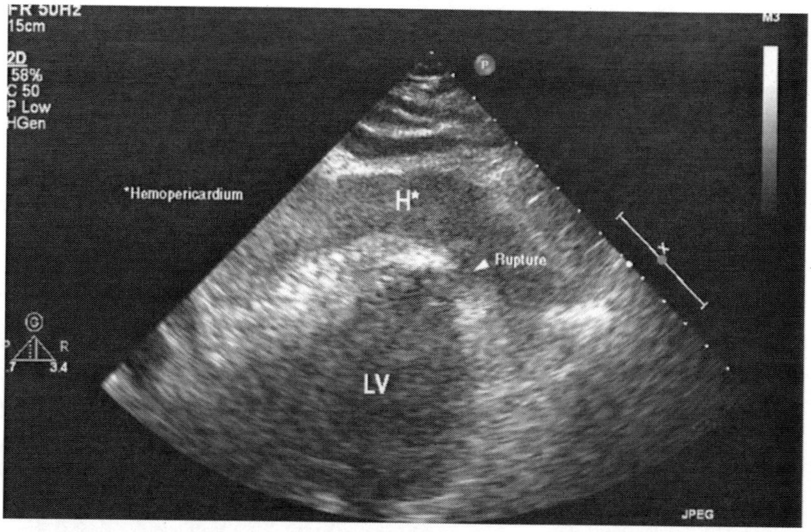

Figure 6. Left Ventricular Free Wall Rupture.

In cases of acute severe MR and ventricular free wall rupture, immediate surgical revascularization along with repair of the exacerbating condition is the preferred treatment option. Often an IABP is necessary for acute stabilization. There is controversy currently on the optimal timing of surgical repair of a VSR, particularly if the patient is stable. If the VSD is associated with an inferior wall infarct, theses lesions are extremely challenging to repair surgically and carry a high operative risk.

Right Ventricle and Cardiogenic Shock

The right ventricle (RV) plays a key role in the development and progression of CS. While isolated RV shock represents only 4% of cases of CS complicating MI, the mortality rate is nearly as high as (left ventricular) LV shock. [9] Therefore it is imperative that one treats isolated RV dysfunction and ischemia as aggressively as they would LV impairment. RV dysfunction limits left ventricular preload and ultimately cardiac output. Initial treatment focuses on volume resuscitation. However, volume should be administered judiciously and should not be infused if no improvement in blood pressure and cardiac output are seen. Forcing volume into an ischemic, noncompliant right ventricle results in shifting of the interventricular septum toward the LV cavity, further impacting the function of the LV. Inotropic therapy is more effective in maintaining the cardiac output. Also, RV infarcts are associated with conduction disturbances. Therefore, maintaining adequate ventricular rate with the placement of a transvenous pacer will improve hemodynamics in the presence of high-grade atrial-ventricular block. Finally, if the patient still has hemodynamic compromise, placement of an intra-aortic balloon pump (IABP) may be needed to improve coronary perfusion and decrease wall stress associated with ischemia.

A noncompliant, ischemic right ventricle elevates the right ventricular end diastolic pressure and right atrial pressure. If a patient has a patent foramen ovale (PFO) this increased pressure may result in right to left shunting through PFO. This condition should be considered and investigated with a transthoracic echo or TEE especially if the patient remains hypoxic despite aggressive measures.

Isolated RV infarcts should be treated as aggressively as LV infarcts due to the high mortality rate observed. An observational study investigated the impact of primary reperfusion therapy on early and late mortality in acute right ventricular infarction. These patients were classified as with or without RV failure and with cardiogenic shock. For patients who presented with acute right ventricular infarct and CS, without any reperfusion strategy the mortality was 80%. When thrombolytics were administered the mortality rate was 100% and with primary PCI the rate decreased to 44%. [10] This data highlights the importance of aggressive, early revascularization for isolated RV infarcts complicated by cardiogenic shock.

Pharmacologic Agents

Early revascularization is the cornerstone of treatment for CS complicated by an acute myocardial infarction. Antithrombotic agents and anticoagulants should be used as recommended in the American College of Cardiology (ACC)/American Heart Association (AHA) guidelines for STEMI and NSTEMI as adjunct therapy for primary PCI.

Cardiac medications which are traditionally recommended for systolic congestive heart failure and for uncomplicated myocardial infarction should be withheld during CS. Beta blockers should be avoided as they may blunt the patient's ability to maintain their cardiac output in the setting of a limited stroke volume. Angiotensin converting enzyme inhibitors (ACEI) and angiotensin receptor blockers (ARBs) should be avoided during cardiogenic shock. Intravenous nitroglycerin should be used with caution when shock is complicated by right ventricular infarcts.

Inotropic and vasopressor agents are important in the initial management of CS patients. Their role is to improve and maintain systolic blood pressure and augment cardiac index while definitive therapy is being pursued. Inotropic agents increase myocardial contractility, increase heart rate, and cause either vasodilatation or constriction depending on the agent utilized. Dobutamine, a selective beta 1-adrenergic receptor agonist can improve myocardial contractility and increase cardiac output. However, Dobutamine may exacerbate hypotension and can precipitate tachyarrhythmias which could worsen underlying ischemia. It is not recommended for use when systolic blood pressure is less than 80 mmHg. Dopamine acts directly on myocardial beta-1 adrenergic receptors and indirectly releases norepinephrine. It has both inotropic and vasopressor effects. Tachycardia and increased peripheral resistance with administration may again exacerbate coronary ischemia.

Norepinephrine is the agent recommended by the ACC/AHA for use with severe hypotension. Norepinephrine is a potent catecholamine with both alpha and beta-1 adrenergic effects. In general, any inotropic agents should be used for as short a time as possible and their use is often limited by precipitating dysrhythmias.

Revascularization

There has been an evolution of modern therapy for acute MI with cardiogenic shock. Early and aggressive revascularization with primary PCI is the preferred treatment strategy for those affected. The current guidelines recommend immediate stabilization and transfer to a PCI-capable facility. The SHOCK trial demonstrated a 13% absolute increase in one year survival if early PCI was undertaken and successful as compared to initial medical stabilization. While the trial suggested lowest mortality was seen when intervention was performed between 0-6 hours after symptom onset, there was still a survival benefit as long as 48 hours from MI and 18 hours after shock onset[7].

Historically, the elderly population (>75 years old) with cardiogenic shock and MI has presented a challenge to the treating cardiologist. Often, these individuals have concominent comorbidities which delayed physicians from recommending an invasive strategy. However, there is recent evidence which strongly implies this population derives mortality benefit from early revascularization. Data from a registry of 166 elderly CS STEMI patients from 2008-2011 was analyzed. This registry found fewer in-hospital deaths and improved one year survival in the early revascularization group[10]. Therefore, unless strong contraindications exist the elderly should be referred for urgent revascularization.

Early revascularization via primary PCI with stenting is the preferred strategy for patients presenting with an acute infarct and CS. However, challenges arise when multivessel coronary disease is found or when left main coronary stenosis is encountered. Meta-analysis of SHOCK registry and US National Registry of Myocardial Infarction attempted to compare outcomes between PCI vs. coronary artery bypass graft (CABG) surgery in the setting of cardiogenic shock. In-hospital mortality in patients was comparable for single vessel disease between the PCI and CABG groups (33.3% CABG vs. 32.9% PCI). However, mortality rates were lower for the CABG group in patients with two and three vessel disease (29.6% CABG vs. 54.9% PCI). [11]

Multivessel PCI in cardiogenic shock was reexamined in a 2012 registry where there is now more widespread usage of coronary stents and glycoprotein IIb-IIIa inhibitors which were limited in the SHOCK registry. The Euro Heart Survey PCI registry evaluated patients with CS and multivessel PCI vs. single vessel infarct related artery PCI. [12] There was no significant mortality benefits noted between the two groups; therefore PCI of non-infarct related arteries in the setting of MI with cardiogenic shock does not seem to have a survival benefit.

As previously stated, left main stenosis is discovered in approximately 29% of patients with MI and CS. The vast majority of these stenoses are not protected by prior bypass with either a mammary artery or saphenous vein graft. Information from the GRACE trial (Global Registry of Acute Coronary Events) examined 8 years of follow up date on 1799 patients requiring unprotected left main revascularization in the setting of a myocardial infarction. This reveals similar survival rates between PCI and CABG in these high risk patients. PCI patients did have a need for further repeat revascularizations but the patients undergoing

CABG had a higher incidence of stroke. [13] Based on this analysis, PCI is currently recommended for unprotected critical left main stenosis in an acute MI and CS.

Mechanical Cardiac Support

Intra-aortic balloon pump (IABP) counterpulsation is a widely available means of providing hemodynamic support in a critically ill patient. Clinicians insert IABPs for the benefits of augmenting coronary perfusion and decreasing afterload and ultimately left ventricular stress. The original SHOCK registry suggested there may be benefit in IABP counterpulsation in the setting of CS with MI. GUSTO-1 (Global Utilization of Steptokinase and Tissue Plasminogen Activator for Occluded Coronary Arteries) trial also reported that IABP use was associated with a trend toward lower 30 day and one year mortality rates in patients who presented in CS complicating an AMI. [14] Critics stated the benefit seen was not related to use of an IABP, but due to significant differences in revascularization rates.

Intraaortic Balloon Support for Myocardial Infarction with Cardiogenic Shock (IABP-SHOCK II) conducted a randomized, prospective, multi-center trial which concluded the use of an IABP did not significantly reduce 30 day mortality compared with the best available medical therapy alone in patients with myocardial infarction and CS in whom early revascularization was performed. 95.8% of all patients underwent primary PCI as treatment for their infarct and 3.5% of patient required emergent CABG. At 30 days 39.7% of patients in the IABP group had died compared to 41.3% of patients in the control group. [15] Also, there were no significant differences between the groups in the secondary end-points as well as no significant differences in the adverse events.

The results of the IABP-SHOCK II trial did not address the use of IABP for ventricular septal rupture and acute severe mitral regurgitation complicating acute myocardial infarction. Kettner et al. retrospectively examined the effect of IABP use on 30 day survival in patients with post infarction VSD or acute mitral regurgitation who develop cardiogenic shock. [16] IABP was inserted in 83% of patients with shock and 57% of those without shock. Their results revealed a 30 day mortality benefit in IABP use in those patients with shock (61% vs. 100%). There was no mortality benefit for using IABP in patients with rupture associated with their MI who do not present in fulminate cardiogenic shock. IABP should be reserved as a temporizing measure while surgical consultation is obtained.

In acute cardiogenic shock, ventricular assist devices (VADs) are another means of providing circulatory support for the failing ventricle. While first utilized in the surgical setting as either a bridge to transplant or as destination therapy, percutaneous assist devices are now able to be placed emergently by the interventional cardiologist. The Tandem Heart removes blood from the left atrium by means of a catheter that is placed after a transeptal puncture. The blood is returned to the circulation through the femoral artery by a centrifugal pump.

IABP vs. Tandem Heart percutaneous VAD (pVAD) was compared in a small trial of cardiogenic shock patients with myocardial infarction. Revascularization was 100% in both cohorts. While mortality rates between the two groups was not significantly different, the hemodynamic profile was improved with the group receiving pVAD as were the rates of limb ischemia. [17] There is no mortality benefit to inserting the Tandem Heart pVAD to the IABP in this population of patients.

Another commonly utilized (pVAD available is the IMPELLA (figure 7). This is inserted with a smaller size sheath into the femoral artery and the rotary pump motor is positioned across the aortic valve. It provides flow of up to 2.5 L/min by aspirating blood from the left ventricle and ejecting it into the aorta. As with the Tandem Heart pVAD, the IMPELLA does not add any mortality benefit in cardiogenic shock when compared to IABP counter-pulsation. [18]

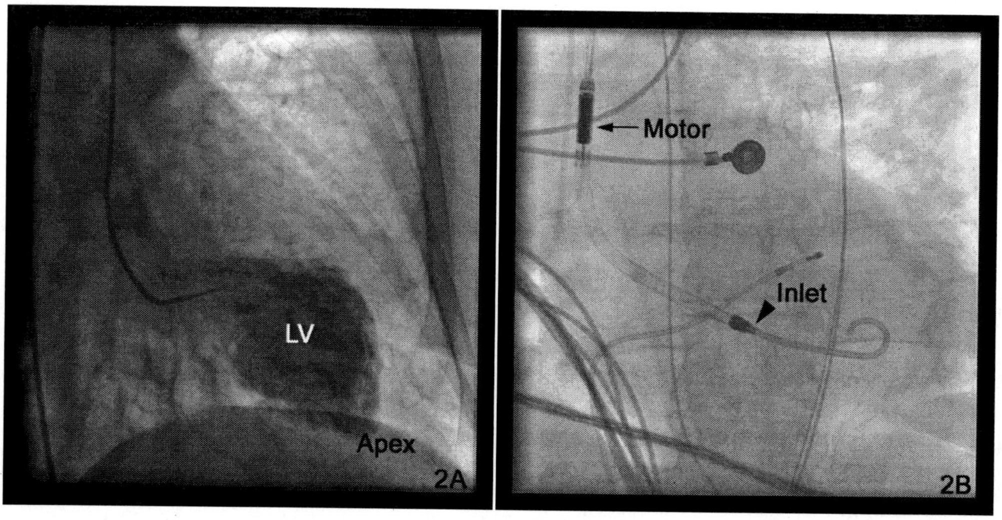

Figure 7. IMPELLA.

Recently a study examined outcomes of patients with CS utilizing IMPELLA prior to initiation of PCI. The investigators studied 154 patients who underwent PCI and IMPELLA 2.5 support from 38 US centers. The primary end-point was survival to discharge and secondary end-points included hemodynamic assessments and complications. Patients who had IMPELLA placed prior to their PCI had a better survival to discharge than patients in whom IMPELLA was placed post PCI (65.1% vs. 40.7%). [19] Complication rates were similar between the two groups. The favorable results were thought to be due to more complete revascularization in the setting of refractory CS when IMPELLA was placed early.

Extracorporeal membrane oxygenation (ECMO) is an invasive and aggressive means for providing cardiac and pulmonary support for a patient not responding to conventional therapies. ECMO replaces the function of both the heart and lungs. De-oxygenated blood is removed from the body and pumped through an oxygenator than returned to the circulation. ECMO can be further classified into veno-venous and veno-arterial. Veno-venous ECMO is utilized with isolated respiratory failure and veno-arterial is reserved for cardiogenic shock. Peripheral ECMO is easier to initiate and can be placed by the interventionalist and the patient may be transported subsequently to a center with staff experienced in this modality.

Conclusion

Cardiogenic shock remains a significant challenge to the clinical physicians. Aggressive medical therapy for both STEMI and NSTEMI patients presenting with CS should be instituted early with a focus on revascularization with primary PCI. Adjunctive mechanical therapies such as IABP, pVAD and ECMO, while not conferring mortality benefit, should still be considered on an individual basis when options for survival have been exhausted.

The authors thank Ms. Barbara Minnick for her expert assistance in image preparation.

References

[1] Kolte D, Khera S, Aronow WSJ, et al: Trends in incidence, management, and outcomes of cardiogenic shock complicating ST-elevation myocardial infarction in the United States. *Am Heart Assoc.* 2014 Jan. 13; 3(1):e000590.

[2] Anderson ML, Peterson ED, Peng SA, et al: Differences in the profile, treatment, and prognosis of patients with cardiogenic shock by myocardial infarction classification: A report from NCDR. *Circ Cardiovasc Qual Outcomes.* 2013 Nov; 6(6): 708-15.

[3] Kohsaka S, Menon V, Lowe AM, Lange M, Dzavik V, Sleeper LA, Hochman JS. Systemic inflammatory response syndrome after acute myocardial infarction complicated by cardiogenic shock. *Arch Intern Med.* 2005; 165:1643-1650.

[4] Zeymer U, Vogt A, Zahn R, Weber MA, Tebbe U, Gottwik M, Bonzel T. Senges J, Neuhaus KL. Predictors of in-hospital mortality in 1333 patients with acute myocardial infarction complicated by cardiogenic shock treated with primary percutaneous coronary intervention: results of the primary PCI registry of the Arbeitsgemeinschaft Leitende Kardiologische Krankenhausarzte. *Eur Heart J.* 2004; 25:322-328.

[5] Janine Poss, Felix Mahfoud, Sara Seiler, et al: FGF-23 is associated with increased disease severity and early mortality in cardiogenic shock. *European Heart Journal: Acute Cardiovascular Care.* September 2013 2:211-218.

[6] Jakl M, Stasek J, Kala P, et al: Acute myocardial infarction complicated by shock: outcome analysis based on initial electrocardiogram. *Scand Cardovasc J.* 2014 Feb; 48(1):13-9.

[7] Hochman JS, Sleeper LA, Webb JG, Sanborn TA, White HD, Talley JD, Buller CE, Jacobs AK, Slater JN, Col J, McKinlay SM, LeJentel TH. Early revascularization in acute myocardial infarction complicated by cardiogenic shock: SHOCK Investigators: Should We Emergently Revascularize Occluded Coronaries for Cardiogenic shock. *N Engl J Med.* 1999, 341:625-634.

[8] Goldberg RJ, Spencer FA, Gore JM. Thirty –year trends (1975-2005) in the magnitude of, management of, and hospital death rates associated with cardiogenic shock in patient with acute myocardial infarction: a population based perspective. *Circulation* 2009; 119:1211-1219.

[9] Jacobs AK, Leopold JA, Bates E, Mendes LA, Sleeper LA, White H, Davidoff R, Boland J, Modur S, Forman R, Hochman JS. Cardiogenic shock caused by right

ventricular infarction: a report from the SHOCK registry. *J Am Coll Cardiol.* 2003; 41:1273-1279.

[10] Lupi-Herrera E, González-Pacheco H, Juárez-Herrera U, et al: Primary reperfusion in acute right ventricular infarction: An observational study. *World J Cardiol.* 2014 Jan 26;6(1):14-22.

[11] Mehta RH, Lopes RD, Ballotta A. Percutaneous coronary intervention or coronary artery bypass surgery for cardiogenic shock and multivessel coronary artery disease? *Am Heart J* 2010; 159:141-7.

[12] Bauer T, Zeymer U, Hochadel M. Use and outcomes of multivessel percutaneous coronary intervention in patients with acute myocardial infarction complicated by cardiogenic shock. *Am J Cardiol* 2012; 109:941- 946.

[13] Lee MS, Bokhoor P, Park SJ. Unprotected left main coronary disease and ST segment myocardial elevation infarction: a contemporary review and argument for percutaneous coronary intervention. *JACC Cardiovasc Interv* 2010; 3791-5.

[14] Anderson RD, Ohman EM, Holmes DR Jr, Col I, Stebbins AI, Bates ER, Stromel RJ, Granger CB, Topol EJ, Califf RM: Use of intra-aortic balloon counterpulsation in patients presenting with cardiogenic shock: observations from the GUSTO-1 Study. Global Utilization of Streptokinase and TPA for Occluded Arteries. *J Am Coll Cardiol* 1997; 30:708-715.

[15] Thiele H and the IABP-SHOCK II Trial Investigators: Intraaortic Balloon Support for Myocardial Infarction with Cardiogenic Shock. N Engl J Med 2012; 367:1287-1296.

[16] Kettner J, Sramko M, Holek M, Pirk J, Kautzner J. Utility of intra-aortic balloon pump support for ventricular septal rupture and acute mitral regurgitation complicating acute myocardial infarction. *Am J Cardiol.* 2013 Dec 1; 112 (11): 1709-13.

[17] Thiele H, Sick P, Boudriot E, Diederich KW, Hambrecht R, Niebauer J, Schuler G. Randomized comparison of intra-aortic balloon support with a percutaneous left ventricular assist device in patients with revascularized acute myocardial infarction complicated by cardiogenic shock. *Eur Heart J* 2005, 26:1276-1283.

[18] Cheng JM, den Uil CA, Hoeks SE, van der Ent M, Jewbali LS, van Domburg RT, Serruys, PW: Percutaneous left ventricular assist device versus intra-aortic balloon pump counterpulsation for treatment of cardiogenic shock: a meta-analysis of controlled trials. *Eur Heart J* 2009, 30:2102-2108.

[19] O'Neill WW, Schreiber T, Wohns DH, et al: The Current Use of Impella 2.5 in Acute Myocardial Infarction Complicated by Cardiogenic Shock: Results from the USpella Registry. *J Interv Cardiol.* 2014 Feb; 27(1):1-11.

In: Myocardial Infarctions
Editor: Pattie Wilkonson

ISBN: 978-1-63321-726-3

Chapter 2

Optical Coherence Tomography Imaging in Acute Myocardial Infarction

Antonios Karanasos[1*], MD, Konstantinos Toutouzas[2], MD, PhD, Jors van der Sijde[1], MD, Nienke van Ditzhuijzen[1], MSc and Evelyn Regar[1], MD, PhD

[1]Thoraxcenter, Erasmus Medical Center, Rotterdam, the Netherlands
[2]1st Department of Cardiology, Athens Medical School, Hippokration Hospital, Athens, Greece

Abstract

Optical coherence tomography (OCT) is a high-resolution intravascular imaging modality able to visualize the micro-environment of the atheromatic plaque and assess intracoronary stents in great detail. As a result, OCT is a valuable research tool for examining the role of morphological characteristics of atheromatic plaque in the progression of coronary artery disease and plaque destabilization, which lead to the clinical manifestation of acute coronary syndromes. Several OCT studies have focused on expanding the current understanding of the pathomechanisms of acute myocardial infarction. Moreover, as OCT is being increasingly used in clinical practice, potential clinical applications of OCT in myocardial infarction are emerging. Despite the lack of established indications for OCT imaging in myocardial infarction thus far, OCT could be potentially of assistance in interventional guidance in several clinical scenarios such as culprit lesion identification, assessment of the underlying mechanisms of stent thrombosis, and guidance of local and systematic antithrombotic therapy. The current chapter summarizes the pathophysiological insights obtained by OCT imaging in acute myocardial infarction, and critically reviews potential areas of clinical application of this imaging modality in myocardial infarction.

* Corresponding author: Antonios Karanasos. Department of Cardiology, Thoraxcenter, Room Bd430, Erasmus Medical Center. Molewaterplein 40, 3015 RD, Rotterdam, the Netherlands. Tel. No.: +3162756155. Fax. No: +31107035046. E-mail: akaranasos@outlook.com.

Introduction

Acute myocardial infarction (AMI) is a major cause of morbidity and mortality. The almost exclusive cause of acute coronary syndromes (ACS), including unstable angina, AMI with or without ST-segment elevation, and sudden cardiac death is atherothrombosis. Pilot pathologic studies have identified the pathophysiologic processes implicated in the destabilization and thrombosis of atheromatic plaques [1-3]. Although these studies have provided us with the basic understanding of the pathogenetic mechanisms of acute coronary syndromes, the *in vivo* processes and natural history of atherothrombosis remain rather obscure, as post-mortem observations tend to represent the far end of the spectrum of clinical manifestations of atherothrombosis. Developments in intracoronary imaging techniques have managed to overcome limitations of angiography -that is restricted to the study of the lumen of the coronary arteries rather than morphological characteristics of the vessel wall-, and have enabled the *in vivo* visualization of plaque morphology [4].

Among these techniques, optical coherence tomography (OCT) plays a prominent role for the study of plaque morphology due to its very high resolution (~15μm), which enables the identification of the majority of the morphological characteristics of stable and complicated atheromatic plaques [5]. Thus, OCT comprises a valuable tool for obtaining *in vivo* insights into the pathomechanisms of ACS, triggered either by native plaques or by stented arterial segments. Furthermore, OCT can be a useful research tool for studying the effect of treatments applied in AMI and monitoring the vascular healing response. Moreover, as OCT is being increasingly used in clinical practice as a tool for interventional guidance, several potential clinical applications of OCT in AMI have emerged, including culprit lesion identification, assessment of the substrate of stent thrombosis and treatment guidance, and evaluation of the effectiveness of local and systematic antithrombotic therapy [6, 7].

Unstable Atherosclerotic Plaque: Insights from Pathology

Pathomechanisms of Acute Coronary Syndromes

Studies in post-mortem specimens of coronary arteries retrieved from sudden cardiac death victims have identified the major pathologic substrates of coronary thrombosis [1]. These include plaque rupture in 60-70% of the cases, plaque erosion in 20-30% of the cases and thrombosis triggered by calcified nodules in 2-5% [2, 3]. Plaque rupture which is the most frequent mechanism of coronary thrombosis consists of disruption of a thin fibrous cap that overlies a large necrotic core, causing the thrombogenic contents of the necrotic core to come in contact with the bloodstream and trigger thrombus formation. Plaque erosion is a less well-understood pathologic entity defined as the presence of thrombosis in the absence of plaque thrombosis, more frequently encountered in younger age individuals of female gender [8]. In the majority of the cases with erosion absence of an endothelial layer is observed at the sites of thrombosis [2]. Calcified nodules is a less common cause of coronary thrombosis, more common among men of older age and is characterized by thrombus accumulation on the site of nodular calcification protruding into the lumen through a disrupted thin fibrous cap.

High-risk or 'Vulnerable' Plaque

The term 'vulnerable plaque' has been introduced for denoting plaques that are in high risk to undergo acute thrombosis [9-11]. Traditionally, this term has been used to characterize plaques that bear morphological resemblance to the aforementioned types of thrombosed plaques. As there is debate on whether calcified nodules without thrombosis can be characterized as 'high-risk' plaques, considering a relatively benign prognosis [12], the major types of plaques that are considered vulnerable are these resembling eroded and ruptured plaques. Regarding the eroded plaques, the lack of specific distinct morphological characteristics in such plaques poses a major obstacle for the ad-hoc identification of plaques prone to develop erosion. In contrast to eroded plaques, plaques undergoing rupture have distinct morphological characteristics, including a large necrotic core, a thin (<65μm in pathology series) and inflamed fibrous cap, high plaque size, neovascularization, inflammatory cell infiltration and spotty calcification [13]. These characteristics are also observed in another type of plaque, called thin cap fibroatheroma (TCFA) which is considered the precursor of the ruptured plaque, and thus the main morphological subtype of 'vulnerable plaque' [13]. Therefore, early identification of such plaques has been a topic of intensive research, as this identification -in combination with timely intervention- prior to the occurrence of plaque rupture leading to the manifestation of an acute event, could potentially comprise a treatment strategy for reducing the morbidity and mortality of coronary disease.

It is, nevertheless important to acknowledge that most of the available data concerning the association of plaque morphology and coronary thrombosis are derived from post-mortem studies. Therefore, despite the substantial insights obtained by these studies regarding the substrates of atherothrombosis, and their contribution in the current understanding of atherosclerotic plaque morphology, these studies are associated with several inherent limitations that preclude firm conclusions about the *in vivo* course and mechanisms of atherothrombosis. The first limitation is the cross-sectional design of these studies that hampers the temporal evaluation of the natural history of plaque morphology and of the responses associated with systematic or local treatment effects. The second limitation is a potential selection bias, given that these studies have focused on deceased patients, thus representing an extreme manifestation of atherothrombosis and therefore findings from these studies are not utterly representative of the actual *in vivo* contribution of these mechanisms in the pathogenesis of ACS. However, technological advances in the field of intracoronary imaging allow to bridge the gap between *post-mortem* and *in vivo* findings and complement current knowledge regarding the mechanisms of atherosclerosis.

In Vivo Assessment of Coronary Plaque Morphology by OCT

Coronary angiography has traditionally been used for the assessment of coronaries, however not allowing the direct visualization of details of the vessel wall morphology. The development of intravascular imaging techniques enables the direct plaque visualization as it is not restricted to the luminal contour, thus further enabling the *in vivo* assessment of the pathogenetic mechanisms of atherothrombosis. Among intravascular imaging modalities,

OCT is the most potent for examining the morphological plaque characteristics associated with acute coronary syndromes, as it can accurately assess the most important aspects of plaque 'vulnerability', including precise measurement of the thickness of the overlying fibrous plaque and a high sensitivity for thrombus detection.

OCT Principle and Image Acquisition in the Cathlab

OCT is an intravascular imaging modality, based on emission and reflectance of near-infrared light from a rotating imaging lens, that can acquire high resolution cross-sectional images of the coronary artery wall [14]. The emitted infrared light waves reflect off the vascular wall and are then received and processed by the OCT imaging system. As the wavelength of light waves is very short, compared to the wavelength of intravascular ultrasound, OCT cannot directly interpret the signal, but uses instead a technique called low-coherence interferometry in order to process the reflected signal. Thereby, OCT can acquire very high axial (~15μm) and lateral (~25 μm) resolution images, but with the disadvantage of a limited penetration with visualization of only the superficial 1–2 mm of the vascular wall, allowing however imaging of the most important elements of plaque vulnerability which are located near the surface of the plaque. Furthermore, during OCT examination it is necessary to temporarily displace blood during imaging, because of the high scattering of light caused by erythrocytes. In currently available systems, this is achieved through angiographic contrast material injection, warmed to 37°C, through the guide catheter manually or automatically by means of a power injector.

Currently available OCT systems are utilizing a short rapid-exchange monorail catheter for mounting of the optical probe, while the optical signal is transmitted by a single-mode fibre, automatically mounted on the catheter. For image acquisition, the OCT catheter is initially advanced with the aid of a conventional guidewire distally to the target segment, and automated pullback of the optical fibre is performed simultaneously with the contrast injection. The pullback of the catheter imaging tip is performed automatically while rotating inside a transparent sheath, allowing for retrieval of consecutive cross-sectional images for a length of 50-70mm from the coronary artery.

OCT Validation: Stable Coronary Plaques and Fibroatheroma

OCT validation studies performed in post-mortem coronary specimens have focused on defining the optical appearance of the morphological characteristics of the plaque [15-19]. These studies have shown that OCT can be used for plaque characterization with an overall good agreement with histology and high reproducibility. OCT can identify normal wall segments and early atherosclerotic lesions [20, 21], while it can perform tissue characterization in advanced atherosclerotic lesions [5]. The major plaque types discernible by OCT are fibrous plaque, appearing as a signal-rich, homogeneous region with low signal attenuation; fibrocalcific plaque, appearing as a signal-poor heterogeneous region, with sharp borders and low signal attenuation; and necrotic core, which appears as a signal-poor region, with diffuse borders and high signal attenuation within a lesion that is covered by a fibrous cap [5, 15]. Fibroatheroma has been defined as a plaque with necrotic core and a fibrous cap.

Importantly, the thickness of the fibrous cap can be measured with precision by OCT [22, 23]. A thin cap fibroatheroma by OCT is defined as a fibroatheroma covered by a thin fibrous cap; the current threshold for defining a cap as thin is the extrapolated by histology value of 65μm, although the optimal threshold remains a matter of debate, that will be discussed more extensively below. Mixed plaques by OCT are characterized as plaques containing more than one plaque morphologies within a single cross-sectional frame. Additional tissue components that can be identified by OCT include macrophages that are characterized by bright reflectance and high signal attenuation, and intimal vasculature that appears as sharply delineated signal-poor voids within the intima [5, 24]. Figure 1 demonstrates the main plaque types and tissue components identified by OCT.

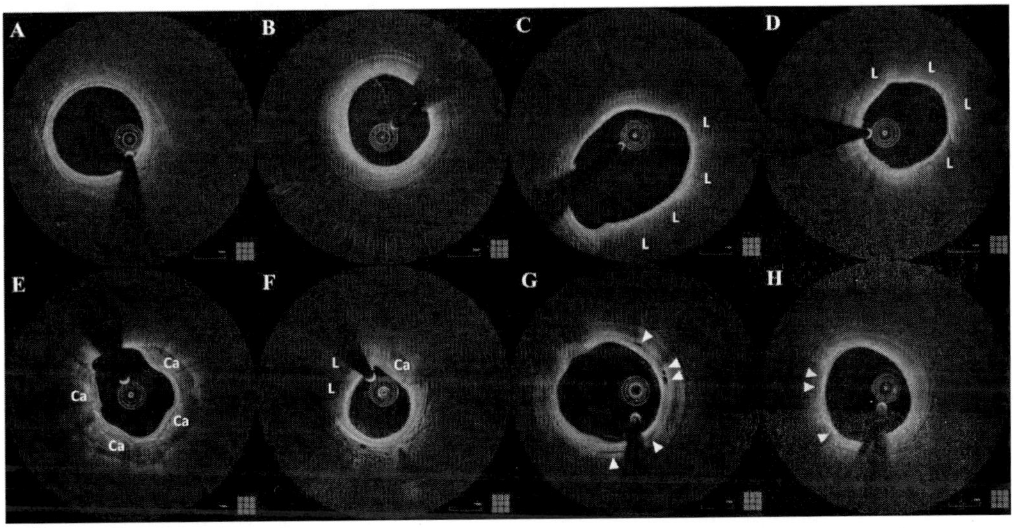

Figure 1. Plaque morphology by OCT.
A. Normal vessel B. Fibrous plaque C. Fibroatheroma (minimum fibrous cap thickness: 120μm) D. Thin cap fibroatheroma (minimum fibrous cap thickness: 40μm) E. Fibrocalcific plaque F. Mixed plaque with necrotic core and calcification G. Intimal microchannels H. Macrophage infiltration. Annotations: L=necrotic core, Ca=calcifications, white arrowheads=microchannels, yellow arrowheads=macrophages.

Thrombosed Coronary Lesions

Importantly, OCT can also be used for tissue characterization in thrombosed plaques. OCT can identify intracoronary thrombus as an intraluminal mass attached to luminal surface or floating within the lumen, and discriminate between two major types of thrombus: red thrombus (red blood cell–rich) with high backscattering and high attenuation, and white thrombus (platelet-rich) that has lower backscattering, is homogeneous and has low attenuation [25]. Plaque rupture can be identified by OCT as a fibroatheroma with fibrous cap disruption over necrotic core, with or without cavity formation [5]. Plaque erosion is defined as a plaque with thrombus and no evidence of cap rupture evaluated in multiple adjacent frames. It is important to note that in some cases, due to high signal attenuation caused by the presence of red thrombus, the presence of plaque rupture can be obscured, and thus in the presence of red thrombus, the diagnosis of erosion by OCT should be considered presumptive. Thrombosis on the grounds of calcified nodules can be identified as evidence of thrombus in conjunction with calcium protruding into the lumen, frequently forming sharp, jutting angles [26]. Figure 2 demonstrates the main thrombosed plaque morphologies identified by OCT.

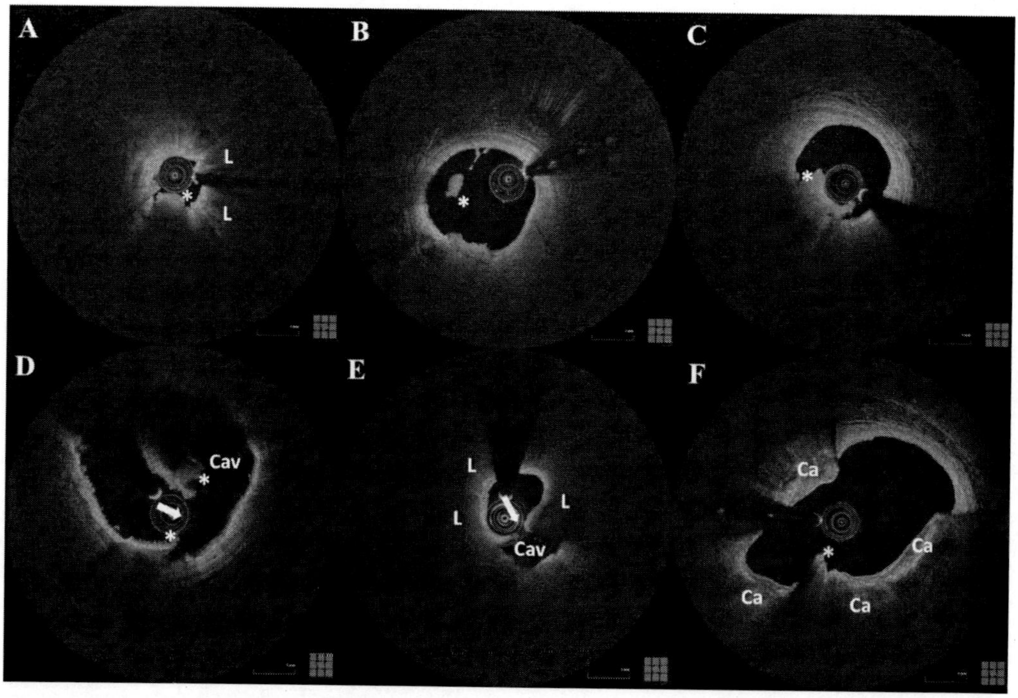

Figure 2. Thrombosed plaque morphology by OCT.
A. Red thrombus B. White thrombus C. Plaque erosion D. Ruptured plaque with large cavity formation E. Ruptured plaque with small cavity formation F. Thrombosed calcified nodules.
Annotations: L=necrotic core, yellow asterisk=red thrombus, white asterisk=white thrombus, Cav=cavity, white arrow=cap disruption, Ca=calcifications.

OCT Insights into the Mechanisms of Plaque Destabilization and Myocardial Infarction

Given the advantages of OCT in characterization of thrombosed plaques, a number of studies have used OCT in order to explore the pathomechanisms of plaque formation, progression and destabilization that will eventually lead to myocardial infarction.

Unstable Plaque Morphology in Culprit Plaques in Patients with ACS

A pilot *in vivo* OCT study focused on the assessment of plaque morphology according to the clinical presentation using three patient groups: patients with stable angina, patients with unstable angina and non-ST-segment elevation myocardial infarction (NSTEMI), and patients with ST-segment elevation myocardial infarction (STEMI) 5 days after thrombolytic therapy administration [27]. Culprit plaques of patients with unstable angina, NSTEMI and STEMI were associated with lower fibrous cap thickness and higher incidence of TCFA compared to stable lesions. A subsequent study confirmed these findings, showing increased incidence of TCFA, thrombus and plaque rupture in AMI patients compared to stable angina [28].

Superior Assessment of pathomechanisms of ACS

OCT has been also used for the assessment of plaque morphology in the acute phase of ACS, including AMI, after achieving sufficient flow restoration by means of aspiration thrombectomy. A variety of morphological characteristics can be visualized in the culprit lesion of myocardial infarction, as a result of the complexity of atherosclerosis often encountered in these settings [29]. Assessment of the culprit lesion in patients with ACS has shown a superior ability of OCT for the detection of plaque rupture, plaque erosion and intracoronary thrombus compared to intravascular ultrasound (IVUS) or coronary angioscopy [30]. Importantly, in this series of 30 patients, thrombus was successfully visualized by OCT in all cases. Furthermore, this superior visualization of ACS pathomechanisms by OCT enables the evaluation of the incidence of these mechanisms in an *in vivo* setting [31]. In a series of 124 patients with ACS, plaque rupture was identified in 44% of the patients, erosion in 31%, thrombosis of calcified nodules in 8%, and other causes -including subocclusive stenosis, dissection and coronary spasm- in 17% of the cases [32]. Despite a possible misclassification of some cases with plaque rupture as plaque erosion, due to shadowing from residual intraluminal thrombus (in 13% of the cases underlying plaque was not fully visualized classifying them as a probable erosion), this study provides an estimate of the relative contribution of each pathomechanism in patients with ACS, indicating that in an *in vivo* setting, plaque rupture could be accountable for less thrombosis events than what has been previously demonstrated in post-mortem studies. Of note, in this study, plaque rupture was more common among STEMI patients, in contrast to erosion that was more common among non-ST elevation ACS patients and calcified nodules that where exclusively observed among patients with non-ST elevation ACS.

Association between Plaque Morphology and Clinical Presentation

Importantly, morphological characteristics of the ruptured plaque can also differ depending on clinical presentation. It has been independently demonstrated by Toutouzas et al. [33] and Ino et al. [34] that among AMI patients with ruptured culprit plaques, morphological characteristics of the ruptured site differ between ST-segment elevation and non-ST-segment elevation acute myocardial infarction. Specifically, ruptured plaques of patients with STEMI are associated with a greater extent of cap disruption compared to ruptured plaques of patients with NSTEMI. Also, patients with STEMI had a smaller minimal lumen area compared to patients with NSTEMI [33], showing the importance of residual lumen for the development of more severe vessel occlusion as in STEMI. This finding was further corroborated by the finding of a lower lumen area in patients with culprit ruptured plaques of ACS versus non-culprit plaques in the same patients that had undergone silent rupture [35]. This difference in lumen area of ruptured plaque, both in the rupture site and the minimal lumen area site of the plaque, was also present in a comparison of asymptomatic patients with silent plaque rupture in OCT examination, with non-ST-segment elevation ACS with culprit lesion plaque rupture [36]. Collectively, these studies provide indirect evidence that the degree of the pre-existing lumen narrowing might contribute to the clinical manifestation following plaque rupture.

Moreover, morphological differences have also been found between culprit ruptured plaques of patients with exercise-triggered ACS and culprit ruptured plaques of patients with rest-onset ACS [37]. Patients with exercise-triggered ACS had a higher cap thickness and higher incidence of rupture at the shoulder of the plaque. Finally, in a study of ACS patients, the finding of culprit lesion rupture as pathomechanism by OCT was associated with lower incidence of prodromal symptoms compared to patients without evidence of culprit plaque rupture (36% versus 84%) [38].

Plaque Morphology in ACS – Assessment of Cap Thickness in Plaque Rupture

Additionally, OCT has provided observations regarding culprit plaque morphology in ACS. In a population comprised by both stable patients and ACS patients, positive remodeling of the culprit lesion was associated with TCFA and morphology and evidence of inflammation [39], a finding also observed in a patient subset consisting exclusively by patients with ACS [40]. These observations are in line with pathologic studies indicating plaque remodeling as a component of plaque vulnerability [13] and *in vivo* IVUS studies showing the association of increased local inflammatory activation in ACS patients with positive remodeling and plaque rupture [41]. Furthermore, OCT has been used for identifying a critical value of cap thickness that characterizes rupture-prone plaques *in vivo*. In autopsy series, ruptured caps have a mean thickness of 23μm ± 19μm with 95% of them being thinner than 64μm [1]. However, it is not known whether the same values apply for OCT, as there is a mean overestimation of cap thickness by OCT in comparison with histology of 24μm ± 44μm [22], and also histologic cross-sections are subject to anisotropic tissue shrinkage potentially underestimating measurements [23, 42]. In the study of Tanaka et al. [37], cap thickness in ruptured plaques ranged from 20μm to 160μm, while in the study of Toutouzas et al. [33], 96% of the caps were thinner than 90μm. Furthermore, cap thickness within the plaque was consistently thinner in the rupture site compared to the minimal lumen area site, where cap thickness was as high as 200μm [33]. In an attempt to define a cut-off value for cap thickness, Yonetsu et al. performed cap thickness measurements in 71 ruptured and 111 non-ruptured plaques [43]. As expected fibrous cap thickness was lower for ruptured plaques, a finding observed both for minimal cap thickness of the entire plaque and for minimal cap thickness measured in fixed intervals within the culprit lesion. In 95% of ruptured plaques in this study, minimal cap thickness was below 80μm, whereas a value of 67μm could discriminate ruptured and non-ruptured plaques with 83% sensitivity and 77% specificity. Therefore, despite the current consensus on the utilization of the histology-derived 65μm cut-off for definition of thin-cap fibroatheroma by OCT, it is important to keep in mind that fibroatheromas with higher cap thickness -up to 100μm or even higher- could still be prone to rupture.

OCT Can Identify Spontaneous Coronary Dissection

In addition to insights about morphology of the ruptured plaques, OCT has been used for the study of the morphology of other causes of acute coronary syndromes such as spontaneous dissection and coronary spasm. Indeed, spontaneous dissection can be imaged by OCT as a separation of the intimal layer with formation of a false lumen at the level of the media [44], with or without intramural hematoma formation [45]. In such cases, OCT can also be used clinically in order to facilitate diagnosis and assist in selecting an appropriate management strategy.

OCT Findings in Spontaneous Coronary Spasm and Recanalized Thrombus

Similarly to spontaneous dissection, coronary spasm is another rare cause of acute coronary syndromes. OCT in this setting has demonstrated a variety of morphological changes in the coronary artery comprising intimal notches [46], and transient separation of the coronary artery wall layers [47, 48], that is sometimes accompanied by micro-thrombosis [49]. Finally, recanalized thrombus can be identified by OCT appearing as multiple intraluminal tissue rims, resembling a 'honeycomb' [50, 51].

Localization of High-risk Plaques in the Coronary Tree

OCT studies have also provided important insights concerning the spatial distribution of high-risk plaques in the coronary tree. It is known by angiographic studies that most STEMI events tend to cluster within the proximal portion of coronary artery [52], a distribution similar to the distribution of coronary atherosclerosis [53]. Pathologic studies have shown that this distribution of occlusions coincides with the distribution of high-risk plaques, where thin cap fibroatheromas and ruptured plaques are localized in focal spots within the proximal third of coronary arteries [54, 55]. Fujii et al. [56] demonstrated in both stable and ACS patients a proximal clustering of both culprit and non-culprit lesion TCFAs, while a small study on ACS patients demonstrated clustering of TCFAs in the proximal segment of the left anterior descending artery (LAD), but an even distribution within the left circumflex artery (LCx) and the right coronary artery (RCA) [37]. In a study of Toutouzas et al. [57, 67] culprit lesions of ACS patients were evaluated by OCT in relation with their spatial distribution in the coronary tree. The distribution of culprit lesions in this study was similar to the distribution described in previous angiographic studies [52]. OCT further demonstrated that among these plaques, culprit plaques located in the proximal 30mm were more often associated with rupture compared to the more distal lesions, indicating that plaque rupture is the main pathomechanism for ACS in these proximal lesions [57]. The distribution of rupture coincided, as expected, with the distribution of thin cap fibroatheromas that were also clustered within the proximal 30mm. Vessel sub-analysis showed that this distribution was evident in the LAD and the LCx, whereas in the RCA there was an even distribution along the coronary artery. A possible explanation for this finding is the presence of multiple side-branches in the proximal segments of the left coronary system, leading to changes in the hemodynamic conditions and development of areas of low shear stress [58, 59], which in turn could lead to the development of unstable plaque phenotypes [60]. This knowledge of the spatial distribution of the high-risk plaques can be potentially useful in the future for the development of preventive treatment strategies [61, 62].

Multiple Coronary Lesion Instability in ACS

Although myocardial infarction is in principle a focal manifestation arising from a single lesion, complex systemic pathophysiologic processes such as inflammation are involved in the pathogenesis, leading to multiple lesion instability [63-65]. Thus, non-culprit lesions of patients with myocardial infarction have a more complex angiographic morphology and are associated with rapid lesion progression and increased event rate at follow-up [66, 67]. This notion is further supported by a recent study, randomizing STEMI patients undergoing primary percutaneous coronary intervention (PCI) of the culprit lesion to additional prophylactic revascularization of non-culprit lesion with >50% stenosis or culprit-only treatment, which demonstrated a reduction in events in the group undergoing prophylactic angioplasty of these non-culprit lesions [68]. These observations have shaped the hypothesis that these non-culprit lesions of ACS have different morphology than lesions of stable patients. Indeed, OCT studies have lent further evidence to this hypothesis, providing a pathophysiological explanation for these clinical observations. Specifically, non-culprit lesions of patients with AMI were demonstrated to have increased incidence of non-culprit lesion TCFA and thrombus compared to non-culprit lesions of patients with stable angina, and a higher incidence of multiple TCFA lesions [28, 69]. Furthermore, a comparison of the non-culprit lesion of ACS patients with lesions of stable patients showed a higher lipid content, a thinner fibrous cap and a higher incidence of macrophage infiltration and thrombus in non-culprit lesions of ACS patients, in conjunction with higher incidence of TCFA [70]. This effect seems to be derived mainly by patients with rupture of the culprit plaque as pathomechanism for the ACS, as in these patients non-culprit lesions are associated with a higher incidence of TCFA and silent rupture compared to patients without plaque rupture in the culprit lesion [71]. Of note, this evidence of multiple lesions instability in AMI is more pronounced in patients with diabetes, where the incidence of non culprit lesion TCFA and rupture is more common than in patients without diabetes [72].

Plaque Morphology and Systemic Inflammation

Systemic inflammatory responses have been implicated as potential contributors for the observed lesion instability. Multiple studies have examined a possible association of systemic inflammation, as assessed by circulating inflammatory biomarkers, and culprit plaque morphology in ACS (Table 1) [28, 40, 73-81]. Among these inflammatory markers, C-reactive protein (CRP) is one of the most well studied biomarkers in ACS, as there is an association of its levels with the extent of angiographic disease and ACS [82]. The majority of studies demonstrate the presence of elevated CRP levels in plaque rupture, TCFA and an inverse correlation of CRP levels with cap thickness [28, 40, 73, 76-78, 80], whereas some smaller sample studies failed to detect such a difference [74, 75]. Some other inflammatory biomarkers such as IL-18, MMP-9 and pentraxin-3 have also been associated with TCFA and plaque rupture, while flow cytometry studies have shown increased expression of PSGL-1 in circulating monocytes in plaque rupture. In contrast, plaque erosion has been associated with increased levels of myeloperoxidase (MPO), a hemoprotein released by activated neutrophils [74, 78]. Finally, this association of inflammatory activation plaque morphology by OCT in ACS has also been observed in conjunction with biomarkers representing the influence of risk factors, such as levels of circulating malondialdehyde-modified low-density lipoprotein and the mean amplitude of glycemic excursion (MAGE) [77, 81]. Overall, this association of high-risk plaque morphology with inflammatory molecules and mechanisms underscores the contribution of inflammation in the pathomechanisms of plaque destabilization in ACS.

Table 1. Association of inflammatory biomarkers and plaque morphology in patients with ACS

Study	Population	Inflammatory marker	**Association with plaque morphology**
Inflammatory biomarkers			
Raffel et al. [80]	32 ACS and 11 SA patients	WBC count	WBC count correlated with cap thickness, macrophage density of the plaque CRP levels higher in TCFA versus non-TCFA lesions
Kashiwagi et al. [40]	47 ACS patients	CRP	CRP levels higher in TCFA versus non-TCFA lesions
Fujii et al. [28]	35 AMI and 20 SA patients	CRP	CRP independent predictor of multiple TCFA in the coronary tree in AMI
Bouki et al. [73]	32 ACS and 14 SA patients	CRP, IL-18	CRP and IL-18 levels higher in TCFA versus non-TCFA lesions CRP and IL-18 levels higher in ruptured plaques versus non-ruptured plaques IL-18 levels lower in plaques with calcification CRP levels independent predictor of ruptured plaque
Li et al. [76]	12 AMI, 23 UA and 11 SA patients	WBC count, CRP, IL-18, TNFα	Cap thickness inversely correlated with WBC count and CRP, IL-18, and TNFα levels WBC count and CRP, IL-18, and TNFα levels higher in TCFA versus non-TCFA lesions No association for any factor with plaque rupture CRP levels independent predictor of TCFA
Nicolli et al. [78]	50 non-ST elevation ACS patients	CRP, MPO, MMP-9, MMP-2, Cystatin-C	CRP and MMP-9 levels higher in plaque rupture compared to erosion and severe stenosis without thrombus MPO levels higher in plaque erosion compared to rupture and severe stenosis without thrombus Cystacin-C levels higher in severe stenosis without thrombus compared to plaque rupture or erosion No association of MMP-2 with plaque morphology

Table 1. (Continued)

Study	Population	Inflammatory marker	**Association with plaque morphology**
Ferrante et al. [74]	25 AMI patients	CRP, MPO	No difference in CRP levels for plaque rupture versus plaque erosion Elevated MPO levels in plaque erosion versus plaque rupture
Koga et al. [75]	28 ACS and 47 SA patients	CRP, pentraxin-3	Levels of pentraxin-3, but not CRP higher in TCFA versus non-TCFA lesions, both in ACS and SA lesions
Ozaki et al. [79]	25 AMI and 20 UA patients	PSGL-1 expression in circulating monocytes	Increased PSGL-1 expression in circulating monocytes in lesions with plaque rupture
Matsuo et al. [77]	53 ACS and 49 SA patients	MDA-LDL, CRP	Higher CRP levels but no difference in MDA-LDL levels in TCFA versus non-TCFA lesions in ACS Significantly higher MDA-LDL levels in ruptured TCFA versus non-ruptured TCFA in ACS
Teraguchi et al. [81]	37 AMI patients	MAGE, circulating monocytes	Increased MAGE in plaque rupture compared to non-ruptured plaque Increased circulating monocytes in plaque rupture

Abbreviations: WBC=white blood cells, CRP=C-reactive protein, IL=interleukin, TNFα=tumor necrosis factor alpha, MPO=myeloperoxidase, MMP= Matrix metalloproteinase, PSGL-1=P-selectin glycoprotein ligand-1, MDA-LDL=malondialdehyde-modified low-density lipoprotein , MAGE= mean amplitude of glycemic excursion.

Culprit lesion Morphology and Outcome of Thrombolysis

Plaque morphology seems also to play an important role in flow restoration after thrombolytic therapy administration. In a series of 55 patients undergoing pharamacological thrombolysis with tenecteplase for the treatment of STEMI, patients with complete flow restoration in the culprit artery after thrombolysis (TIMI flow grade III) had significant differences in plaque morphology with patients with TIMI flow grade 0-II in the culprit lesion [83]. In specific, culprit plaques of patients without complete flow restoration were associated with increased lipid content, thinner fibrous cap, and presented with rupture more often than patients with complete flow restoration. Fibrous cap thickness was the most important factor, having a significant correlation with flow velocity in the culprit artery, as expressed by the corrected TIMI frame count, and being the only factor independently associated with TIMI flow grade. This observation is in line with the finding of improved reperfusion in patients pre-treated with statins [84], a factor known to increase coronary plaque stability [85]. Although the reason behind this observation is not entirely clear, increased thrombogenicity due to an exaggerated inflammatory reaction has been speculated to play an important role

[83]. Furthermore, the residual thrombus pattern after successful administration of thrombolytic therapy in STEMI has also been examined with reference to the pathomechanism of the ACS [86]. In patients with a ruptured culprit lesion, the residual thrombus burden one day after fibrinolysis, as assessed by OCT, was higher than in patients with erosion of the culprit lesion. Ruptured culprit plaques had predominantly white thrombus at the site of the rupture with red thrombus being evenly distributed over the entire culprit lesion length, while in plaques with erosion, white thrombus was mainly found and red thrombus was sparse. Collectively, these findings suggest that underlying plaque morphology in STEMI is a major determinant of the response to thrombolytic therapy.

Myocardial Infarction after Stent Implantation: OCT Insights

An important advantage of OCT is that it can be used for assessing the pathophysiological substrate of ACS in stented arteries, namely stent thrombosis. Although the utilization of stents in PCI, mainly drug-eluting stents, has been a major advancement leading to a reduction of the short-term complications, it has also introduced the need for a long-term vigilance, as events from the stented lesion emerge as late as 15 or more after implantation [87, 88].

Pathologic Findings in Late and Very Late Stent Thrombosis: Impaired Healing and Neoatherosclerosis

The reason behind this ongoing late stent failure is not completely understood, contrary to acute stent thrombosis where procedural factors appear to play a major role [89]. Pathologic studies were the first to identify factors associated with late stent thrombosis [90, 91]. While first studies in bare metal stents (BMS) hinted to the underlying plaque as an important contributor in the pathogenesis, subsequent studies in drug-eluting stents (DES) revealed a very high incidence of uncovered and malapposed struts in patients with events implicating an impaired healing response as the main pathogenetic factor [91]. This impaired healing response was mainly observed in first-generation DES and attributed to a vessel wall toxicity induced by the released drug in the case of paclitaxel-eluting stents or by the polymer in the case of sirolimus-eluting stents [92]. Consequently, poor strut endothelialization was considered a risk factor for stent thrombosis, and considering the ~10μm resolution of OCT, several OCT studies have focused on exploring the association of impaired healing with stent thrombosis [93]. Simultaneously, *in vivo* OCT observations together with pathologic studies demonstrated a variety in the neointimal patterns observed at the follow-up after stent implantation, resembling components of native atherosclerosis [94-98]. Moreover, OCT observations demonstrating neointimal disruption, in analogy to plaque rupture in native atherosclerosis, have raised questions about the exact role of this mechanism in the pathogenesis of very late stent thrombosis [87].

Neoatherosclerosis with Plaque Rupture as Mechanism of Stent Failure

Several studies have studied the OCT findings in patients with late and very late stent thrombosis, in an attempt to identify the pathomechanisms (Table 2) [99-109]. Despite minor differences in the incidences of each pathomechanism, these studies collectively demonstrate a very high prevalence of plaque rupture as a pathomechanism for very late BMS thrombosis, a process observed at a very late follow-up of BMS [106], and two different mechanisms contributing almost equally [109, 110] in late and very late DES thrombosis: neointimal plaque rupture, and impaired healing response with incomplete stent apposition and low rates of coverage (Figure 3). Neointimal rupture is a mechanism occurring mainly at longer intervals since stent implantation [109, 111], in neointimal regions with high necrotic core content and thin fibrous cap [107], similarly to what is observed in native atherosclerosis, but also with a very high incidence of macrophage infiltration [107].

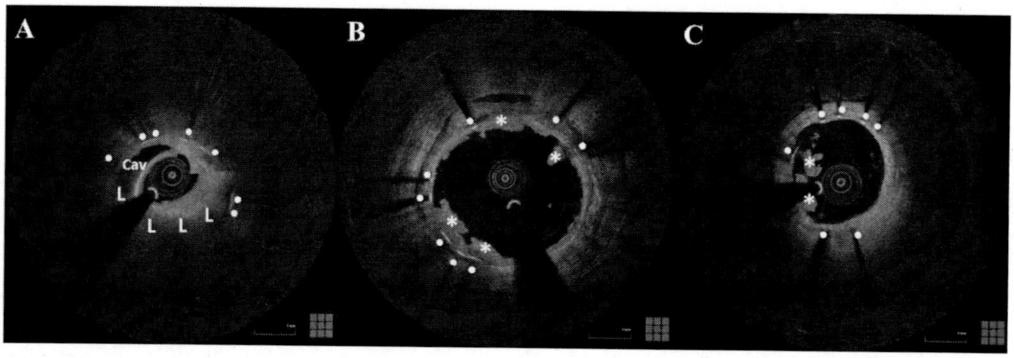

Figure 3. Different pathomechanisms of stent thrombosis.
A. Neointimal rupture with in-stent cavity formation B. Thrombus attached to malapposed struts C. Thrombus attached to an uncovered strut.
Annotations: L=necrotic core, white bullets=stent struts, white asterisk=white thrombus, Cav=cavity.

Delayed Healing and Incomplete Stent Apposition: High Prevalence but Unclear Prognostic Value

Regarding the second mechanism, impaired healing, all studies in DES focusing in patients with events demonstrate a very high incidence of uncovered and malapposed struts, considerably higher than the one reported in control subjects without thrombosis [102, 104], control subjects with stent restenosis [101], or even patients with stent thrombosis due to neointimal rupture [5, 110]. Importantly, these findings are exaggerated within the stent in segments where thrombus is found versus segments without thrombus [104]. Conversely, this association has not been prospectively demonstrated in any study, raising questions about the prognostic significance of such findings [93, 112]. Finally, a third more rare mechanism is also identified in some cases, consisting of a native plaque rupture at the edges of a stent triggering thrombosis within the stented segment [105, 110]. Regarding bioresorbable vascular scaffolds (BVS), the first reports of scaffold thrombosis are appearing [113], although the exact pathomechanisms are yet be identified for these devices.

Table 2. Optical coherence tomography findings in late and very late stent thrombosis

Study	n	DES type	Interval (months)	Uncovered struts(%)	Patients with uncovered struts	Malapposed struts(%)	Patients with malapposed struts	Neointimal rupture	Edge rupture
Ko et al. [99]	18 DES	14 SES/ 3 PES/ 1 EES	40±20	N/A	50%	N/A	39%	22.2%	
Davlouros et al. [100)	7 DES	N/A	8 (3-62)	32%	100%	33%	N/A	BMS 70%/ DES 0%	
Miyazaki et al. [101]	6 DES	5 SES/ 1 PES	37±12	29%	100%	7%	67%	33%	
Guagliumi et al. [102]	18 DES	6 SES/ 10 PES/ 1 EES/ 1 ZES	21 (6-60)	12.3%	84%	10%	78%	11.1%	
Alfonso et al. [105]	8 BMS/ 7 DES	N/A	43±51	N/A	60%	N/A	40%	6.7%	13.3%
Kang et al. [103]	6 BMS/ 27 DES	N/A	74 (46-90)	N/A	17% BMS/ 56% DES	N/A	0% BMS/ 52% DES	BMS 100%/ DES 63%	
Amabile et al. [109]	12 BMS/ 8 DES	N/A	90 (16-210)	32% in 10 cases without rupture	N/A	N/A	N/A	10%	
Parodi et al. [104]	17	N/A	N/A	14%	>10% in 29%	6,7%	>10% in 24%	N/A	
Karanasos et al. [108]	7 BMS/ 32 DES	7 SES/ 19 PES/ 6 EES	63 (21-200)	N/A	66%	N/A	33%	41%	5.1%

Abbreviations: DES=drug eluting stents, BMS=bare metal stent, SES=sirolimus eluting stents, PES=paclitaxel eluting stent, EES=everolimus eluting stents, ZES=zotarolimus eluting stents.

Assessment of the Treatment Effect by OCT

Acute Effects of Stent Implantation in AMI

As OCT is a valuable modality to assess the acute vascular trauma and residual thrombus after stenting [114, 115], but also evaluate stent expansion and apposition [116], it has been used in order to assess the effects of treatment strategies in myocardial infarction [6, 7]. Several studies have investigated the acute results of stent implantation in AMI. Kim et al. examined the acute vascular healing response in 24 patients with stent implantation for the treatment of myocardial infarction, focusing mainly on the incidence of acute incomplete stent apposition (ISA) [117]. The investigators found a very high incidence of incomplete strut apposition ranging for 10% to 28% on a strut-level basis, depending on the type of stent use. When this was assessed on a stent level, the incidence of incomplete stent apposition was 67%, 83%, and 100%, respectively, depending on whether a >10% malapposed struts, >5% malapposed struts, or any malapposed struts definition of incomplete stent apposition was used [117]. In the APPOSITION II trial [118], OCT was used to assess the vascular healing response after implantation of a self-expanding versus a balloon-expandable stent. The use of a self-expanding stent was associated with improved stent apposition (stent-level ISA with >5% malapposed struts definition: 13.9% for self-expanding versus 37.1% for balloon-expandable) and less vascular trauma compared to a balloon expandable stent without significant differences in lumen or stent area. On a strut-level basis, a lower percentage of malapposed stent struts was observed in the self-expanding group than in the balloon-expandable group (2.20 ± 3.92% verus 5.99 ± 7.28%). Importantly, at a three-day follow-up, there were no self-expanding stents with >5% malapposed struts in the self-expanding group, while there was no significant difference over time in the percentage of malapposed struts for the balloon-expandable group.

Evaluation of the Efficacy of Local Antithrombotic Strategies

As OCT can detect and quantify the residual thrombus after stenting [115, 119], it can be also used for the evaluation of various adjunctive therapies aiming at the reduction of distal embolization (Figure 4). The TROFI study was a randomized study that investigated the impact of thrombectomy on the residual flow area (lumen area – prolapse and thrombus area) after 2nd generation stent implantation in myocardial infarction [120]. Only a modest trend was found for higher minimal flow area in the group of thrombectomy, whereas there were no significant differences in morphometric measurements of stent and lumen, residual thrombus or incomplete stent apposition [120]. Similarly, in NSTEMI patients, the use of aspiration thrombectomy failed to significantly reduce intracoronary thrombus burden, prior to stent implantation [121]. Parodi et al. randomized 80 AMI patients to rheolytic versus aspiration thrombectomy, showing only a trend for lower residual thrombus after rheolytic thrombectomy versus aspiration thrombectomy; however, other markers of reperfusion were better in the rheolytic thrombectomy arm, leading to reduced incidence of malapposed struts at a 6-month follow-up [122]. Another adjunctive treatment for AMI evaluated by OCT is local delivery of IIb/IIIa by means of a dedicated catheter. A comparison of this approach versus intracoronary administration of IIb/IIIa showed a higher reduction of thrombus burden with the local treatment [123], while future studies will aim to investigate what is the impact of this adjunctive treatment in combination with thrombectomy on the residual thrombus burden after stent implantation by OCT [124]. Finally, a small observational study has evaluated potential differences in thrombus burden by OCT among different antiplatelet regimes, however, small numbers preclude the extraction of conclusions [125].

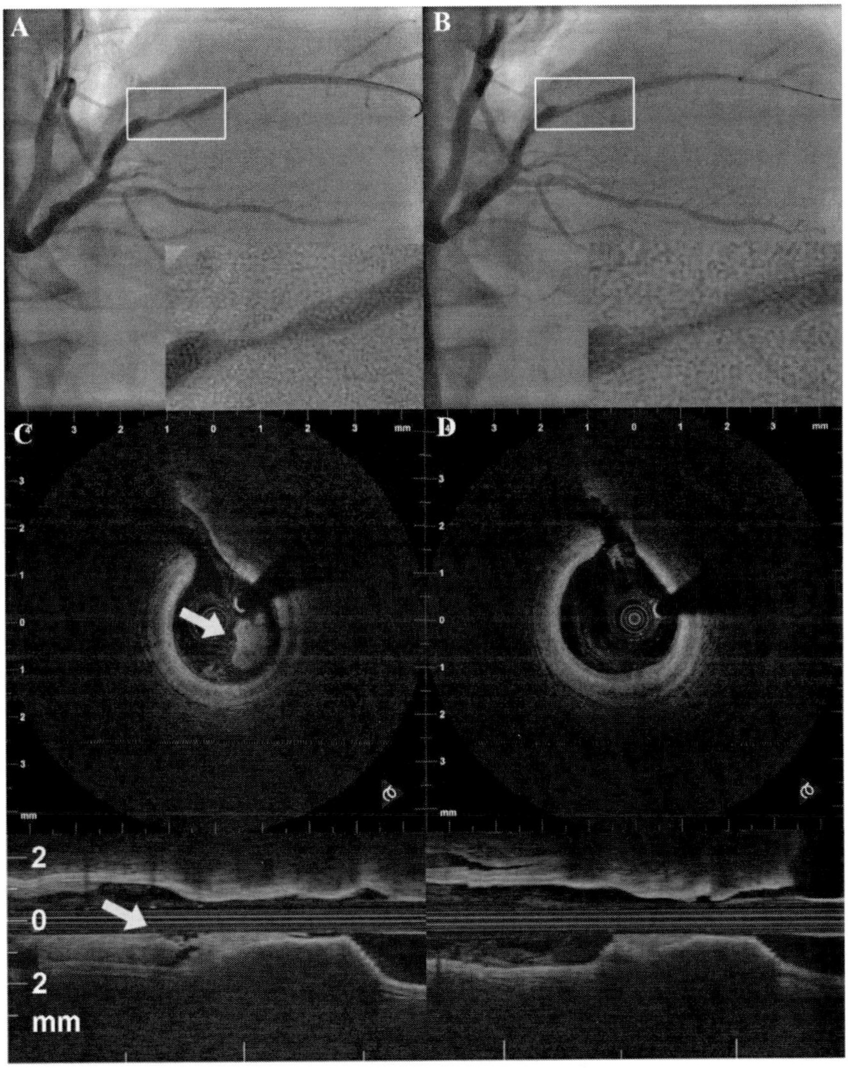

Figure 4. Assessment of thrombectomy result.
A. Coronary angiography of the right posterolateral branch of a patient with myocardial infarction. B. OCT reveals significant thrombus burden (yellow arrow). C. Angiography after manual thrombus aspiration. D. OCT shows reduction of the thrombus burden, confirming the effectiveness of thrombus aspiration. Reproduced from Karanasos et al., Curr Cardiovasc Imaging Rep. 2012;5:206-220 [6].

Chronic Arterial Healing Response after Stent Implantation in AMI

Additionally to the acute assessment of intervention, OCT has been used for the assessment of the chronic artery healing response after stent implantation, a factor implicated in the pathogenesis of late events. Gonzalo et al. [126] first demonstrated an impaired healing response at a mid-term follow-up of stents implanted for STEMI compared to stents implanted for stable and unstable angina, with higher rates of uncovered and malapposed struts. This finding was also encountered at the very late (~5 years) OCT follow-up of SIRTAX study, where stent implantation during acute coronary syndrome versus stable angina was associated with higher rate of uncovered struts [127]. This impaired healing response is more pronounced in first-generation DES compared to BMS [128]. These rates appear to be low for second-generation DES and not to be affected by the use of thrombectomy at the baseline procedure [129]. Of note, the amount of coverage in the follow-up of these stents was correlated with the amount of the residual intraluminal material post-stenting showing the important role of thrombus as a mediator of the healing response [129].

Bioresorbable Scaffolds in AMI

As bioresorbable vascular scaffolds are being increasingly used for the treatment of coronary artery disease, AMI patients appear as a patient population that could have higher benefit from the implanatation of these devices [130]. However, given the limited data available on BVS implantation in thrombosed lesions, OCT appears as a useful tool for the study of the acute vascular response [131]. The BVS-STEMI-first study examined the acute vascular response after BVS implantation in 49 patients with myocardial infarction, 31 of whom had an OCT study of the culprit lesion [132]. The OCT findings were consistent with a good procedural result, without significant lumen compromise or stent underexpansion, a mean percentage of malapposed struts per patient of 2.80 ± 3.90%, and an incidence of scaffolds with >5% malapposed struts of 22.6%. Importantly, despite a high strut thickness of the BVS, a low incidence of angiographic signs of distal embolization was found, while OCT assessment of the tissue prolapse/residual thrombus after scaffold implantation was at similar levels with what has been reported for metal stents [115]. Similar conclusions were reached by an independent study, Prague-19 [133], that also showed good scaffold expansion and apposition in 21 STEMI patients treated with BVS. Although these reports demonstrate that BVS could potentially be a promising treatment for STEMI, data is still fairly limited and OCT studies of the mid- and long-term healing response will be able to give further insight on the effects of such an approach [134-136]

Potential Utility of OCT in Interventional Guidance in Myocardial Infarction

Optimization of Stent Expansion – Reduction of Residual Thrombus Burden

As OCT is being increasingly used in clinical practice, the concept of OCT-guided procedures emerges as an approach for improving the outcome of invasive treatment of coronary artery disease. However, in contrast to IVUS, where numerous studies have investigated the impact of IVUS-guided strategies, only limited data are available for OCT. The main body of evidence for OCT guidance comes from the CLI-OPCI study [137], a non-randomized registry where the outcomes of 335 'all-comer' patients -including ACS patients- undergoing OCT-guided PCI, and the one-year outcomes were compared with the outcomes of 335 matched patients undergoing angiography-guided PCI during the same period. The primary endpoint of 1-year cardiac mortality and myocardial infarction was lower for OCT-guided PCI, both for crude and propensity-matched data, mainly due to a high incidence of events in the angio-guided group [137]. Despite the observational nature of this study, this is the first study that demonstrates a potential benefit from OCT guidance in PCI. Conceptually, such a benefit could be higher for patients with ACS, considering the ability of OCT to detect and quantify thrombus, and simultaneously assess the underlying pathomechanism. The use of OCT in stent thrombosis was discussed earlier; however OCT can also be used in this setting for the assessment of the efficacy of thrombus-reducing strategies as aspiration thrombectomy and rheolytic thrombectomy [138]. A similar assessment can also be performed after stent implantation in AMI caused by native plaque, in order to reduce the residual thrombus burden. Di Giorgio et al. demonstrated the feasibility of OCT-guided additional balloon dilation in patients with residual in-stent thrombus after PCI in AMI comparing it with no further intervention [139]. Eighty patients were sequentially divided in 2 equal groups treated with the two different strategies. The use of OCT-guided post-dilation was associated with an increase in stent and lumen area, and a decrease in residual thrombus area, without however any significant differences between the OCT-guided group and the control group in OCT morphometric measurements or angiographic markers of distal embolization [139].

Culprit Lesion Identification in ACS Patients with (Near-)normal Coronaries

Another intriguing potential application for OCT is its use for culprit lesion identification in acute coronary syndromes, without an evident culprit lesion or with doubtful findings such as haziness in the angiogram (Figure 5) [140, 141]. Non-invasive imaging studies have demonstrated that occult atherosclerosis is the cause of ACS in the majority of such cases [142]. Despite a potential utility of such non-invasive approaches in secondary risk stratification of these patients, the lack of guidance during the procedure precludes potential invasive treatment of these lesions and can lead to a mean infarct mass by magnetic resonance imaging of ~10g [142]. Therefore, intravascular imaging by OCT can be used in such scenarios, as it can identify the underlying pathophysiological substrate in the acute phase, and also identify thrombus that constitutes *per se* a potential target for intervention. So far, several anecdotal reports regarding the utility of OCT in culprit lesion identification in AMI or unstable angina have been published [143-147], but larger series are needed in order to evaluate the potential utility of this modality in this setting.

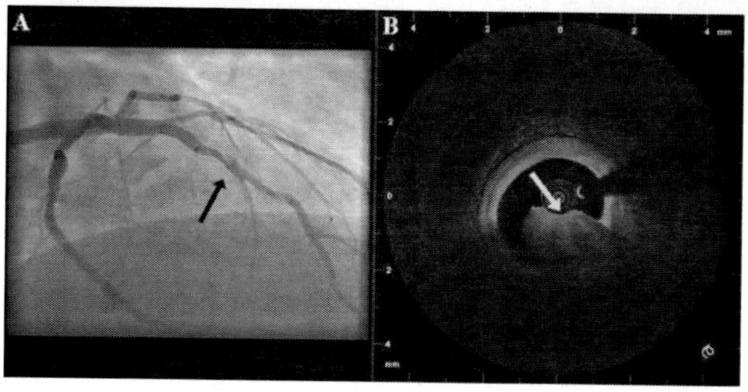

Figure 5. Culprit lesion identification by OCT.Evaluation by OCT of a patient with acute coronary syndrome and haziness in the coronary angiogram. OCT revealed the presence of thrombus. Reproduced from Karanasos et al., Curr Cardiovasc Imaging Rep. 2012;5:206-220 [6].

Assessment of Need for Stent Implantation in AMI Patients Treated with Thrombectomy

Finally, OCT could potentially indicate selection of a less invasive strategy in selected cases of patients with myocardial infarction. Recently, several small series have demonstrated the concept of treatment of the culprit lesion of myocardial infarction with flow restoration by means of thrombectomy, avoiding stent implantation in the acute phase, and evaluation of the need for stent implantation several days after the acute event [148-150]. OCT could be used in this setting for evaluation of the morphology and appraisal of the need for stent implantation either during the acute phase or during the deferred catheterization. Cervinka et al. used OCT for assessing the need of stent implantation in STEMI patients treated by thrombectomy [151]. Among 100 consecutive patients with STEMI treated with thrombus aspiration and IIb/IIIa administration, 20 patients with TIMI flow grade ≥2, absence of ongoing symptoms and presence of a mainly thrombotic stenosis by OCT were treated conservatively without stent implantation. The clinical follow-up showed no major adverse cardiovascular events for either group, while follow-up angiogram and OCT-study at 1 week and 9 months after the event in the thrombectomy-only treated patients showed the presence of non-stenotic lesions (<50% stenosis) with healing of rupture by 9 months [151]. Other investigators have suggested that the presence of plaque erosion and the absence of significant stenosis could constitute a potential criterion for selecting patients that can be treated with thrombectomy alone [152], and the feasibility of such an approach was demonstrated in a highly selected series of 31 patients [153]. Nonetheless, evidence about such approaches is still fairly limited and restricted to proof-of-concept studies, and bigger randomized studies using more objective OCT criteria are warranted to validate the feasibility and potential benefit of such approaches.

Future Directions

From the body of evidence discussed above, it becomes evident that OCT is an imaging modality that has provided useful insights into the pathomechanisms of acute coronary syndromes and that holds promise for application in clinical practice, where it could potentially improve interventional outcomes in patients with acute coronary syndromes. However, it should be kept in mind that the majority of the studies performed up to date are cross-sectional observational studies with small numbers of patients, focused mainly at generating hypotheses about the pathobiology of atherosclerosis and the potential fields for clinical application of OCT. Therefore, the performance of larger studies aiming at 1) obtaining a better understanding of the natural history of atherosclerosis, the exact mechanisms of plaque progression and destabilization, and treatments that can have an impact on the reduction of the mortality and morbidity of acute coronary syndromes, and 2) evaluating whether OCT can improve patient-oriented outcomes when used for interventional guidance in such settings will be able to define the role of OCT in research and clinical practice.

Several technological developments that could help us achieve these goals are already under way. These technological advances are moving both in the direction of improving plaque characterization using the current technology and in the direction of development of new technologies based on OCT imaging. Towards the first direction, algorithms for the automated measurement of cap thickness can provide a fast and volumetric measure of this critical component of plaque vulnerability, while simultaneously increasing reproducibility of such measurements [154-156], whereas systems for automated tissue characterization in atherosclerotic plaques can be used for a faster, more objective evaluation of atherosclerotic plaque morphology [157-160]. Towards the second direction, the development of ultra-high-speed OCT imaging systems will allow the complete high-resolution assessment of long arterial segments within a heartbeat [161], further allowing the full biomechanical assessment of the hemodynamic environment in the coronary arteries [58, 162]. Furthermore, new imaging systems with resolution comparable to electronic microscopy able to identify (sub-) cellular structures [163], or providing information regarding the collagen content of atherosclerotic plaques [164, 165], or hybrid systems incorporating the ability for detection of molecules targeted with probes simultaneously with plaque imaging [166], are currently under development and are expected to increase our understanding of the pathobiologic processes of acute coronary syndromes.

Conclusion

The development of OCT has allowed us to gain important *in vivo* insights in the mechanisms of atherosclerotic plaque progression and destabilization leading to the manifestation of acute coronary syndromes. Plaque morphology in acute coronary syndromes, the relationship of plaque characteristics with thrombosis and thrombolysis, the role of inflammation in plaque destabilization and the mechanisms of myocardial infarction after stent implantation are some of the areas in which OCT has increased our understanding. This better understanding of atherosclerosis can help in the development of new treatment strategies aiming at an early identification of high-risk plaques and timely intervention that could result in a reduction of the morbidity and mortality of acute coronary syndromes. Meanwhile, the use of OCT as a clinical tool is still an area under investigation. Small-scale clinical studies and reports have demonstrated the potential of OCT as a means for interventional guidance in acute coronary syndromes. Although several potential fields of application have been identified, such as culprit lesion identification and evaluation of the need for local or systematic antithrombotic therapies or for stent implantation, the role of OCT in this setting has yet to be established; future larger scale studies that can show clinical benefit from the use of OCT will ultimately help in establishing appropriate clinical indications for OCT guidance.

References

[1] Burke AP, Farb A, Malcom GT, Liang YH, Smialek J, Virmani R. Coronary risk factors and plaque morphology in men with coronary disease who died suddenly. *N. Engl. J. Med.* 1997;336:1276-1282.

[2] Falk E, Nakano M, Bentzon JF, Finn AV, Virmani R. Update on acute coronary syndromes: The pathologists' view. *Eur Heart J.* 2013;34:719-728.

[3] Virmani R, Kolodgie FD, Burke AP, Farb A, Schwartz SM. Lessons from sudden coronary death a comprehensive morphological classification scheme for atherosclerotic lesions. *Arterioscler. Thromb. Vasc. Biol.* 2000;20:1262-1275.

[4] Toutouzas K, Stathogiannis K, Synetos A, Karanasos A, Stefanadis C. Vulnerable atherosclerotic plaque: From the basic research laboratory to the clinic. *Cardiology.* 2012;123:248-253.

[5] Tearney GJ, Regar E, Akasaka T, Adriaenssens T, Barlis P, Bezerra HG, Bouma B, Bruining N, Cho JM, Chowdhary S, Costa MA, de Silva R, Dijkstra J, Di Mario C, Dudek D, Falk E, Feldman MD, Fitzgerald P, Garcia-Garcia HM, Gonzalo N, Granada JF, Guagliumi G, Holm NR, Honda Y, Ikeno F, Kawasaki M, Kochman J, Koltowski L, Kubo T, Kume T, Kyono H, Lam CC, Lamouche G, Lee DP, Leon MB, Maehara A, Manfrini O, Mintz GS, Mizuno K, Morel MA, Nadkarni S, Okura H, Otake H, Pietrasik A, Prati F, Raber L, Radu MD, Rieber J, Riga M, Rollins A, Rosenberg M, Sirbu V, Serruys PW, Shimada K, Shinke T, Shite J, Siegel E, Sonoda S, Suter M, Takarada S, Tanaka A, Terashima M, Thim T, Uemura S, Ughi GJ, van Beusekom HM, van der Steen AF, van Es GA, van Soest G, Virmani R, Waxman S, Weissman NJ, Weisz G. Consensus standards for acquisition, measurement, and reporting of intravascular optical coherence tomography studies: A report from the international working group for intravascular optical coherence tomography standardization and validation. *J Am Coll Cardiol.* 2012;59:1058-1072.

[6] Karanasos A, Ligthart J, Witberg K, van Soest G, Bruining N, Regar E. Optical coherence tomography: Potential clinical applications. *Curr Cardiovasc Imaging Rep.* 2012;5:206-220.

[7] Regar E, van Soest G, Bruining N, Constantinescu AA, van Geuns RJ, van der Giessen W, Serruys PW. Optical coherence tomography in patients with acute coronary syndrome. *EuroIntervention.* 2010;6 Suppl G:G154-160.

[8] Kramer MC, Rittersma SZ, de Winter RJ, Ladich ER, Fowler DR, Liang YH, Kutys R, Carter-Monroe N, Kolodgie FD, van der Wal AC, Virmani R. Relationship of thrombus healing to underlying plaque morphology in sudden coronary death. *J Am Coll Cardiol.* 2010;55:122-132.

[9] Muller JE, Stone PH, Turi ZG, Rutherford JD, Czeisler CA, Parker C, Poole WK, Passamani E, Roberts R, Robertson T, et al. Circadian variation in the frequency of onset of acute myocardial infarction. *N Engl J Med.* 1985;313:1315-1322.

[10] Naghavi M, Libby P, Falk E, Casscells SW, Litovsky S, Rumberger J, Badimon JJ, Stefanadis C, Moreno P, Pasterkamp G, Fayad Z, Stone PH, Waxman S, Raggi P, Madjid M, Zarrabi A, Burke A, Yuan C, Fitzgerald PJ, Siscovick DS, de Korte CL, Aikawa M, Airaksinen KE, Assmann G, Becker CR, Chesebro JH, Farb A, Galis ZS, Jackson C, Jang IK, Koenig W, Lodder RA, March K, Demirovic J, Navab M, Priori SG, Rekhter MD, Bahr R, Grundy SM, Mehran R, Colombo A, Boerwinkle E, Ballantyne C, Insull W, Jr., Schwartz RS, Vogel R, Serruys PW, Hansson GK, Faxon DP, Kaul S, Drexler H, Greenland P, Muller JE, Virmani R, Ridker PM, Zipes DP, Shah PK, Willerson JT. From vulnerable plaque to vulnerable patient: A call for new definitions and risk assessment strategies: Part ii. *Circulation.* 2003;108:1772-1778.

[11] Naghavi M, Libby P, Falk E, Casscells SW, Litovsky S, Rumberger J, Badimon JJ, Stefanadis C, Moreno P, Pasterkamp G, Fayad Z, Stone PH, Waxman S, Raggi P, Madjid M, Zarrabi A, Burke A, Yuan C, Fitzgerald PJ, Siscovick DS, de Korte CL, Aikawa M, Juhani Airaksinen KE, Assmann G, Becker CR, Chesebro JH, Farb A, Galis ZS, Jackson C, Jang IK, Koenig W, Lodder RA, March K, Demirovic J, Navab M, Priori SG, Rekhter MD, Bahr R, Grundy SM, Mehran R, Colombo A, Boerwinkle E, Ballantyne C, Insull W, Jr., Schwartz RS, Vogel R, Serruys PW, Hansson GK, Faxon DP, Kaul S, Drexler H, Greenland P, Muller JE, Virmani R, Ridker PM, Zipes DP, Shah PK, Willerson JT. From vulnerable plaque to vulnerable patient: A call for new definitions and risk assessment strategies: Part i. *Circulation.* 2003;108:1664-1672.

[12] Xu Y, Mintz GS, Tam A, McPherson JA, Iniguez A, Fajadet J, Fahy M, Weisz G, De Bruyne B, Serruys PW, Stone GW, Maehara A. Prevalence, distribution, predictors, and outcomes of patients with calcified nodules in native coronary arteries: A 3-vessel intravascular ultrasound analysis from providing regional observations to study predictors of events in the coronary tree (prospect). *Circulation.* 2012;126:537 545.

[13] Virmani R, Burke AP, Farb A, Kolodgie FD. Pathology of the vulnerable plaque. *J. Am. Coll. Cardiol.* 2006;47:C13-C18.

[14] Regar E, Ligthart J, Bruining N, van Soest G. The diagnostic value of intracoronary optical coherence tomography. *Herz.* 2011;36:417-429.

[15] Yabushita H, Bouma BE, Houser SL, Aretz HT, Jang IK, Schlendorf KH, Kauffman CR, Shishkov M, Kang DH, Halpern EF, Tearney GJ. Characterization of human atherosclerosis by optical coherence tomography. *Circulation.* 2002;106:1640-1645.

[16] Rieber J, Meissner O, Babaryka G, Reim S, Oswald M, Koenig A, Schiele TM, Shapiro M, Theisen K, Reiser MF, Klauss V, Hoffmann U. Diagnostic accuracy of optical coherence tomography and intravascular ultrasound for the detection and characterization of atherosclerotic plaque composition in ex-vivo coronary specimens: A comparison with histology. *Coron Artery Dis.* 2006;17:425-430.

[17] Manfrini O, Mont E, Leone O, Arbustini E, Eusebi V, Virmani R, Bugiardini R. Sources of error and interpretation of plaque morphology by optical coherence tomography. *Am J Cardiol.* 2006;98:156-159.

[18] Kawasaki M, Bouma BE, Bressner J, Houser SL, Nadkarni SK, MacNeill BD, Jang IK, Fujiwara H, Tearney GJ. Diagnostic accuracy of optical coherence tomography and

integrated backscatter intravascular ultrasound images for tissue characterization of human coronary plaques. *J Am Coll Cardiol.* 2006;48:81-88.

[19] Kume T, Akasaka T, Kawamoto T, Watanabe N, Toyota E, Neishi Y, Sukmawan R, Sadahira Y, Yoshida K. Assessment of coronary arterial plaque by optical coherence tomography. *Am J Cardiol.* 2006;97:1172-1175.

[20] Kume T, Akasaka T, Kawamoto T, Watanabe N, Toyota E, Neishi Y, Sukmawan R, Sadahira Y, Yoshida K. Assessment of coronary intima--media thickness by optical coherence tomography: Comparison with intravascular ultrasound. *Circ J.* 2005;69:903-907.

[21] Zimarino M, Prati F, Stabile E, Pizzicannella J, Fouad T, Filippini A, Rabozzi R, Trubiani O, Pizzicannella G, De Caterina R. Optical coherence tomography accurately identifies intermediate atherosclerotic lesions--an *in vivo* evaluation in the rabbit carotid artery. *Atherosclerosis.* 2007;193:94-101.

[22] Kume T, Akasaka T, Kawamoto T, Okura H, Watanabe N, Toyota E, Neishi Y, Sukmawan R, Sadahira Y, Yoshida K. Measurement of the thickness of the fibrous cap by optical coherence tomography. *Am Heart J.* 2006;152:755 e751-754.

[23] Cilingiroglu M, Oh JH, Sugunan B, Kemp NJ, Kim J, Lee S, Zaatari HN, Escobedo D, Thomsen S, Milner TE, Feldman MD. Detection of vulnerable plaque in a murine model of atherosclerosis with optical coherence tomography. *Catheter Cardiovasc Interv.* 2006;67:915-923.

[24] van Soest G, Regar E, Goderie TP, Gonzalo N, Koljenovic S, van Leenders GJ, Serruys PW, van der Steen AF. Pitfalls in plaque characterization by OCT: Image artifacts in native coronary arteries. *JACC Cardiovasc Imaging.* 2011;4:810-813.

[25] Kume T, Akasaka T, Kawamoto T, Ogasawara Y, Watanabe N, Toyota E, Neishi Y, Sukmawan R, Sadahira Y, Yoshida K. Assessment of coronary arterial thrombus by optical coherence tomography. *Am. J. Cardiol.* 2006;97:1713-1717.

[26] Karanasos A, Ligthart JM, Witberg KT, Regar E. Calcified nodules: An underrated mechanism of coronary thrombosis? *JACC Cardiovasc Imaging.* 2012;5:1071-1072.

[27] Jang I-K, Tearney GJ, MacNeill B, Takano M, Moselewski F, Iftima N, Shishkov M, Houser S, Aretz HT, Halpern EF, Bouma BE. *In vivo* characterization of coronary atherosclerotic plaque by use of optical coherence tomography. *Circulation.* 2005;111:1551-1555.

[28] Fujii K, Masutani M, Okumura T, Kawasaki D, Akagami T, Ezumi A, Sakoda T, Masuyama T, Ohyanagi M. Frequency and predictor of coronary thin-cap fibroatheroma in patients with acute myocardial infarction and stable angina pectoris a 3-vessel optical coherence tomography study. *J. Am. Coll. Cardiol.* 2008;52:787-788.

[29] Toutouzas K, Karanasos A, Stefanadis C. Multiple plaque morphologies assessed by optical coherence tomography in a patient with acute coronary syndrome. *Heart.* 2010;96:1335-1336.

[30] Kubo T, Imanishi T, Takarada S, Kuroi A, Ueno S, Yamano T, Tanimoto T, Matsuo Y, Masho T, Kitabata H, Tsuda K, Tomobuchi Y, Akasaka T. Assessment of culprit lesion morphology in acute myocardial infarction: Ability of optical coherence tomography compared with intravascular ultrasound and coronary angioscopy. *J. Am. Coll. Cardiol.* 2007;50:933-939.

[31] Gonzalo N, Tearney GJ, van Soest G, Serruys P, Garcia-Garcia HM, Bouma BE, Regar E. Witnessed coronary plaque rupture during cardiac catheterization. *JACC Cardiovasc Imaging*. 2011;4:437-438.

[32] Jia H, Abtahian F, Aguirre AD, Lee S, Chia S, Lowe H, Kato K, Yonetsu T, Vergallo R, Hu S, Tian J, Lee H, Park S-J, Jang Y-S, Raffel OC, Mizuno K, Uemura S, Itoh T, Kakuta T, Choi S-Y, Dauerman HL, Prasad A, Toma C, McNulty I, Zhang S, Yu B, Fuster V, Narula J, Virmani R, Jang I-K. *In vivo* diagnosis of plaque erosion and calcified nodule in patients with acute coronary syndrome by intravascular optical coherence tomography. *J. Am. Coll. Cardiol.* 2013;62:1748-1758.

[33] Toutouzas K, Karanasos A, Tsiamis E, Riga M, Drakopoulou M, Synetos A, Papanikolaou A, Tsioufis C, Androulakis A, Stefanadi E, Tousoulis D, Stefanadis C. New insights by optical coherence tomography into the differences and similarities of culprit ruptured plaque morphology in non-st-elevation myocardial infarction and st-elevation myocardial infarction. *Am. Heart J.* 2011;161:1192-1199.

[34] Ino Y, Kubo T, Tanaka A, Kuroi A, Tsujioka H, Ikejima H, Okouchi K, Kashiwagi M, Takarada S, Kitabata H, Tanimoto T, Komukai K, Ishibashi K, Kimura K, Hirata K, Mizukoshi M, Imanishi T, Akasaka T. Difference of culprit lesion morphologies between st-segment elevation myocardial infarction and non-st-segment elevation acute coronary syndrome: An optical coherence tomography study. *JACC Cardiovasc Interv.* 2011;4:76-82.

[35] Tian J, Ren X, Vergallo R, Xing L, Yu H, Jia H, Soeda T, McNulty I, Hu S, Lee H, Yu B, Jang I-K. Distinct morphological features of ruptured culprit plaque for acute coronary events compared to those with silent rupture and thin-cap fibroatheroma: A combined optical coherence tomography and intravascular ultrasound study. *J. Am. Coll. Cardiol.* 2014;63:2209-2216.

[36] Shimamura K, Ino Y, Kubo T, Nishiguchi T, Tanimoto T, Ozaki Y, Satogami K, Orii M, Shiono Y, Komukai K, Yamano T, Matsuo Y, Kitabata H, Yamaguchi T, Hirata K, Tanaka A, Imanishi T, Akasaka T. Difference of ruptured plaque morphology between asymptomatic coronary artery disease and non-st elevation acute coronary syndrome patients: An optical coherence tomography study. *Atherosclerosis*.

[37] Tanaka A, Imanishi T, Kitabata H, Kubo T, Takarada S, Tanimoto T, Kuroi A, Tsujioka H, Ikejima H, Ueno S, Kataiwa H, Okouchi K, Kashiwaghi M, Matsumoto H, Takemoto K, Nakamura N, Hirata K, Mizukoshi M, Akasaka T. Morphology of exertion-triggered plaque rupture in patients with acute coronary syndrome: An optical coherence tomography study. *Circulation*. 2008;118:2368-2373.

[38] Kato M, Dote K, Sasaki S, Kagawa E, Nakano Y, Watanabe Y, Higashi A, Itakura K, Ochiumi Y, Takiguchi Y. Presentations of acute coronary syndrome related to coronary lesion morphologies as assessed by intravascular ultrasound and optical coherence tomography. *Int. J. Cardiol.* 2013;165:506-511.

[39] Raffel OC, Merchant FM, Tearney GJ, Chia S, Gauthier DD, Pomerantsev E, Mizuno K, Bouma BE, Jang I-K. *In vivo* association between positive coronary artery remodelling and coronary plaque characteristics assessed by intravascular optical coherence tomography. *Eur Heart J.* 2008;29:1721-1728.

[40] Kashiwagi M, Tanaka A, Kitabata H, Tsujioka H, Matsumoto H, Arita Y, Ookochi K, Kuroi A, Kataiwa H, Tanimoto T, Ikejima H, Takarada S, Kubo T, Hirata K, Nakamura N, Mizukoshi M, Imanishi T, Akasaka T. Relationship between coronary arterial

remodeling, fibrous cap thickness and high-sensitivity c-reactive protein levels in patients with acute coronary syndrome. *Circ. J.* 2009;73:1291-1295.

[41] Toutouzas K, Synetos A, Stefanadi E, Vaina S, Markou V, Vavuranakis M, Tsiamis E, Tousoulis D, Stefanadis C. Correlation between morphologic characteristics and local temperature differences in culprit lesions of patients with symptomatic coronary artery disease. *J Am Coll Cardiol.* 2007;49:2264-2271.

[42] Barlis P, Serruys PW, Gonzalo N, van der Giessen WJ, de Jaegere PJ, Regar E. Assessment of culprit and remote coronary narrowings using optical coherence tomography with long-term outcomes. *Am. J. Cardiol.* 2008;102:391-395.

[43] Yonetsu T, Kakuta T, Lee T, Takahashi K, Kawaguchi N, Yamamoto G, Koura K, Hishikari K, Iesaka Y, Fujiwara H, Isobe M. *In vivo* critical fibrous cap thickness for rupture-prone coronary plaques assessed by optical coherence tomography. *Eur Heart J.* 2011;32:1251-1259.

[44] Alfonso F, Paulo M, Gonzalo N, Dutary J, Jimenez-Quevedo P, Lennie V, Escaned J, Bañuelos C, Hernandez R, Macaya C. Diagnosis of spontaneous coronary artery dissection by optical coherence tomography. *J. Am. Coll. Cardiol.* 2012;59:1073-1079.

[45] Johnson TW, Smith D, Strange JW, Bucciarelli-Ducci C, Lowe R, Baumbach A. Spontaneous multivessel coronary intramural hematoma: An insight with OCT. *JACC Cardiovasc Imaging.* 2012;5:1070-1071.

[46] Tanaka A, Shimada K, Tearney GJ, Kitabata H, Taguchi H, Fukuda S, Kashiwagi M, Kubo T, Takarada S, Hirata K, Mizukoshi M, Yoshikawa J, Bouma BE, Akasaka T. Conformational change in coronary artery structure assessed by optical coherence tomography in patients with vasospastic angina. *J. Am. Coll. Cardiol.* 2011;58:1608-1613.

[47] Kohno H, Sueda S, Sakaue T. Separation of the intima-media complex from the adventitia during spontaneous coronary artery spasm documented by intracoronary optical coherence tomography. *Int. J. Cardiol.* 2012;154:e4-5.

[48] Vizzi V, Johnson TW, Jenkins N, Strange JW, Baumbach A. Dynamic separation of coronary artery medial and adventitial layers with vasospasm: New insights using oct. *Int. J. Cardiol.* 2013;167:2344-2345.

[49] Park H-C, Choi SI, Lee JU, Kim S-G, Shin J, Kim H-J. Morphological findings in typical variant angina presenting as acute coronary syndrome using optical coherence tomography. *J Interv Cardiol.* 2013;26:491-500.

[50] Kang S-J, Nakano M, Virmani R, Song H-G, Ahn J-M, Kim W-J, Lee J-Y, Park D-W, Lee S-W, Kim Y-H, Lee CW, Park S-W, Park S-J. Oct findings in patients with recanalization of organized thrombi in coronary arteries. *JACC Cardiovasc Imaging.* 2012;5:725-732.

[51] Toutouzas K, Karanasos A, Stathogiannis K, Synetos A, Tsiamis E, Papadopoulos D, Stefanadis C. A honeycomb-like structure in the left anterior descending coronary artery: Demonstration of recanalized thrombus by optical coherence tomography. *JACC Cardiovasc Interv.* 2012;5:688-689.

[52] Wang JC, Normand S-LT, Mauri L, Kuntz RE. Coronary artery spatial distribution of acute myocardial infarction occlusions. *Circulation.* 2004;110:278-284.

[53] Hochman JS, Phillips WJ, Ruggieri D, Ryan SF. The distribution of atherosclerotic lesions in the coronary arterial tree: Relation to cardiac risk factors. *Am. Heart J.* 1988;116:1217-1222.

[54] Cheruvu PK, Finn AV, Gardner C, Caplan J, Goldstein J, Stone GW, Virmani R, Muller JE. Frequency and distribution of thin-cap fibroatheroma and ruptured plaques in human coronary arteries: A pathologic study. *J. Am. Coll. Cardiol.* 2007;50:940-949.

[55] Kume T, Okura H, Yamada R, Kawamoto T, Watanabe N, Neishi Y, Sadahira Y, Akasaka T, Yoshida K. Frequency and spatial distribution of thin-cap fibroatheroma assessed by 3-vessel intravascular ultrasound and optical coherence tomography: An ex vivo validation and an initial *in vivo* feasibility study. *Circ. J.* 2009;73:1086-1091.

[56] Fujii K, Kawasaki D, Masutani M, Okumura T, Akagami T, Sakoda T, Tsujino T, Ohyanagi M, Masuyama T. Oct assessment of thin-cap fibroatheroma distribution in native coronary arteries. *JACC Cardiovasc Imaging*. 2010;3:168-175.

[57] Toutouzas K, Karanasos A, Riga M, Tsiamis E, Synetos A, Michelongona A, Papanikolaou A, Triantafyllou G, Tsioufis C, Stefanadis C. Optical coherence tomography assessment of the spatial distribution of culprit ruptured plaques and thin-cap fibroatheromas in acute coronary syndrome. *EuroIntervention*. 2012;8:477-485.

[58] Chatzizisis YS, Jonas M, Coskun AU, Beigel R, Stone BV, Maynard C, Gerrity RG, Daley W, Rogers C, Edelman ER, Feldman CL, Stone PH. Prediction of the localization of high-risk coronary atherosclerotic plaques on the basis of low endothelial shear stress: An intravascular ultrasound and histopathology natural history study. *Circulation*. 2008;117:993-1002.

[59] Cunningham KS, Gotlieb AI. The role of shear stress in the pathogenesis of atherosclerosis. *Lab. Invest.* 2005;85:9-23.

[60] Koskinas KC, Feldman CL, Chatzizisis YS, Coskun AU, Jonas M, Maynard C, Baker AB, Papafaklis MI, Edelman ER, Stone PH. Natural history of experimental coronary atherosclerosis and vascular remodeling in relation to endothelial shear stress: A serial, *in vivo* intravascular ultrasound study. *Circulation*. 2010;121:2092-2101.

[61] Karanasos A, Simsek C, Serruys P, Ligthart J, Witberg K, van Geuns RJ, Sianos G, Zijlstra F, Regar E. Five-year optical coherence tomography follow-up of an everolimus-eluting bioresorbable vascular scaffold: Changing the paradigm of coronary stenting? *Circulation*. 2012;126:e89-91.

[62] Wykrzykowska JJ, Diletti R, Gutierrez-Chico JL, van Geuns RJ, van der Giessen WJ, Ramcharitar S, Duckers HE, Schultz C, de Feyter P, van der Ent M, Regar E, de Jaegere P, Garcia-Garcia HM, Pawar R, Gonzalo N, Ligthart J, de Schepper J, van den Berg N, Milewski K, Granada JF, Serruys PW. Plaque sealing and passivation with a mechanical self-expanding low outward force nitinol vshield device for the treatment of ivus and OCT-derived thin cap fibroatheromas (TCFAs) in native coronary arteries: Report of the pilot study vshield evaluated at cardiac hospital in rotterdam for investigation and treatment of TCFA (SECRITT). *EuroIntervention*. 2012;8:945-954.

[63] Toutouzas K, Drakopoulou M, Markou V, Karabelas I, Vaina S, Vavuranakis M, Tsiamis E, Tsioufis C, Androulakis A, Stefanadis C. Correlation of systemic inflammation with local inflammatory activity in non-culprit lesions: Beneficial effect of statins. *Int. J. Cardiol.* 2007;119:368-373.

[64] Toutouzas K, Drakopoulou M, Mitropoulos J, Tsiamis E, Vaina S, Vavuranakis M, Markou V, Bosinakou E, Stefanadis C. Elevated plaque temperature in non-culprit de novo atheromatous lesions of patients with acute coronary syndromes. *J. Am. Coll. Cardiol.* 2006;47:301-306.

[65] Toutouzas K, Drakopoulou M, Vaina S, Stefanadis C. Significance of characterization of non-culprit lesions: An underscored clinical problem. *Atherosclerosis.* 2007;195:236-241.

[66] Goldstein JA, Demetriou D, Grines CL, Pica M, Shoukfeh M, O'Neill WW. Multiple complex coronary plaques in patients with acute myocardial infarction. *N. Engl. J. Med.* 2000;343:915-922.

[67] Tsiamis E, Toutouzas K, Synetos A, Karambelas J, Karanasos A, Demponeras C, Drakopoulou M, Stefanadi E, Tsioufis C, Tousoulis D, Stefanadis C. Prognostic clinical and angiographic characteristics for the development of a new significant lesion in remote segments after successful percutaneous coronary intervention. *Int. J. Cardiol.* 2010;143:29-34.

[68] Wald DS, Morris JK, Wald NJ, Chase AJ, Edwards RJ, Hughes LO, Berry C, Oldroyd KG. Randomized trial of preventive angioplasty in myocardial infarction. *N Engl J Med.* 2013;369:1115-1123.

[69] Kubo T, Imanishi T, Kashiwagi M, Ikejima H, Tsujioka H, Kuroi A, Ishibashi K, Komukai K, Tanimoto T, Ino Y, Kitabata H, Takarada S, Tanaka A, Mizukoshi M, Akasaka T. Multiple coronary lesion instability in patients with acute myocardial infarction as determined by optical coherence tomography. *Am. J. Cardiol.* 2010;105:318-322.

[70] Kato K, Yonetsu T, Kim S-J, Xing L, Lee H, McNulty I, Yeh RW, Sakhuja R, Zhang S, Uemura S, Yu B, Mizuno K, Jang I-K. Nonculprit plaques in patients with acute coronary syndromes have more vulnerable features compared with those with non-acute coronary syndromes: A 3-vessel optical coherence tomography study. *Circ Cardiovasc Imaging.* 2012;5:433-440.

[71] Vergallo R, Ren X, Yonetsu T, Kato K, Uemura S, Yu B, Jia H, Abtahian F, Aguirre AD, Tian J, Hu S, Soeda T, Lee H, McNulty I, Park S-J, Jang Y, Prasad A, Lee S, Zhang S, Porto I, Biasucci LM, Crea F, Jang I-K. Pancoronary plaque vulnerability in patients with acute coronary syndrome and ruptured culprit plaque: A 3-vessel optical coherence tomography study. *Am. Heart J.* 2014;167:59-67.

[72] Fukunaga M, Fujii K, Nakata T, Shibuya M, Miki K, Kawasaki D, Masutani M, Kawabata-Lee M, Ohyanagi M, Masuyama T. Multiple complex coronary atherosclerosis in diabetic patients with acute myocardial infarction: A three-vessel optical coherence tomography study. *EuroIntervention.* 2012;8:955-961.

[73] Bouki KP, Katsafados MG, Chatzopoulos DN, Psychari SN, Toutouzas KP, Charalampopoulos AF, Sakkali EN, Koudouri AA, Liakos GK, Apostolou TS. Inflammatory markers and plaque morphology: An optical coherence tomography study. *Int. J. Cardiol.* 2012;154:287-292.

[74] Ferrante G, Nakano M, Prati F, Niccoli G, Mallus MT, Ramazzotti V, Montone RA, Kolodgie FD, Virmani R, Crea F. High levels of systemic myeloperoxidase are associated with coronary plaque erosion in patients with acute coronary syndromes: A clinicopathological study. *Circulation.* 2010;122:2505-2513.

[75] Koga S, Ikeda S, Yoshida T, Nakata T, Takeno M, Masuda N, Koide Y, Kawano H, Maemura K. Elevated levels of systemic pentraxin 3 are associated with thin-cap fibroatheroma in coronary culprit lesions: Assessment by optical coherence tomography and intravascular ultrasound. *JACC Cardiovasc Interv.* 2013;6:945-954.

[76] Li QX, Fu QQ, Shi SW, Wang YF, Xie JJ, Yu X, Cheng X, Liao YH. Relationship between plasma inflammatory markers and plaque fibrous cap thickness determined by intravascular optical coherence tomography. *Heart*. 2010;96:196-201.

[77] Matsuo Y, Kubo T, Okumoto Y, Ishibashi K, Komukai K, Tanimoto T, Ino Y, Kitabata H, Hirata K, Imanishi T, Akagi H, Akasaka T. Circulating malondialdehyde-modified low-density lipoprotein levels are associated with the presence of thin-cap fibroatheromas determined by optical coherence tomography in coronary artery disease. *Eur Heart J Cardiovasc Imaging*. 2013;14:43-50.

[78] Niccoli G, Montone RA, Cataneo L, Cosentino N, Gramegna M, Refaat H, Porto I, Burzotta F, Trani C, Leone AM, Severino A, Crea F. Morphological-biohumoral correlations in acute coronary syndromes: Pathogenetic implications. *Int. J. Cardiol.* 2014;171:463-466.

[79] Ozaki Y, Imanishi T, Teraguchi I, Nishiguchi T, Orii M, Shiono Y, Shimamura K, Ishibashi K, Tanimoto T, Yamano T, Ino Y, Yamaguchi T, Kubo T, Akasaka T. Association between p-selectin glycoprotein ligand-1 and pathogenesis in acute coronary syndrome assessed by optical coherence tomography. *Atherosclerosis*. 2014;233:697-703.

[80] Raffel OC, Tearney GJ, Gauthier DD, Halpern EF, Bouma BE, Jang I-K. Relationship between a systemic inflammatory marker, plaque inflammation, and plaque characteristics determined by intravascular optical coherence tomography. *Arterioscler. Thromb. Vasc. Biol.* 2007;27:1820-1827.

[81] Teraguchi I, Imanishi T, Ozaki Y, Tanimoto T, Orii M, Shiono Y, Shimamura K, Ishibashi K, Yamano T, Ino Y, Yamaguchi T, Hirata K, Kubo T, Akasaka T. Impact of glucose fluctuation and monocyte subsets on coronary plaque rupture. *Nutr Metab Cardiovasc Dis*. 2014;24:309-314.

[82] Drakopoulou M, Toutouzas K, Stefanadi E, Tsiamis E, Tousoulis D, Stefanadis C. Association of inflammatory markers with angiographic severity and extent of coronary artery disease. *Atherosclerosis*. 2009;206:335-339.

[83] Toutouzas K, Tsiamis E, Karanasos A, Drakopoulou M, Synetos A, Tsioufis C, Tousoulis D, Davlouros P, Alexopoulos D, Bouki K, Apostolou T, Stefanadis C. Morphological characteristics of culprit atheromatic plaque are associated with coronary flow after thrombolytic therapy: New implications of optical coherence tomography from a multicenter study. *JACC Cardiovasc Interv*. 2010;3:507-514.

[84] Mytas D, Zairis M, Karanasos A, Kosma L, Arsenos P, Tentolouris C, Pitsavos C, Foussas S, Stefanadis C, Cokkinos D. Effect of statin pretreatment on the outcome of ST-segment elevation myocardial infarction in patients without prior history of coronary artery disease. *Hellenic J Cardiol*. 2013;54:422-428.

[85] Takarada S, Imanishi T, Ishibashi K, Tanimoto T, Komukai K, Ino Y, Kitabata H, Kubo T, Tanaka A, Kimura K, Mizukoshi M, Akasaka T. The effect of lipid and inflammatory profiles on the morphological changes of lipid-rich plaques in patients with non-ST-segment elevated acute coronary syndrome: Follow-up study by optical coherence tomography and intravascular ultrasound. *JACC Cardiovasc Interv*. 2010;3:766-772.

[86] Hu S, Yonetsu T, Jia H, Karanasos A, Aguirre AD, Tian J, Abtahian F, Vergallo R, Soeda T, Lee H, McNulty I, Kato K, Yu B, Mizuno K, Toutouzas K, Stefanadis C, Jang I-K. Residual thrombus pattern in patients with ST-segment elevation myocardial

infarction caused by plaque erosion versus plaque rupture after successful fibrinolysis: An optical coherence tomography study. *J. Am. Coll. Cardiol.* 2014;63:1336-1338.

[87] Karanasos A, Ligthart JM, Regar E. In-stent neoatherosclerosis: A cause of late stent thrombosis in a patient with "full metal jacket" 15 years after implantation: Insights from optical coherence tomography. *JACC Cardiovasc Interv*. 2012;5:799-800.

[88] Yamaji K, Kimura T, Morimoto T, Nakagawa Y, Inoue K, Soga Y, Arita T, Shirai S, Ando K, Kondo K, Sakai K, Goya M, Iwabuchi M, Yokoi H, Nosaka H, Nobuyoshi M. Very long-term (15 to 20 years) clinical and angiographic outcome after coronary bare metal stent implantation. *Circ Cardiovasc Interv*. 2010;3:468-475.

[89] Cheneau E, Leborgne L, Mintz GS, Kotani J, Pichard AD, Satler LF, Canos D, Castagna M, Weissman NJ, Waksman R. Predictors of subacute stent thrombosis: Results of a systematic intravascular ultrasound study. *Circulation*. 2003;108:43-47.

[90] Farb A, Burke AP, Kolodgie FD, Virmani R. Pathological mechanisms of fatal late coronary stent thrombosis in humans. *Circulation*. 2003;108:1701-1706.

[91] Finn AV, Joner M, Nakazawa G, Kolodgie F, Newell J, John MC, Gold HK, Virmani R. Pathological correlates of late drug-eluting stent thrombosis: Strut coverage as a marker of endothelialization. *Circulation*. 2007;115:2435-2441.

[92] Nakazawa G, Finn AV, Vorpahl M, Ladich ER, Kolodgie FD, Virmani R. Coronary responses and differential mechanisms of late stent thrombosis attributed to first-generation sirolimus- and paclitaxel-eluting stents. *J Am Coll Cardiol*. 2011;57:390-398.

[93] Gutierrez-Chico JL, Alegria-Barrero E, Teijeiro-Mestre R, Chan PH, Tsujioka H, de Silva R, Viceconte N, Lindsay A, Patterson T, Foin N, Akasaka T, di Mario C. Optical coherence tomography: From research to practice. *Eur Heart J Cardiovasc Imaging*. 2012.

[94] Inoue K, Abe K, Ando K, Shirai S, Nishiyama K, Nakanishi M, Yamada T, Sakai K, Nakagawa Y, Hamasaki N, Kimura T, Nobuyoshi M, Miyamoto TA. Pathological analyses of long-term intracoronary palmaz-schatz stenting; is its efficacy permanent? *Cardiovasc. Pathol.* 2004;13:109-115.

[95] Nakazawa G, Otsuka F, Nakano M, Vorpahl M, Yazdani SK, Ladich E, Kolodgie FD, Finn AV, Virmani R. The pathology of neoatherosclerosis in human coronary implants bare-metal and drug-eluting stents. *J. Am. Coll. Cardiol.* 2011;57:1314-1322.

[96] Gonzalo N, Serruys PW, Okamura T, van Beusekom HM, Garcia-Garcia HM, van Soest G, van der Giessen W, Regar E. Optical coherence tomography patterns of stent restenosis. *Am Heart J*. 2009;158:284-293.

[97] Hou J, Qi H, Zhang M, Ma L, Liu H, Han Z, Meng L, Yang S, Zhang S, Yu B, Jang IK. Development of lipid-rich plaque inside bare metal stent: Possible mechanism of late stent thrombosis? An optical coherence tomography study. *Heart*. 2010;96:1187-1190.

[98] Tanimoto S, Aoki J, Serruys PW, Regar E. Paclitaxel-eluting stent restenosis shows three-layer appearance by optical coherence tomography. *EuroIntervention*. 2006;1:484.

[99] Ko Y-G, Kim D-M, Cho JM, Choi SY, Yoon JH, Kim J-S, Kim B-K, Choi D, Jang Y, Hong M-K. Optical coherence tomography findings of very late stent thrombosis after drug-eluting stent implantation. *Int J Cardiovasc Imaging*. 2012;28:715-723.

[100] Davlouros PA, Karantalis V, Xanthopoulou I, Mavronasiou E, Tsigkas G, Toutouzas K, Alexopoulos D. Mechanisms of non-fatal stent-related myocardial infarction late following coronary stenting with drug-eluting stents and bare metal stents. Insights from optical coherence tomography. *Circ. J.* 2011;75:2789-2797.

[101] Miyazaki S, Hiasa Y, Takahashi T, Yano Y, Minami T, Murakami N, Mizobe M, Tobetto Y, Nakagawa T, Chen P-M, Ogura R, Miyajima H, Yuba K, Hosokawa S, Kishi K, Ohtani R. *In vivo* optical coherence tomography of very late drug-eluting stent thrombosis compared with late in-stent restenosis. *Circ. J.* 2012;76:390-398.

[102] Guagliumi G, Sirbu V, Musumeci G, Gerber R, Biondi-Zoccai G, Ikejima H, Ladich E, Lortkipanidze N, Matiashvili A, Valsecchi O, Virmani R, Stone GW. Examination of the *in vivo* mechanisms of late drug-eluting stent thrombosis: Findings from optical coherence tomography and intravascular ultrasound imaging. *JACC Cardiovasc Interv.* 2012;5:12-20.

[103] Kang S-J, Lee CW, Song H, Ahn J-M, Kim W-J, Lee J-Y, Park D-W, Lee S-W, Kim Y-H, Mintz GS, Park S-W, Park S-J. OCT analysis in patients with very late stent thrombosis. *JACC Cardiovasc Imaging*. 2013;6:695-703.

[104] Parodi G, La Manna A, Di Vito L, Valgimigli M, Fineschi M, Bellandi B, Niccoli G, Giusti B, Valenti R, Cremonesi A, Biondi-Zoccai G, Prati F. Stent-related defects in patients presenting with stent thrombosis: Differences at optical coherence tomography between subacute and late/very late thrombosis in the mechanism of stent thrombosis (most) study. *EuroIntervention*. 2013;9:936-944.

[105] Alfonso F, Dutary J, Paulo M, Gonzalo N, Perez-Vizcayno MJ, Jimenez-Quevedo P, Escaned J, Banuelos C, Hernandez R, Macaya C. Combined use of optical coherence tomography and intravascular ultrasound imaging in patients undergoing coronary interventions for stent thrombosis. *Heart*. 2012;98:1213-1220.

[106] Karanasos A, Witberg K, Ligthart J, Toutouzas K, Daemen J, Van Soest G, Gnanadesigan M, Van Mieghem N, Zijlstra F, Regar E. In-stent neoatherosclerosis: Are first generation drug eluting stents different than bare metal stents? An optical coherence tomography study. *Progress in Biomedical Optics and Imaging - Proceedings of SPIE*. 2013;8565.

[107] Karanasos A, Ligthart J, Witberg K, Toutouzas K, Daemen J, Van Soest G, Gnanadesigan M, Van Geuns RJ, De Jaegere P, Regar E. Association of neointimal morphology by optical coherence tomography with rupture of neoatherosclerotic plaque very late after coronary stent implantation. *Progress in Biomedical Optics and Imaging - Proceedings of SPIE*. 2013;8565.

[108] Karanasos A, Ligthart J, Toutouzas K, Witberg K, van Geuns RJ, Van Mieghem N, Schultz C, Duckers H, De Jaegere P, Regar E. TCT-304 Neoatherosclerosis and impaired vascular healing are associated with clinical presentation late after coronary stent implantation. An optical coherence tomography study. *(abstract) J. Am. Coll. Cardiol.* 2012;60.

[109] Amabile N, Souteyrand G, Ghostine S, Combaret N, Slama MS, Barber-Chamoux N, Motreff P, Caussin C. Very late stent thrombosis related to incomplete neointimal coverage or neoatherosclerotic plaque rupture identified by optical coherence tomography imaging. *Eur Heart J Cardiovasc Imaging*. 2014;15:24-31.

[110] Karanasos A, Witberg K, Van Geuns RJ, Schultz C, Van Mieghem N, De Jaegere P, Bruining N, Zijlstra F, Regar E. Morphological characteristics by optical coherence

tomography of ruptured neoatherosclerotic plaques in patients with very late stent thrombosis. *(abstract) Eur Heart J.* 2012;33:176-176.

[111] Karanasos A, Ligthart J, Schultz C, Van Geuns RJ, Van Mieghem N, De Jaegere P, Daemen J, Zijlstra F, Regar E. Clinical and angiographic predictors of neointimal rupture as a culprit for very late stent thrombosis. Insights from optical coherence tomography. *(abstract) Eur Heart J.* 2012;33:399-399.

[112] Im E, Kim BK, Ko YG, Shin DH, Kim JS, Choi D, Jang Y, Hong MK. Incidences, predictors, and clinical outcomes of acute and late stent malapposition detected by optical coherence tomography after drug-eluting stent implantation. *Circ Cardiovasc Interv.* 2014;7:88-96.

[113] Karanasos A, van Geuns RJ, Zijlstra F, Regar E. Very late bioresorbable scaffold thrombosis after discontinuation of dual antiplatelet therapy. *Eur Heart J.* 2014;35:1781-1781

[114] Gonzalo N, Serruys PW, Okamura T, Shen ZJ, Onuma Y, Garcia-Garcia HM, Sarno G, Schultz C, van Geuns RJ, Ligthart J, Regar E. Optical coherence tomography assessment of the acute effects of stent implantation on the vessel wall: A systematic quantitative approach. *Heart.* 2009;95:1913-1919.

[115] Magro M, Regar E, Gutiérrez-Chico JL, Garcia-Garcia H, Simsek C, Schultz C, Zijlstra F, Serruys PW, van Geuns RJ. Residual atherothrombotic material after stenting in acute myocardial infarction--an optical coherence tomographic evaluation. *Int. J. Cardiol.* 2013;167:656-663.

[116] Karanasos A, Regar E. Standing on solid ground?: Reassessing the role of incomplete strut apposition in drug-eluting stents. *Circ Cardiovasc Interv.* 2014;7:6-8.

[117] Kim U, Kim JS, Lee JM, Son JW, Kim J, Ko YG, Choi D, Jang Y. The initial extent of malapposition in st-elevation myocardial infarction treated with drug-eluting stent: The usefulness of optical coherence tomography. *Yonsei Med J.* 2010;51:332-338.

[118] van Geuns R-J, Tamburino C, Fajadet J, Vrolix M, Witzenbichler B, Eeckhout E, Spaulding C, Reczuch K, La Manna A, Spaargaren R, García-García HM, Regar E, Capodanno D, Van Langenhove G, Verheye S. Self-expanding versus balloon-expandable stents in acute myocardial infarction: Results from the APPOSITION II study: Self-expanding stents in ST-segment elevation myocardial infarction. *JACC Cardiovasc Interv.* 2012;5:1209-1219.

[119] Muramatsu T, García-García HM, Lee IS, Bruining N, Onuma Y, Serruys PW. Quantitative optical frequency domain imaging assessment of in-stent structures in patients with st-segment elevation myocardial infarction: Impact of imaging sampling rate. *Circ. J.* 2012;76:2822-2831.

[120] Onuma Y, Thuesen L, van Geuns R-J, van der Ent M, Desch S, Fajadet J, Christiansen E, Smits P, Holm NR, Regar E, van Mieghem N, Borovicanin V, Paunovic D, Senshu K, van Es G-A, Muramatsu T, Lee I-S, Schuler G, Zijlstra F, Garcia-Garcia HM, Serruys PW, Investigators T. Randomized study to assess the effect of thrombus aspiration on flow area in patients with st-elevation myocardial infarction: An optical frequency domain imaging study--TROFI trial. *Eur Heart J.* 2013;34:1050-1060.

[121] Wieringa WG, Lexis CPH, Diercks GFH, Lipsic E, Tan E-S, Schurer RAJ, van der Werf HW, van den Heuvel AFM, Suurmeijer AJH, Zijlstra F, de Smet BJGL, Pundziute G. The feasibility of optical coherence tomography guided thrombus

aspiration in patients with non-st-elevation myocardial infarction after initial conservative therapy--a pilot study. *Int. J. Cardiol.* 2013;168:4981-4982.

[122] Parodi G, Valenti R, Migliorini A, Maehara A, Vergara R, Carrabba N, Mintz GS, Antoniucci D. Comparison of manual thrombus aspiration with rheolytic thrombectomy in acute myocardial infarction. *Circ Cardiovasc Interv*. 2013;6:224-230.

[123] Prati F, Capodanno D, Pawlowski T, Ramazzotti V, Albertucci M, La Manna A, Di Salvo M, Gil RJ, Tamburino C. Local delivery versus intracoronary infusion of abciximab in patients with acute coronary syndromes. *JACC Cardiovasc Interv*. 2010;3:928-934.

[124] Prati F, Di Vito L, Ramazzotti V, Imola F, Pawlowski T, Materia L, Tavazzi L, Biondi-Zoccai G, Albertucci M. Randomized trial of standard versus clearway-infused abciximab and thrombectomy in myocardial infarction: Rationale and design of the coctail ii study. *J Cardiovasc Med (Hagerstown)*. 2013;14:364-371.

[125] Abtahian F, Yonetsu T, Vergallo R, Jia H, Kato K, Tian J, Hu S, McNulty I, Jang I-K. Ticagrelor immediately prior to stenting is associated with smaller residual thrombus in patients with acute coronary syndrome. *Int. J. Cardiol.* 2013;168:3099-3101.

[126] Gonzalo N, Barlis P, Serruys PW, Garcia-Garcia HM, Onuma Y, Ligthart J, Regar E. Incomplete stent apposition and delayed tissue coverage are more frequent in drug-eluting stents implanted during primary percutaneous coronary intervention for ST-segment elevation myocardial infarction than in drug-eluting stents implanted for stable/unstable angina: Insights from optical coherence tomography. *JACC Cardiovasc Interv*. 2009;2:445-452.

[127] Räber L, Zanchin T, Baumgartner S, Taniwaki M, Kalesan B, Moschovitis A, Garcia-Garcia HM, Justiz J, Pilgrim T, Wenaweser P, Meier B, Jüni P, Windecker S. Differential healing response attributed to culprit lesions of patients with acute coronary syndromes and stable coronary artery after implantation of drug-eluting stents: An optical coherence tomography study. *Int. J. Cardiol.* 2014;173:259-267.

[128] Guagliumi G, Costa MA, Sirbu V, Musumeci G, Bezerra HG, Suzuki N, Matiashvili A, Lortkipanidze N, Mihalcsik L, Trivisonno A, Valsecchi O, Mintz GS, Dressler O, Parise H, Maehara A, Cristea E, Lansky AJ, Mehran R, Stone GW. Strut coverage and late malapposition with paclitaxel-eluting stents compared with bare metal stents in acute myocardial infarction: Optical coherence tomography substudy of the harmonizing outcomes with revascularization and stents in acute myocardial infarction (HORIZONS-AMI) trial. *Circulation*. 2011;123:274-281.

[129] García-García HM, Muramatsu T, Nakatani S, Lee IS, Holm NR, Thuesen L, van Geuns R-J, van der Ent M, Borovicanin V, Paunovic D, Onuma Y, Serruys PW. Serial optical frequency domain imaging in stemi patients: The follow-up report of TROFI study. *Eur Heart J Cardiovasc Imaging*. 2014.

[130] Gori T, Schulz E, Hink U, Wenzel P, Post F, Jabs A, Munzel T. Early outcome after implantation of ABSORB bioresorbable drug-eluting scaffolds in patients with acute coronary syndromes. *EuroIntervention*. 2014;9:1036-1041.

[131] Karanasos A, Regar E, Geeve P, van Mieghem NM. Bioresorbable scaffold in myocardial infarction: Has the time come? *Int J Cardiol*. 2013;167:e17-19.

[132] Diletti R, Karanasos A, Muramatsu T, Nakatani S, Van Mieghem NM, Onuma Y, Nauta ST, Ishibashi Y, Lenzen MJ, Ligthart J, Schultz C, Regar E, de Jaegere PP, Serruys PW, Zijlstra F, van Geuns RJ. Everolimus-eluting bioresorbable vascular

scaffolds for treatment of patients presenting with ST-segment elevation myocardial infarction: BVS STEMI first study. *Eur Heart J*. 2014;35:777-786.

[133] Kočka V, Malý M, Toušek P, Buděšínský T, Lisa L, Prodanov P, Jarkovský J, Widimský P. Bioresorbable vascular scaffolds in acute st-segment elevation myocardial infarction: A prospective multicentre study 'Prague 19'. *Eur Heart J*. 2014;35:787-794.

[134] Karanasos A, van Mieghem N, Diletti R, Onuma Y, Nauta S, Felix C, Daemen J, Kauer F, de Jaegere P, Serruys P, Regar E, Zijlstra F, van Geuns R. Oct assessment of the mid-term vascular healing response following everolimus-eluting bioresorbable scaffold implantation in myocardial infarction. The bioresorbable scaffolds STEMI-first OCT study. (abstract). *EuroIntervention*. 2014;EuroPCR abstracts 2014:Euro14A-MA072.

[135] Simsek C, Karanasos A, Magro M, Garcia-Garcia HM, Onuma Y, Regar E, Boersma E, Serruys P, van Geuns R-J. Long-term invasive follow-up of the everolimus-eluting bioresorbable vascular scaffold: Five-year results of multiple invasive imaging modalities. *EuroIntervention*. 2014;in press.

[136] Karanasos A, Gnanadesigan M, van Ditzhuijzen N, simsek c, Freire R, Dijkstra J, Van Soest G, Zijlstra F, van Geuns R, Regar E. Optical coherence tomography assessment of the 5-year vascular healing response following implantation of the everolimus-eluting bioresorbable vascular scaffold (abstract). *Journal of the American College of Cardiology*. 2014;63.

[137] Prati F, Di Vito L, Biondi-Zoccai G, Occhipinti M, La Manna A, Tamburino C, Burzotta F, Trani C, Porto I, Ramazzotti V, Imola F, Manzoli A, Materia L, Cremonesi A, Albertucci M. Angiography alone versus angiography plus optical coherence tomography to guide decision-making during percutaneous coronary intervention: The centro per la lotta contro l'infarto-optimisation of percutaneous coronary intervention (CLI-OPCI) study. *EuroIntervention*. 2012;8:823-829.

[138] Van Mieghem NM, Kauer F, Regar E. Rheolytic versus aspiration thrombectomy in acute ST-segment elevation myocardial infarction judged by OCT. *EuroIntervention*. 2010;5.

[139] Di Giorgio A, Capodanno D, Ramazzotti V, Imola F, Mallus MT, Stazi F, Paoletti G, Biondi-Zoccai G, Tamburino C, Prati F. Optical coherence tomography guided in-stent thrombus removal in patients with acute coronary syndromes. *Int J Cardiovasc Imaging*. 2013;29:989-996.

[140] Planer D, Mehran R, Ohman EM, White HD, Newman JD, Xu K, Stone GW. Prognosis of patients with non-ST-segment-elevation myocardial infarction and nonobstructive coronary artery disease: Propensity-matched analysis from the acute catheterization and urgent intervention triage strategy trial. *Circ Cardiovasc Interv*. 2014;7:285-293.

[141] Lanza GA, Crea F. Acute coronary syndromes without obstructive coronary atherosclerosis: The tiles of a complex puzzle. *Circ Cardiovasc Interv*. 2014;7:278-281.

[142] Aldrovandi A, Cademartiri F, Arduini D, Lina D, Ugo F, Maffei E, Menozzi A, Martini C, Palumbo A, Bontardelli F, Gherli T, Ruffini L, Ardissino D. Computed tomography coronary angiography in patients with acute myocardial infarction without significant coronary stenosis. *Circulation*. 2012;126:3000-3007.

[143] Karanasos A, Tsiamis E, Stefanadis C. Myocardial infarction caused by ostial right coronary artery thrombus in the absence of atheromatosis. *J Invasive Cardiol.* 2012;24:E188-189.

[144] Toutouzas K, Karanasos A, Stefanadis C. Pitfalls of angiography in the assessment of atherosclerosis: The role of optical coherence tomography. *J Invasive Cardiol.* 2012;24:246-247.

[145] Stefano GT, Bezerra HG, Attizzani G, Chamie D, Mehanna E, Yamamoto H, Costa MA. Utilization of frequency domain optical coherence tomography and fractional flow reserve to assess intermediate coronary artery stenoses: Conciliating anatomic and physiologic information. *Int J Cardiovasc Imaging*. 2011;27:299-308.

[146] Van Mieghem NM, Ligthart J, Manintveld OC, Regar E. Acute coronary syndrome in 3 dimensions: The culprit exposed. *J. Am. Coll. Cardiol.* 2011;58.

[147] McCabe JM, Croce KJ. Optical coherence tomography. *Circulation*. 2012;126:2140-2143.

[148] Kramer MC, Verouden NC, Li X, Koch KT, van der Wal AC, Tijssen JG, de Winter RJ. Thrombus aspiration alone during primary percutanous coronary intervention as definitive treatment in acute ST-elevation myocardial infarction. *Catheter Cardiovasc Interv*. 2012;79:860-867.

[149] Escaned J, Echavarria-Pinto M, Gorgadze T, Gonzalo N, Armengol F, Hernandez R, Jimenez-Quevedo P, Nunez-Gil IJ, Perez-Vizcayno MJ, Alfonso F, Banuelos C, Ibañez B, Garcia E, Fernandez Ortiz A, Macaya C. Safety of lone thrombus aspiration without concomitant coronary stenting in selected patients with acute myocardial infarction. *EuroIntervention*. 2013;8:1149-1156.

[150] Kelbæk H, Engstrøm T, Ahtarovski KA, Lønborg J, Vejlstrup N, Pedersen F, Holmvang L, Helqvist S, Saunamäki K, Jørgensen E, Clemmensen P, Kløvgaard L, Tilsted H-H, Raungaard B, Ravkilde J, Aaroe J, Eggert S, Køber L. Deferred stent implantation in patients with ST-segment elevation myocardial infarction: A pilot study. *EuroIntervention*. 2013;8:1126-1133.

[151] Cervinka P, Spaček R, Bystroň M, Kvašňák M, Kupec A, Cervinková M, Kala P. Optical coherence tomography-guided primary percutaneous coronary intervention in ST-segment elevation myocardial infarction patients: A pilot study. *Can J Cardiol.* 2014;30:420-427.

[152] Braunwald E. Coronary plaque erosion: Recognition and management. *JACC Cardiovasc Imaging*. 2013;6:288-289.

[153] Prati F, Uemura S, Souteyrand G, Virmani R, Motreff P, Di Vito L, Biondi-Zoccai G, Halperin J, Fuster V, Ozaki Y, Narula J. OCT-based diagnosis and management of STEMI associated with intact fibrous cap. *JACC Cardiovasc Imaging*. 2013;6:283-287.

[154] Chamié D, Wang Z, Bezerra H, Rollins AM, Costa MA. Optical coherence tomography and fibrous cap characterization. *Curr Cardiovasc Imaging Rep*. 2011;4:276-283.

[155] Zahnd G, Karanasos A, van Soest G, Regar E, Niessen WJ, Gijsen F, van Walsum T. Semi-automated quantification of fibrous cap thickness in intracoronary optical coherence tomography. *Information processing in computer-assisted interventions*. Springer; 2014:78-89.

[156] Wang Z, Chamie D, Bezerra HG, Yamamoto H, Kanovsky J, Wilson DL, Costa MA, Rollins AM. Volumetric quantification of fibrous caps using intravascular optical coherence tomography. *Biomed Opt Express*. 2012;3:1413-1426.

[157] Ughi GJ, Adriaenssens T, Sinnaeve P, Desmet W, D'Hooge J. Automated tissue characterization of *in vivo* atherosclerotic plaques by intravascular optical coherence tomography images. *Biomed Opt Express*. 2013;4:1014-1030.

[158] Gnanadesigan M, van Soest G, White S, Scoltock S, Ughi GJ, Baumbach A, van der Steen AFW, Regar E, Johnson TW. Effect of temperature and fixation on the optical properties of atherosclerotic tissue: A validation study of an *ex-vivo* whole heart cadaveric model. *Biomed Opt Express*. 2014;5:1038-1049.

[159] Regar E, Gnanadesigan M, Van der Steen AF, van Soest G. Quantitative optical coherence tomography tissue-type imaging for lipid-core plaque detection. *JACC Cardiovasc Interv*. 2013;6:891-892.

[160] van Soest G, Goderie T, Regar E, Koljenovic S, van Leenders GL, Gonzalo N, van Noorden S, Okamura T, Bouma BE, Tearney GJ, Oosterhuis JW, Serruys PW, van der Steen AF. Atherosclerotic tissue characterization *in vivo* by optical coherence tomography attenuation imaging. *J Biomed Opt*. 2010;15:011105.

[161] Wang T, Wieser W, Springeling G, Beurskens R, Lancee CT, Pfeiffer T, van der Steen AFW, Huber R, van Soest G. Intravascular optical coherence tomography imaging at 3200 frames per second. *Opt Lett*. 2013;38:1715-1717.

[162] Karanasos A, Schuurbiers J, Gnanadesigan M, van Ditzhuijzen N, Dijkstra J, Van Soest G, Zijlstra F, van Geuns R, Wentzel J, Regar E. Association of wall shear stress with vascular healing response by oct 5 years after bioresorbable scaffold implantation (abstract). *Journal of the American College of Cardiology*. 2014;63.

[163] Liu L, Gardecki JA, Nadkarni SK, Toussaint JD, Yagi Y, Bouma BE, Tearney GJ. Imaging the subcellular structure of human coronary atherosclerosis using micro-optical coherence tomography. *Nat. Med.* 2011;17:1010-1014.

[164] Villiger M, Zhang EZ, Nadkarni S, Oh WY, Bouma BE, Vakoc BJ. Artifacts in polarization-sensitive optical coherence tomography caused by polarization mode dispersion. *Opt Lett*. 2013;38:923-925.

[165] Nadkarni SK, Pierce MC, Park BH, de Boer JF, Whittaker P, Bouma BE, Bressner JE, Halpern E, Houser SL, Tearney GJ. Measurement of collagen and smooth muscle cell content in atherosclerotic plaques using polarization-sensitive optical coherence tomography. *J Am Coll Cardiol*. 2007;49:1474-1481.

[166] Yoo H, Kim JW, Shishkov M, Namati E, Morse T, Shubochkin R, McCarthy JR, Ntziachristos V, Bouma BE, Jaffer FA, Tearney GJ. Intra-arterial catheter for simultaneous microstructural and molecular imaging *in vivo*. *Nat Med*. 2011;17:1680-1684.

In: Myocardial Infarctions
Editor: Pattie Wilkonson

ISBN: 978-1-63321-726-3

Chapter 3

Psychosocial Risk Factors in Cardiovascular Disease

Carla Favoccia[1*], Giada Pietrabissa[2,3], Gianluca Castelnuovo[2,3], Gian Mauro Manzoni[4], Mariella Montano[1], Gianandrea Bertone[1], Annamaria Titon[1], Ferruccio Nibbio[1] and Luca Gondoni[1]

[1]Cardiac Rehabilitation Unit, Istituto Auxologico Italiano IRCCS, Saint Joseph Hospital, Verbania, Italy

[2]Psychology Research Laboratory, Istituto Auxologico Italiano IRCCS, Saint Joseph Hospital, Verbania, Italy

[3]Department of Psychology, Catholic University, Milan, Italy

[4]Faculty of Psychology, eCampus University, Novedrate, Como, Italy

Abstract

Introduction: according to the literature, psychosocial factors significantly contribute to both pathogenesis and expression of coronary artery disease (CAD). Depression, anxiety, anger and hostility, social isolation and stressful life-style represent the main contributing factors both to higher prevalence of unhealthy behaviors (poor diet, physical inactivity, alcohol use or smoking) and adverse pathophysiological mechanisms, such as neuroendocrine and platelet activation.

Material and method: over the past few decades, there has been an increasing interest in investigating the relationship between psychosocial risk factors and cardiovascular disease, leading to a growing pool of clinical and epidemiological data on the subject. Specifically, a large case–control trial, involving 52 countries, has identified nine potentially modifiable risk factors for CAD, among which psychosocial factors have been included and divided into two general categories: chronic stressors and emotional factors. These are believed to exacerbate the development of cardiovascular disease by two mechanisms: 1) encouraging unhealthy behaviors and increasing the non-compliance

* Carla Favoccia, MD. Cardiac Rehabilitation Unit, Istituto Auxologico Italiano IRCCS, Saint Joseph Hospital, Verbania, Italy. University of Pavia, c/o Fondazione IRCCS Policlinico S. Matteo, V.le Golgi, 19, 27100 Pavia, Italy. Phone: +3402718198. E-mail: carla.favoccia@gmail.com.

to treatments; and 2) eliciting physiological responses that may lead to insufficient oxygen delivery to the heart muscle, threatening heart rhythms, more vulnerable plaque, and the potential for blood clotting. Etiological controlled studies also confirmed this relationship.

In this work, we outline the psychosocial domains significantly considered associated with increased risk of cardiovascular morbidity and mortality. We also discuss critical pathophysiological mechanisms and pathways that, operating in a synergistic and integrative way, promote related clinical manifestations. Also, the impact of cardiac rehabilitation programs on psychological-related cardiovascular events is discussed.

Discussion: the importance of psychosocial variables in the development, clinical manifestations, and prognosis of patients with heart disease received increased attention in recent years. However, the influence of psychosocial risk factors in cardiovascular disease remains under-estimated when compared with the conventional ones. To recognize this relationship and to offers an important target for cardiovascular education, counseling and behavioral interventions, even after controlling for major risk factors. Cardiac rehabilitation programs considering a multidisciplinary approach are then widely recommended for the management of risk factors, nutritional, psychological, behavioral and social aspects potentially affecting patient outcomes.

Conflicts of interest and Source of Funding: None declared

“The gods are just, and of our pleasant vices
Make instruments to plague us.”

King Lear, V.iii.193 William Shakespeare

Introduction

There are many convincing data supporting the relationship between cardiovascular risk and psychosocial factors. Despite existent actions of prevention, the incidence of coronary artery disease (CAD) still remains largely unexplained. Consequently, clinical researchers are currently considering new elements potentially involved in the pathophysiology of cardiovascular damage and psychosocial risk factors (PSRF) have been largely investigated. According to Rozansky and his collaborators PSRF can be divided into 5 clusters (1) depression, (2) anxiety, (3) personality factors and character traits (e.g., hostility), (4) social isolation, as well as (5) sub-acute and chronic life stress [1]. The pathophysiological link between psychosocial risk factors and CAD can be determined both by direct effects on the endothelium and indirect effects on the cardiovascular system [2]. In addition, numerous case studies confirm patients with psychosocial disorders being more susceptible to develop traditional risk factors such as hypertension, diabetes and dyslipidemia [3]. Since the 17th century, coronary artery disease has been considered having psychosomatic nature, reflecting the realities of living in modern society, such as stress, lack of time, competitiveness and ambition. Then, CAD is currently interpreted as product of the interaction between social influences and other etiological factors as part of a broad bio-psycho-social model [4]. In fact, although biological, psychological and social factors are all necessary, none of them is by itself sufficient to produce cardiovascular disease, and treatment recommendations consider the therapist addressing biological, experiential and social factors. In addition, many studies have investigated both the influence of psychosocial factors on CAD and the role of cardiovascular disease in developing psychopathology, documenting a bidirectional relationship. In fact, psychological factors can affect certain health related behaviors and even act as obstacles for adherence to treatment which in turn may influence the risk of CAD. Whether they represent actors or bystanders is not clear yet. Also, in the up-to-date practice of Cardiac Rehabilitation (CR), psychosocial services are growing in importance and European guidelines intensively encourage psycho-educational activities which increase the likelihood of permanent lifestyle changes [3].

This contribution represents a two voice dialog between Cardiologists and Psychologists.

Starting with providing an overview of the current state-of-the-art on the topics, we discuss the pathophysiological link between psychosocial factors and CAD as well as both present and future psychological interventions or strategies aim at reducing stress and depression in cardiac patients.

Understanding Cardiovascular Disease

Cardiovascular disease is one of the main causes of morbidity and mortality in the western countries. Due to the multifactorial etiology of the disease and the several risk factors determining its development, a complete knowledge of the pathogenesis of CAD has not been reached yet.

To this aim, the Framingham study first introduced the concept of "risk factor" as potentially responsible for increasing the risk for coronary event in the long term, assessing the relationship between CAD and certain clinical situations [5].

Risk factors have been initially divided into two groups, the modifiable ones, such as diabetes mellitus, hypertension, dyslipidemia and unhealthy lifestyle (incorrect diet, physical inactivity and smoking) and the non-modifiable, among which increasing age, male gender and genetic predisposition represent the main ones (Table 1) [4].

Table 1. Risk factors associated with Cardiovascular Diseases

Major modifiable risk factors	**Other modifiable risk factors**
- High Blood pressure	- Low socioeconomic status (SES)
- Abnormal blood lipids	- Mental ill-health (depression)
- Tobacco Use	- Psychosocial stress
- Physical inactivity	- Alcohol use
- Obesity	- Use of certain medication
- Unhealthy diet	- Lipoprotein(a)
- Diabetes mellitus	- Left ventricular hypertrophy (LVH)
Non-modifiable risk factors	**"Novel" risk factors**
- Advancing age	- Excess homocysteine in blood
- Heredity or family history	- Inflammatory markers (C-reactive protein)
- Gender	- Abnormal blood coagulation (elevate blood levels of fibrinogen)
- Ethnicity or race	

However, traditional risk factors alone do not fully explain the growing incidence of the disease and there is increasing awareness that psychosocial attributes may act as mediators, and even directly as causal factors for CAD [6]. The American guidelines for the prevention of cardiovascular disease do not properly take into account psychosocial risk factors as implicated into pathogenesis of CAD while European guidelines describe them referring to low socio-economic status, work-related stress, financial difficulties, family problems, depression, anxiety and hostility. Also, psychological stress is increasingly recognized as highly affecting cardiovascular disease [2].

Thus, psychosocial attributes may contribute to worsen both the clinical course and prognosis, and the need of including psychological treatments into the Cardiac Rehabilitation program came to light [7].

When we discuss cardiovascular risk factors we generally refer to conditions that increase the risk of having a coronary event in the long term. We have a scant knowledge of the factors that cause the acute events. Beyond the plaque characteristics, the blood dynamics and other chronic conditions we have recognized a set of stressors that might have an implication in the process: among them we find stress (whatever the cause), catecholamine surge (which is also implicated in the takotsubo cardiomyopathy), and depression.

Psychosocial Risk Factor for Cardiovascular Disease

A psychosocial risk factor can be defined as a measurement that potentially relates psychological phenomena to the social environment and/or to pathophysiological changes [8].

However, by their very nature and being extremely subjected to cultural influences, these variables are understandably difficult to define objectively, especially when compared with other "traditional" and biomedical risk factors. They typically rely on individual self-reporting and frequently consist of several related elements [9]. The definitions of psychosocial factors promoting adverse cardiac events vary in different studies: nevertheless, they are generally broadly divided into two general categories: *emotional factors* and *chronic stressors* [6, 10, 11].

Emotional factors include affective disorders such as major depression and anxiety disorders as well as hostility and anger. Chronic stressors include factors such as low social support, low socioeconomic status, work stress, marital stress, and caregiver strain.

Emotional Factors

Depression

Of all the emotion-related factors that have been studied with respect to heart disease, depression has been most consistently linked with the development and prognosis of cardiovascular syndrome to the point of appearing more common among patients suffering from CAD than the general population [12].

By 2020, the World Health Organization (WHO) predicts that both CAD and depression will be the two major causes of disability-adjusted life years in developed countries [13, 14].

Depression represents a state of prolonged sadness and/or anhedonia (inability to take pleasure in life) that can affect a person's thoughts, behavior, feelings and sense of well-being. Symptoms vary from mild (subclinical) to classic major depression and suicidal ideation.

It is intuitive to consider depression as a consequence of heart diseasc, but several studies show that this relationship can be bidirectional, with depression also increasing the risk for CAD and mortality [15]. However, it is important to note that scientific literature has often focused on symptom of depression rather than on depressive disorders meeting diagnostic criteria.

Patients with depression are more likely to sustain unhealthy lifestyle and poor medication adherence, which adversely impact on treatment outcomes [16] and low mood is also related to poor secondary prevention behaviors, like exercise, dieting and quitting smoking in patients suffering from heart diseases. Maintaining healthy habits and being in a good physical shape has been shown essential for reducing the risk of heart disease and this is true even for people who don't have metabolic syndrome (MetS), a cluster of conditions (increased blood pressure, a high blood sugar level, excess body fat around the waist and abnormal cholesterol levels) that occur together, increasing the risk of heart disease, stroke and diabetes. In fact, even metabolically healthy overweight and obese people can develop heart problems.

Specifically, obesity in its own right is associated with an increased risk of heart attack representing, particularly among women, an independent predictor of CAD [17, 18].

Hence, the effects of depression in both initially healthy individuals and patients with known CAD have been largely evaluated, showing depression having a role in promoting CAD events in both cohorts [1].

Due to compelling evidence that depression affects cardiac mortality and morbidity, lifestyle, and medical adherence, screening for depression can possibly improve clinical outcomes in primary care setting [19] and help identifying CAD patients at risk for poor secondary prevention outcomes [20]. Symptoms of depression are not simple to differentiate from indicators of physical illness, such as lack of energy and sleep disturbance, but non depressed cardiac patients generally do not present signs of psychiatric emotional distress such as crying, sense of worthlessness or suicidal ideation [21]. Also, symptoms of depression are sometimes less specific and more mild in the non-cardiac population [15].

Furthermore, adding to the argument of screening is the evidence that treatment of depression is complicated and may involve close monitoring and switching of medications before patients achieve full remission. Also, the time of onset of the depressive symptoms provides information that guide the course of the treatment, and people with longstanding, preexisting depression require a different psychotherapeutic technique when compared with people in their first episode of depression.

The Canadian Cardiac Randomized Evaluation of Antidepressant and Psychotherapy Efficacy (CREATE) [22] and the Enhancing Recovery in Coronary Heart Disease (ENRICHD) studies [23] did not find the use of psychotherapy, (i.e. interpersonal psychotherapy and cognitive behavioral therapy) substantially useful, highlighting the importance of using antidepressants in treating depressive symptoms. Psychopharmacological treatment, preferably an SSRI, has been shown appropriate in patients with CAD but fear for cardiotoxicity [24] and concerns about the fact that reducing emotional distress in the short-term may actually improve long-term mortality in patients still persist [25].

Anxiety

Independently from depression [26-28], evidence suggests anxiety also having an adverse impact on prognosis in CAD patients, although its role as an etiological risk factor is less clear because of researches typically focus on only one or two manifestations of the construct. Anxiety has been conceptualized as a stable personality trait (trait anxiety), a symptom elicited through provocation (state anxiety), and a psychiatric disorder [29] and it is generally characterized by a *subjective experience of dread and foreboding occurring in conjunction with unpleasant feeling of somatic tension, nervousness, apprehension and worry, with activation of the autonomic nervous system* [30]. Although multiple manifestations of anxiety often coexist within the same individual, this is not typically captured in empirical research [29].

Also, studies examining the risk of cardiovascular outcomes associated with anxiety disorders appear scant or conflicting [1, 28] and the number of researches finding a strong association between phobias and sudden cardiac death is currently limited to three: the Northwick Park Heart Study [31], the Health Professionals Follow-up Study [32] and the Normative Aging Study [33].

Primary categories of anxiety disorders that have been investigated are generalized anxiety disorder, Panic Disorder and Post-Traumatic Stress Disorder.

People who are having a *panic attack* often interpret their symptoms as being heart related. The attack is characterized by intense fear, with rapid development of frightening and distressing symptoms within 10 minutes, without warning and often for no apparent reason. People having panic attacks can experience symptoms such as sensation that heart is beating irregularly (palpitations), sweating, trembling, shortness of breath, feeling of shocking, chest pain, nausea, dizziness, depersonalization, feeling of losing control or going crazy, fear of dying, tingling and hot flushes. Cardiac patients who develop symptoms of anxiety are in a difficult blind: to ignore chest pain is dangerous, yet it is difficult and sometimes impossible to discern the difference between chest pain caused by anxiety or ischemia heart disease.

Emotional adjusting, depression as well as intense and persistent anxiety are also experienced by 20-40% of heart patients up to several years after the event, often giving rise to *Post-Traumatic Stress Disorder* (PTSD). Doerfler et al. found PTSD being highly associated with increased mortality among patients suffering from heart diseases [34], and a systematic review has shown presence of PTSD in seven out of nine studies [35].

However, methodological differences make it difficult to undertake between-study comparison, then to evaluate both prevalence rates of PTSD among heart patients and timing of the psychopathology onset, currently estimated between 3 to 6 month post-Myocardial Infarction (MI) [15, 36]. *It is possible to talk about PTSD when, in response to a life-threatening event, a person experiences marked distress and functional impairment [37] accompanied by sentiment of severe helplessness, fear or horror* [38].

Symptoms criteria cluster into three category: re-experiencing of symptoms (in dreams or through flashbacks), avoidance of reminders of the traumatic event and emotional numbing (generating inability of experience positive emotions) as well as psychological hyperarousal, suggesting the individuals' body being in a constant state of alertness. Changes in heart rate and respiration may suggest the possibility of death, and people usually start avoiding physical effort [34]. Having strong impact on medical outcomes regardless disease severity [35], PTSD also influences the use of emergency medical services for "feeling another heart attack", leading to increased health care costs [36]. Women are more likely to develop PTSD following a traumatic experience when compared to men [39], although more research is needed in order to determine whether gender *per se* constitutes a risk factor for developing PTSD [40]. PTSD also results in social withdrawal, which in turn affects social relationship and support [41] as well as return to work [36].

The prevalence of anxiety among hospitalized cardiac patients is high, with about 16% of men and 24% of women undergoing Cardiac Rehabilitation having a state anxiety score comparable with psychiatric patients [42]. Despite their high prevalence, anxiety, PTSD and depression are rarely recognized and diagnosed by medical professionals, thus hindering screening and effective interventions which are warranted because of their negative impact on morbidity, mortality and quality of life. Patients reporting significant levels of PTSD, anxiety or depressive symptoms should be referred to a mental health professional for attending psychotherapy, pharmacotherapy or a combination of both. Cognitive-Behavioral Therapy (CBT), taking into account the interrelation of thinking, emotion and behavior, represents the gold standard treatment in CR programs and it is generally well-accepted by patients [43, 44]. Also, considering the efficacy of SSRIs in treating PTSD and depression in physically healthy individuals, no reason is assumed to deny these drugs from cardiac patients when they are relatively safe and likely to offer important benefits [45].

Anger and Hostility

Epidemiological studies have also considered anger/hostility as other emotional factors associated with CAD. Initially identified as having a Type A behavior pattern (TABP) by the cardiologists Friedman and Rosenman [46, 47], a person characterized by hostility, intense ambition, competitive drive, constant preoccupation with deadlines or sense of time urgency, was considered to be more likely for developing coronary heart disease. However, these original findings were not supported by subsequent researches [48] and a meta-analysis of prospective studies between 1966 and 1998 failed to show an association between TABP and CAD.

Some researchers therefore changed their focus investigating whether anger, hostility, and related constructs would be more closely linked to the development of CAD. In fact, despite having different meanings, these terms are often confused [49].

Briefly, *hostility is typically described as a negative attitude or cognitive trait directed toward others* while *anger represents an emotional state that consists of feelings that vary from mild irritation to intense fury or rage, and aggressiveness as a verbal or physical pattern.*

The first quantitative systematic review [50] on the topic shows anger and hostility being significantly associated with 20% increased risk of CAD events in healthy populations and slightly poor prognosis in individuals with existing CAD. Frequent anger episodes related to anger and hostility traits might accelerate recurrence of CAD [51], then interventions aimed at preventing heart diseases should focus on the psychological management of anger and hostility. Also, the effect of anger and hostility has been shown more relevant in healthy men than women. However, the role of psychological factors in both the onset and progression of heart diseases should be studied in concert rather than using an individual risk factor approach; anger and hostility do not comprise only one behavioral construct, as the authors posited, and interview-based methods, through observed interpersonal interactions [52], provide better measure of multidimensional constructs then patient-reported scales, which require self-awareness of hostility and tend to be influenced by reporting bias [53].

Psychosocial Stressors

Psychosocial stressors as potentially modifiable risks factors are also increasingly recognized as important issues in cardiovascular disease even if this link is not well understood.

In fact, measurement of stress is complex, difficult to define objectively on a large scale and both cultural and ethnic influences may affect how stress is perceived and reported [54].

The concept of psychological stress has also evolved over time, and is now defined as *feeling tension, anxiety or irritability; or as having sleeping difficulties as a result of conditions at home or at work.*

Stress responses usually arise when demands or people exceed their psychological resources or adaptive capacity, and individual differences exist in how well people cope with challenges or losses in their lives. Demands or stressors can take the form of (1) *long-term challenges*, comprising chronic work-related stress and factors in private life, such as marital problem and financial difficulties, (2) *acute life events,* such as individual stressors (i.e. bereavement, social isolation or job loss) or acute population stressors (i.e. earthquakes, terrorist attacks and sporting events) as well as (3) *daily minor harassments* such as traffic problem while commuting [55, 56].

Despite a report published by the National Heart Foundation of Australia (NHFA) concluded that neither a strong nor a consistent evidence of a causal association between work-related stressors and CAD are present, [57], there is plausible evidence for work stress having a biological impact [8].

Stress at work, one of the most widely used variables in quantifying psychosocial stress, has been linked with CAD in both prospective and retrospective studies [54, 58] and has been shown to double the risk for developing metabolic syndrome [59].

Most of the literature evaluating the effects of work stress generally refers to individuals' perceptions rather than external ratings of work stress, such as job strain and effort-reward imbalance, organizational justice and shifting work [60-62], while the association between the development of CAD and job (in)security, job satisfaction and working hours is mixed.

Specifically, two main epidemiological models describing the construct of job strain have been shown to significantly predict cardiovascular mortality and recurrent CAD events [63, 64]: the *Karasek model*, in which job strain is the result of a combination of high job demand and low job decision latitude [65] and the *effort-reward imbalance model*, according with the mismatch between high effort, low rewards and individuals' exhaustive coping style (or over-commitment) leads to adverse health effects [61]. Much of the available evidence regarding job strain as a CAD risk factor comes from western societies, in both men and women [64, 66-69]

Also, *low social support* and *lack of economic resources* seem to contribute in increasing the risk of adverse prognosis in cardiac patients and these factors are especially difficult to achieve. One of the most comprehensive review suggested a 50% increased likelihood of survival for participants with stronger social relationships, with no gender difference [70], and a more recent study evaluating people either at risk of or with existing atherosclerosis showed that people who lived alone were at higher risk of cardiovascular death than those who lived with someone [71]. Unmarried CAD patients without confidants and with low household income have been shown to be at high risk of cardiovascular death over a 5-year period [72].

Data from prospective studies have also shown associations between marital problems, widowhood, death of a child, and caring for a sick spouse at home, as increasing risk for heart diseases [55].

Stress can also influence CAD indirectly, by increasing unhealthy behaviors. One of the largest cohort study in the field, for example, has shown smokers being more likely to have over 20 cigarettes per day if experiencing work-stress related, while in the Copenhagen City Heart Study individuals with high compared with low stress level were less likely to quit smoking, more likely to become physically inactive and less likely to stop drinking alcohol [55, 73]. Since some psychosocial stressors result from economic, political and social forces over which the clinician has little control, behavioral and pharmacological interventions aimed at modifying psychosocial risks have been carried out, with mixed results.

Therefore prospective investigations are needed in order to determine which intervention best suits the different individual needs. Moreover, what is deemed to be culturally appropriate in one country may not be in another and this emphasizes the importance of addressing interventions on psychosocial variables in a wide reaching manner.

A Literature Review

The evidence linking psychosocial risk factor and CAD has been widely analyzed by a number of studies. Epidemiologic evidence amassed in the past indicates depressive symptoms independently predicting the incidence of CAD. In fact, it has long been recognized that mild forms of depression are present in up to two thirds of patients hospitalized after an acute myocardial infarction, and major depression generally affecting 15% of CAD patients [74]. Also, etiological investigations suggest that the presence of depression doubles the risk of developing new CAD. Moreover, the INTERHEART study, a large case control study involving 52 different countries [11], has identified nine potentially modifiable risk factors for CAD: (1) smoking, history, (2) hypertension or (3) diabetes, (4) waist circumference, (5) dietary patterns, (6) physical activity, (7) alcohol consumption, (8) blood apolipoproteins (Apo) and (9) psychosocial factors.. Despite substantial differences between regions, ethnic groups and gender were present, authors concluded that, due to the strong association between psychosocial factors, such as stress at work or stress in general, and increased risk of myocardial infarction, actively intervening on these would result in reduced risk for developing heart disease [54].

In addition, the SUPRIM study quantitatively investigated quality of life and PSRF among patients in their first year after a CAD events showing these variables having important implications on rehabilitation programs. Pointing out the efficacy of Cognitive

Behavioral Therapy in decreasing the risk of recurrent CAD and recurrent acute myocardial infarction, the study also underlined psychosocial risk factors being important to address in secondary prevention [75].

The CARDIA prospective observational study has examined the role of time urgency, achievement striving, hostility, depression and anxiety as long term psychosocial risk factors for hypertension in young adults, finding urgency and hostility specifically linked with a proportional increase of hypertension in a long term . [76].

Moreover, several prospective studies have described the relationship between the endothelial dysfunction and CAD, analyzing the link between CAD and the level of brachial artery Flow Mediated Dilatation (FMD), the level of circulating Endothelial function Progenitor Cells (EPCs) or the level of endothelium dependent vasodilator Methacholine (MCh) and Sodium Nitroprusside (SNP) endothelial independent vasodilatation. The EPCs are immature cells that participate in the repair of vascular endothelium damage and contribute to neovascularization and re-endothelization. The FMD is a common non-invasive assessment of vascular endothelial function. Poitras et al. have studied these variables during mental stress condition; demonstrating the existence of strong correlation between endothelial variables and CAD [77]. Mental stress is an interesting model for studying the interactions between brain and heart. Indeed, ischemia induced by mental stress has peculiar features that differentiate it from the exercise induced ischemia: particularly, while heart rate and systolic blood pressure increase less than during exercise, diastolic blood pressure and systemic vascular resistance tend to increase more [78] and this can be caused by a different pathway of activation of the central nervous system.

Chen et al. evaluated the relationship between the circulating EPCs and FMD index and both depression and STRESS levels unstable angina patients suffering from major psychiatric disorders. The number of circulating EPCs increased in patients with unstable angina and acute infarction, and reduced in those with stable angina like in patients suffering from major depression. FMD low levels are related to low risk of cardiac events. Unstable angina patients without major psychiatric disorders, high depression or stress score results showed attenuated FMD and EPCs levels. Also the use of drugs resulted associated with improved FMD [79]. Eriksson et al. have described how MCh has reduced resistance vessel vasodilatation during mental arithmetics. Such effect is prevented by the infusion of beta blockers or neurogenic blockers [80]. These data suggest that endothelial dysfunction may be one of the mechanisms that contribute to the development of CAD in patients with depression and stress [77].

Other studies have described the relationship between depression, anxiety and recurrent cardiac events in patients with CAD. Park et al. showed patients with high levels of depression or anxiety being at increased risk for developing CAD after percutaneous coronary intervention (PCI). and psycho-educational support aim at addressing these variables being useful for improving health outcomes [81]. Analyzing angina patients presenting depression or anxiety, authors showed that, in addition to an increased risk of CAD [82], angina symptoms together with depression or anxiety can worsen both quality of life and cardiac prognosis[83]. Further investigations have taken into consideration the relationship between CAD and socioeconomic status, personality types, stress handling and emotional intelligence.

Once again, type D (distress) personality has been often observed in CAD patients [84], and persons characterized by type-A behavior pattern (hard-driving, competitive, impatient, persistent sense of time urgency) were considered more prone to develop diabetes or hypertension, as well as to more frequently present history of smoking when compared to the control group [85]. Furthermore, patients suffering for psychological problems, have been considered particularly predisposed to develop Post-Traumatic Stress Disorder (PTDS), a potential cause for re-infarctions and mortality [86]. Other studies shows low socioeconomic status amplifying mental stress, which in turn represents an important risk factor for CAD [87]. Prevention is better than cure; therefore, considering the increased role of PSRF in both predisposing the development of CAD and determining worsens cardiac prognosis, it becomes necessary to suddenly recognize them promoting preventive and effective actions.

Physiopathology

Psychosocial risk factors cause a number of physiological changes such as raised blood pressure, increase of insulin resistance and endothelial dysfunction. The effect of psychosocial factors on CAD can be grouped into two broad categories, indirect factors and direct factors, which are not to be considered as two separate phenomena in their own right, but always as entities depending on each other. (Table 2).

Table 2. Physiopathology. The effect of psychosocial factors on CAD

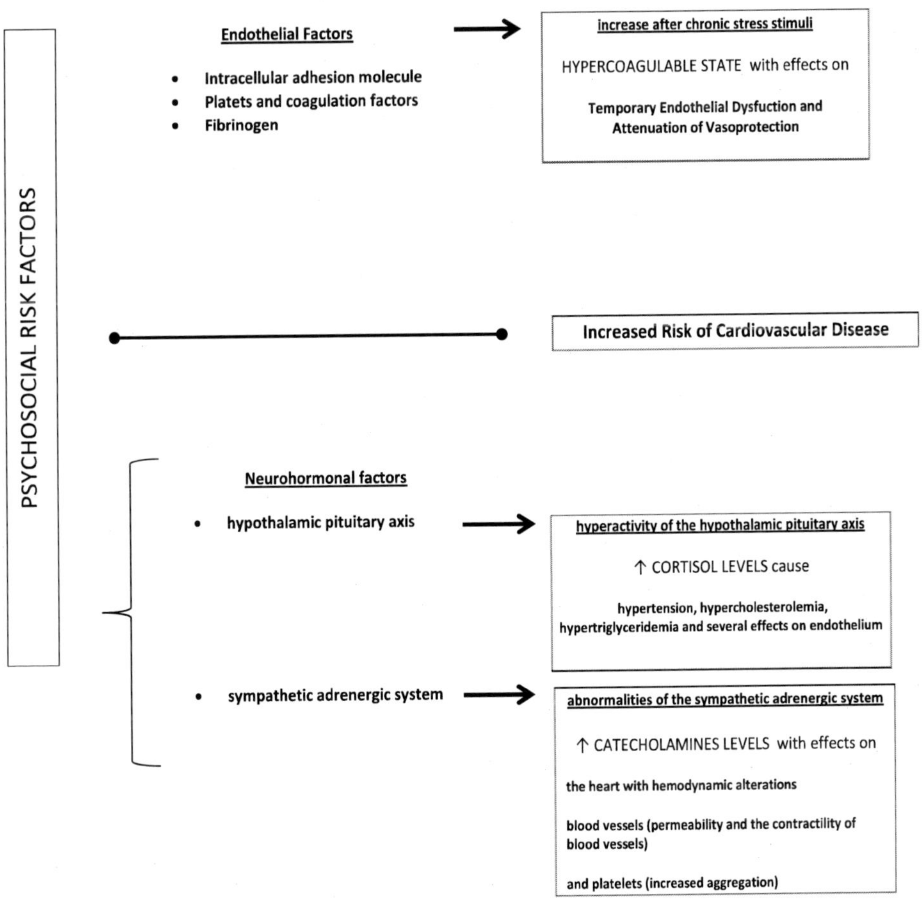

Endothelial Factors

Endothelial factors are released after acute and chronic stress and could be classified in 3 groups: the intracellular adhesion molecule, the platelets and coagulation factors and the fibrinogen. Before describing each of them it is necessary to understand the role of the functional endothelium.

The functional endothelium is a dynamic tissue responsible for many functions including vasodilatation, and it influences vascular structure determining the nature of the interaction between the blood and the vessel wall. It promotes vasoprotection, inhibiting vascular smooth cell migration and producing proliferation and the adhesion of platelets and myocytes to the walls of the blood vessels [88, 89]. The endothelial dysfunction seems to precede the development of atherosclerosis in which plays a significant role.

The intracellular adhesion molecules, such as monocyte chemoattractant proteins, pro inflammatory cytokines and chemokines, increase after chronic stress stimuli leading to prolonged endothelial dysfunction [90]. These molecules could determine abnormalities in cellular adhesion, migration and proliferation resulting in a persistent pro atherosclerotic environment [91].

Platelets play a relevant role during the all stages of plaque development as well as in the acute coronary syndromes. Platelet activation is increased in depression [92]. Increased workload is also associated with increased platelet aggregability, a hypercoagulable state with increases in factor VII and VIII and can also lead to impaired fibrinolysis causing damage to the endothelium and the promotion of plaque [93]. Also fibrinogen is associated with workload. A recent Belgian study described that workers with low job control have exaggerated fibrinogen response to mental stress compared to high job control workers [94]. However other studies did not confirm this relationship [95].

In addition, there are data which show that, in case of high job strain, there is an increase of inflammatory markers such as C Reactive Protein [96, 97]. Pro inflammatory cytokines are involved in the genesis of endothelial damage and may be responsible for some of the somatic features of depression, causing anorexia, malaise, weight loss and sleep disturbances as well as a hemodynamic hyperactivity contributing to CAD in some individuals [98].

Neurohormonal Factors

The response to emotional stress is mediated through the stimulation of hypothalamic neurons that send messages to other brain centers. The sympathetic nervous system outflow to the heart and blood vessels originates in the vasomotor center of the brain. The hypothalamic pituitary axis and sympathetic adrenomedullary systems are the primary biological systems activated during the stress response. The hypothalamic pituitary axis under stress produces the corticotrophin releasing factor (CRF) with a consequent increase of the Adrenocorticotropic Hormone (ACTH), beta endorphin, and other corticosteroid products from the anterior pituitary. These hormones act on the adrenal cortex causing the release of glucocorticoid hormones such as cortisol [99]. The hyperactivity of the hypothalamic pituitary axis leads to an increase of corticosteroid hormones, favors hypertension, hypercholesterolemia and hypertriglyceridemia and has several effects on endothelium and its healing abilities [100-102]. Cortisol hyper-secretion is found in subjects with depression, work stress, hostility as well as in subjects of lower social economic status [1, 2, 103].

The majority of the patients affected with depression show abnormalities of the sympathetic adrenergic system. The regulatory centers of the central nervous system neurons are stimulated by the production of hypothalamic CRF which activates preganglionic sympathetic neurons which in turn stimulate the heart and the adrenal medullary axis, causing elevations of epinephrine and norepinephrine levels [104]. The release of catecholamines from the sympathetic adrenergic system contributes to the development of CAD through various effects on the heart (hemodynamic alterations such as tachycardia and increased contractility), on blood vessels (permeability and the contractility of blood vessels) and platelets (increased aggregation) [105].

Heart rate is determined by the intrinsic activity of the sino-atrial node (SAN), which is controlled by the dynamic interplay of sympathetic and parasympathetic activities. In normal individuals vagal (parasympathetic) tones prevails under resting conditions when the vagal pathway fires rapid and continuous signals to the SAN: even if there is a high inter-individual variability in resting vagal tone, it is believed that a high vagal tone is a sign of good autonomic flexibility and therefore an appropriate response to external stimuli. Heart rate variability (HRV) is a sensitive and well validated instrument for measuring vagal tone and the balance between sympathetic and parasympathetic systems. It explores two domains: in time domain, the measure that is most frequently utilized is the standard deviation of RR intervals of sinus rhythm beats (SDNN) [106, 107]. The rhythm is regulated by the hypothalamus, the limbic system and the brainstem and neurotransmitters like acetylcholine, noradrenaline, serotonin and dopamine. HRV analysis in the frequency domain provides us with information about very low, low and high frequency bands. The analysis of spectral power at low and very low frequencies describes the interplay between the sympathetic and vagal tone whereas the high-frequency band mainly represents the activity of the vagal tone as modulated by respiratory activity: a reduction in HRV high frequency power with increased CAD mortality, particularly in subjects with frequent premature ventricular contractions was observed in depressed patients as well as in patients with or acute or chronic life stressors.

Work stress is associated with decreased HRV and is a one of the major pathways that is involved in reducing HRV. In addition several daily activities may reduce HRV such as smoking, lack of physical exercise, poor diet. Further studies are necessary in order to clarify the role of the autonomic nervous system in health and disease [108, 109].

Other Factors Involved

Traditional risk factors more frequently characterize patients with psychosocial disorders. Depressed and anxious individuals are at greater risk for developing high blood pressure, diabetes and metabolic syndrome. The majority of them are likely to maintain an unhealthy lifestyle, which includes smoking and physical inactivity as well as high fat intake with a non-balanced diet. Diabetic patients suffering from depression are more likely than their non-depressed counter parts to develop CAD [110]. Socially isolated people more often resulted having lower income, higher hostility ratings, greater incidence of cigarette smoking and poor diet than others. [98].

Mental stress reduces diastolic function and may lead to congestive heart failure with preserved systolic function. Whether the brain natriuretic hormone mediates the relationship of mental stress with diastolic function is still unknown [111].

Meeting the Psychological Needs of Cardiac Patients

Cardiac Rehabilitation programs provide a valuable opportunity to identify and support patients regaining strength, preventing condition from worsening, reducing risk factors as well as increasing individuals' adherence to therapy and advices and enhancing their quality of life through customized program of exercise and education [112].

In fact, individuals, have personal and unique experiences of the disease, which is strictly connected to his/her broadest existential context, including not only external happening, but also and above all, the world of meanings that the heart patients attribute to the event.

The Word Health Organization (WHO) [113] defines CR as "*the sum of activities required to influence favorably the underlying cause of disease, as well to ensure the patients the best possible physical, mental and social conditions so that they may, by their own efforts, preserve, or resume when lost, as normal a place as possible in the life of the community*" (p. 5, 1993).

Clinical data support the positive effects upon patients' psychological outcomes of cardiac rehabilitation programmes offering group exercise, education and individual interventions.

However, in the systematic review and meta-synthesis of qualitative studies purposed by Neubeck et al. [114], attention has been given to both obstacles and barriers usually faced by people and influencing their decision of attending CR: (1) *Service and system level barriers* include physician recommendation, interaction with the healthcare team, and misconceptions surrounding CR; (2) *practical barriers*: transport and parking, cost, and language; (3) *personal barriers* are wrong beliefs and perception of both heart disease and CR, and belief in ability to control CVDs factors and consequences, which may be effectively targeted by clinical health psychology interventions; (4) Also, culturally and linguistically are present. "*Those who were most likely to attend (CR) were also most likely to believe Cardiovascular Heart Disease (CHD) was caused by biomedical risk factors and that they had some control over it. Those who were least likely to attend believed that CHD was caused by psychosocial factors and that they had little or no control over it*" (p. 8, 2012).

The fundamental importance of psychological support in CR has also been underlined by Grande and Badura [115] who, like the American Heart Association [116], stated that cardiac rehabilitation programs should consist of a multifaceted and multidisciplinary approach to overall cardiovascular risk reduction, and that programs consisting in exercise training alone should not be considered cardiac rehabilitation at all. In the up-to-date practice of CR, psychosocial services are growing in importance and role [117, 118] and European guidelines [119], intensively encourage psycho-educational activities increasing the likelihood of permanent lifestyle changes.

Offering a range of psychological treatments might be an effective way of meeting cardiac patients' psychological needs and specific psychological interventions included: psycho-education sessions addressing behavioral risk factors and adjustment, brief individual therapy, group workshops and individual therapy, mainly focused on CBT, for anxiety, depression and adjustment to adverse life events [120]. (Table 3).

Table 3. Psychological Interventions according to individual needs (adapted form Child et al., 2010)

Patient NEEDS	INTERVENTIONS
High	Individual Therapy
Moderate	Group Workshops/Brief individual therapy
Mild	Psycho-education sessions

However, due to the complex etiology of the disorder, as well as the multitude of complications that maintain and exacerbate it, important difficulties have been underlined with regard to long-term efficacy of interventions [121-123]. To develop strategies capable of enhancing patients' motivation and compliance to both actively take part in CR program and to maintain the achieved results over time has become a cornerstone all CR programs [124, 125].

In clinical health psychology, different methods have been developed with the aim of favoring health behavior change and preventing relapses, and a particularly promising technique is represented by Motivational Interviewing (MI) [126-132] which is defined as a client-centered yet directive method for enhancing intrinsic motivation to change by exploring and resolving client's ambivalence [133, 134].

By the use of a guiding style, which lies between and incorporates elements of directing and following styles, as well as reflective listening and open-ended questions strategies, the provider invites the persons to verbally carry across their own arguments and barriers for changing, to explore how their current health behavior may conflict with their own goals and values and to prepare strategies that optimally promotes their action competence, enhancing individuals' resources and self-efficacy and avoiding a medical-based didactic approach, too often cause of resistance in patients [135].

Eliciting "change talk" (opposed to the concept of "resistance to change") and commitment for change, people are persuaded to modify their behavior(s) in the way they speak, also increasing confidence in achieving their personal goals. In fact, research findings indicates that change is more likely to be long-lasting in patients who attribute their changes to their own efforts [136] and the more someone talks about change, the more likely they are to change. In addition, web-based and Internet-based technologies may allow the creation of collaborative outpatient rehabilitation programs, providing patients with a remote and continuous psychological-medical support, education and monitoring [137-140].

Conclusion

The cardiac event, in addition to physically impacting individual health, leads the subject to deal with a series of transformations affecting the representation of the self, of the disease and of his/her social and familiar role, with the activation of emotional-affective dynamics too often counterproductive for allowing the adaptation to a new lifestyle. Also, psychosocial issues related to family, couple and sexual dimensions as well as regarding the individuals' tendency to social isolation, may arise. All these factors, often interrelated, understandably affect patients' attitude, behavior, and degree of compliance to treatments.

PSRF have a great impact on the general population, especially in industrialized countries, where stress is highly prevalent. They may increase the risk of developing CAD and at the same time can worsen the prognosis of patients operated on after myocardial infarction or angina or post angina, often resulting in low compliance to therapy thus favoring new episodes of CAD.

Psychological interventions for heart patients, therefore, must become part of an integrated system of actions aimed at considering the individual in its entirety.

The cardiac rehabilitation team strives to deliver a menu-driven program to patients and the psychologist's sessions are one of the main components, together with the ones held by nurses, doctors, physiotherapists and dietitians.

The psychological intervention in CR program is relevant in as much as it significantly contributes to achieving the goals of rehabilitation, reducing the risk for relapses and improving patient compliance to treatment. Of course, hospital timetables, setting and routine constitutes structural impediments that both the therapist and the patient must face, specifically with respect to the typical urgency for inpatients (and heart patients in particular) of feeling better, both physically and psychologically. Once again, it is of fundamental importance to build, together with the client, a customized action, in which he/she can take an active role, can set and share specific objectives and may enhance user's personal resources.

References

[1] Rozanski, A., J.A. Blumenthal, and J. Kaplan, Impact of psychological factors on the pathogenesis of cardiovascular disease and implications for therapy. *Circulation,* 1999. 99(16): p. 2192-217.

[2] Steptoe, A. and M. Kivimaki, Stress and cardiovascular disease. *Nat Rev Cardiol,* 2012. 9(6): p. 360-70.

[3] Hare, D.L., et al., Depression and cardiovascular disease: a clinical review. *Eur Heart J,* 2014. 35(21): p. 1365-1372.

[4] Adkins, D.L., A.C. Voorhies, and T.A. Jones, Behavioral and neuroplastic effects of focal endothelin-1 induced sensorimotor cortex lesions. *Neuroscience,* 2004. 128(3): p. 473-86.

[5] Wolf, P.A., R.D. Abbott, and W.B. Kannel, Atrial fibrillation as an independent risk factor for stroke: the Framingham Study. *Stroke,* 1991. 22(8): p. 983-8.

[6] Neylon, A., et al., A global perspective on psychosocial risk factors for cardiovascular disease. *Prog Cardiovasc Dis,* 2013. 55(6): p. 574-81.

[7] Perk, J., et al., European Guidelines on cardiovascular disease prevention in clinical practice (version 2012). The Fifth Joint Task Force of the European Society of Cardiology and Other Societies on Cardiovascular Disease Prevention in Clinical Practice (constituted by representatives of nine societies and by invited experts). *Eur Heart J,* 2012. 33(13): p. 1635-701.

[8] Hemingway, H. and M. Marmot, Evidence based cardiology: psychosocial factors in the aetiology and prognosis of coronary heart disease. Systematic review of prospective cohort studies. *BMJ,* 1999. 318(7196): p. 1460-7.

[9] Manzoni, G.M., G. Castelnuovo, and R. Proietti, Assessment of psychosocial risk factors is missing in the 2010 ACCF/AHA guideline for assessment of cardiovascular risk in asymptomatic adults. *Journal of the American College of Cardiology,* 2011. 57: p. 1569-70.

[10] Rozanski, A., et al., The epidemiology, pathophysiology, and management of psychosocial risk factors in cardiac practice: the emerging field of behavioral cardiology. *J Am Coll Cardiol,* 2005. 45(5): p. 637-51.

[11] Yusuf, S., et al., Effect of potentially modifiable risk factors associated with myocardial infarction in 52 countries (the INTERHEART study): case-control study. *Lancet,* 2004. 364(9438): p. 937-52.

[12] Thombs, B.D., et al., Prevalence of depression in survivors of acute myocardial infarction. *J Gen Intern Med,* 2006. 21(1): p. 30-8.

[13] Murray, C.J.L. and A.D. Lopez, *The Global Burden of Disease: A Comprehensive Assessment of Mortality and Disability from Diseases, Injuries and Risk Factors in 1990 and Projected to 20201996,* Cambridge, MA: Harvard University Press on behalf of the World Health Organization and the World Bank.

[14] Murray, C.J. and A.D. Lopez, Global mortality, disability, and the contribution of risk factors: Global Burden of Disease Study. *Lancet,* 1997. 349(9063): p. 1436-42.

[15] Lesperance, F., et al., Five-year risk of cardiac mortality in relation to initial severity and one-year changes in depression symptoms after myocardial infarction. *Circulation,* 2002. 105(9): p. 1049-53.

[16] Khawaja, I.S., et al., Depression and coronary artery disease: the association, mechanisms, and therapeutic implications. *Psychiatry (Edgmont),* 2009. 6(1): p. 38-51.

[17] Hubert, H.B., et al., Obesity as an independent risk factor for cardiovascular disease: a 26-year follow-up of participants in the Framingham Heart Study. *Circulation,* 1983. 67(5): p. 968-77.

[18] Kamarck, T.W., et al., Exaggerated blood pressure responses during mental stress are associated with enhanced carotid atherosclerosis in middle-aged Finnish men: findings from the Kuopio Ischemic Heart Disease Study. *Circulation,* 1997. 96(11): p. 3842-8.

[19] Pignone, M.P., et al., Screening for depression in adults: a summary of the evidence for the U.S. Preventive Services Task Force. *Ann Intern Med,* 2002. 136(10): p. 765-76.

[20] Covey, L.S., A.H. Glassman, and F. Stetner, Major depression following smoking cessation. *Am J psychiatry,* 1997. 154(2): p. 263-5.

[21] Freeland, K.E., et al., Undiagnosis of depression in patients wit coronary heart disesase: the role of nonspecific symptoms. *Int J Psychiatry Med.,* 1992(22): p. 221-229.

[22] Lesperance, F., et al., Effects of citalopram and interpersonal therapy on depression in patients with coronary artery disease: the Canadian Cardiac Randomized Evaluation of

Antidepressant and Psychotherapy Efficacy (CREATE) trial. *JAMA Psychiatry,* 2007(297): p. 367-379.

[23] Enhancing Recovery in Coronary Heart Disease (ENRICHD) study intervention: rationale and design. *Psychosom Med,* 2001. 63(5): p. 747-55.

[24] Feinstein, R.E., et al., A national survey of cardiovascular physician's beliefs and clinical care practices when diagnosing and treating depression in patients with cardiovascular disease. *Cardiol Rev.,* 2006. 14: p. 164-169.

[25] Denollet, J. and D.L. Brutsaert, Reducing emotional distress improves prognosis in coronary heart disease: 9-year mortality in a clinical trial of rehabilitation. *Circulation,* 2001. 104(17): p. 2018-23.

[26] Rothenbacher, D., et al., Symptoms of anxiety and depression in patients with stable coronary heart disease: prognostic value and consideration of pathogenetic links. *Eur J Cardiovasc Prev Rehabil,* 2007. 14(4): p. 547-54.

[27] Shibeshi, W.A., Y. Young-Xu, and C.M. Blatt, Anxiety worsens prognosis in patients with coronary artery disease. *J Am Coll Cardiol,* 2007. 49(20): p. 2021-7.

[28] Kubzansky, L.D., et al., Anxiety and coronary heart disease: a synthesis of epidemiological, psychological, and experimental evidence. *Ann Behav Med,* 1998. 20(2): p. 47-58.

[29] Dornelas, E.A., *Psychotherapy with Cardiac Patients. Behavioral cardiology in practice.* 2008, Washington , DC: American Psychological Association.

[30] Spielberger, C.D. and R.L. Rickman, *Assessment of state and trait anxiety in cardiovascular disorders, in Anxiety and the heart,* D.G. Byrne and R.H. Rosenman, Editors. 1990, Hemisphere: New York. p. 73-92.

[31] Haines, A.P., J.D. Imeson, and T.W. Meade, Phobic anxiety and ischaemic heart disease. *Br Med J* (Clin Res Ed), 1987. 295(6593): p. 297-9.

[32] Kawachi, I., et al., Prospective study of phobic anxiety and risk of coronary heart disease in men. *Circulation,* 1994. 89(5): p. 1992-7.

[33] Kawachi, I., et al., Symptoms of anxiety and risk of coronary heart disease. The Normative Aging Study. *Circulation,* 1994. 90(5): p. 2225-9.

[34] Doerfler, L.A. and J.A. Paraskos, Anxiety, posttraumatic stress disorder, and depression in patients with coronary heart disease: a practical review for cardiac rehabilitation professionals. *J Cardiopulm Rehabil,* 2004. 24(6): p. 414-21.

[35] Pedersen, S.S., Post-traumatic stress disorder in patients with coronary artery disease: a review and evaluation of the risk. *Scandinavian Journal of Psychology,* 2001. 42: p. 445-451.

[36] Kutz, I., et al., Posttraumatic stress disorder in myocardial infarction patients: prevalence study. *Isr J Psychiatry Relat Sci,* 1994. 31: p. 160-191.

[37] Barlow, D.H., Anxiety and its disorders2002, New York: Guildford.

[38] APA, *Diagnostic and Statistica Manual of Mental Disorders. 4th ed - Text Revision2000*, Washington: American Psychiatric Association.

[39] Breslau, N., et al., Sex differences in posttraumatic stress disorder. Arch Gen Psychiatry, 1997. 54(11): p. 1044-8.

[40] Wolfe, J. and R. Kimerling, *Gender issues in the assessment of posttraumatic stress disorder., in Assessing psychological trauma and PTSD,* J.P. Wilson and T.M. Kean, Editors. 1997, The Guildford Press: New York.

[41] Joseph, S., et al., Crisis support and psychiatric symptomatology in adult survivors of the Jupiter cruise ship disaster. *Br J Clin Psychol,* 1992. 31 (Pt 1): p. 63-73.

[42] Eng, H.S., et al., Anxiety and depression in patients with coronary heart disease: a study in a tertiary hospital. *Iran J Med Sci,* 2011. 36(3): p. 201-6.

[43] Foa, E.B. and E.A. Meadows, Psychosocial treatments for posttraumatic stress disorder: a critical review. *Annu Rev Psychol,* 1997. 48: p. 449-80.

[44] Keane, T.M., *Psychological and behavioral treatments for post-traumatic stress disorder, in A guide to Treatment that Work,* P.E. Nathan and J.M. Gorman, Editors. 1998, Oxford: New York. p. 398-407.

[45] Ballenger, J.C., et al., Consensus statement on depression, anxiety, and cardiovascular disease. *J Clin Psychiatry,* 2001. 62 Suppl 8: p. 24-7.

[46] Friedman, M. and R.H. Rosenman, Association of specific overt behavior pattern with blood and cardiovascular findings; blood cholesterol level, blood clotting time, incidence of arcus senilis, and clinical coronary artery disease. *JAMA Psychiatry,* 1959. 169: p. 1286-96.

[47] Rosenman, R.H. and M. Friedman, Association of specific behavior pattern in women with blood and cardiovascular findings. *Circulation,* 1961(24): p. 1173-84.

[48] Everson-Rose, S.A. and T.T. Lewis, Psychosocial factors and cardiovascular disease. *Annu Rev Public Health,* 2005. 26: p. 469 -500.

[49] Martin, R., D. Watson, and C.K. Wan, A three-factor model of trait anger: dimensions of affect, behavior, and cognition. *J Person,* 2000(68): p. 869-97.

[50] Chida, Y. and A. Steptoe, The Association of Anger and Hostility With Future Coronary Heart Disease. A Meta-Analytic Review of Prospective Evidence. *Journal of the American College of Cardiology,* 2009. 53(11): p. 936-946.

[51] Strike, P.C. and A. Steptoe, Behavioral and emotional triggers of acute coronary syndromes: a systematic review and critique. *Psychosom Med,* 2005. 67(2): p. 179-86.

[52] Barefoot, J.C., *Developments in the Measurement of Hostility1992*, Washington DC: American Psychological Association.

[53] Davidson, K. and P. Hall, Potential for hostility and faking-good in high-hostile men. *J Behav Med,* 1997. 20(1): p. 47-54.

[54] Rosengren, A., et al., Association of psychosocial risk factors with risk of acute myocardial infarction in 11119 cases and 13648 controls from 52 countries (the INTERHEART study): case-control study. *Lancet,* 2004. 364(9438): p. 953-62.

[55] Steptoe, A. and M. Kivimaki, Stress and cardiovascular disease. *Nat. Rev. Cardiol.,* 2012. 9: p. 360-370.

[56] Bunker, S.J., et al., "Stress" and coronary heart disease: psychosocial risk factors. *Med J Aust,* 2003. 178(6): p. 272-6.

[57] Stress and cardiovascular disease: a report from the National Heart Foundation of Australia. Stress Working Party. *Med J Aust,* 1988. 148(10): p. 510-4.

[58] Marmot, M.G., et al., Contribution of job control and other risk factors to social variations in coronary heart disease incidence. *Lancet,* 1997. 350(9073): p. 235-9.

[59] Chandola, T., E. Brunner, and M. Marmot, Chronic stress at work and the metabolic syndrome: prospective study. *BMJ,* 2006(332): p. 521-525.

[60] Karasek, R.A. and T. Theorell, *Healthy work: stress, productivity and the reconstruction of working life1990,* New York: Basic Books.

[61] Siegrist, J., Adverse health effects of high-effort/low-reward conditions. *J Occup Health Psychol,* 1996. 1(1): p. 27-41.
[62] Slopen, N., et al., Job strain, job insecurity, and incident cardiovascular disease in the Women's Health Study: results from a 10-year prospective study. *PLoS One,* 2012. 7(7): p. e40512.
[63] Peter, R., et al., Psychosocial work environment and myocardial infarction: improving risk estimation by combining two complementary job stress models in the SHEEP Study. *J Epidemiol Community Health,* 2002. 56(4): p. 294-300.
[64] Kivimaki, M., et al., Work stress and risk of cardiovascular mortality: prospective cohort study of industrial employees. *BMJ,* 2002. 325(7369): p. 857.
[65] Karasek, R., et al., Job decision latitude, job demands, and cardiovascular disease: a prospective study of Swedish men. *Am J Public Health,* 1981. 71(7): p. 694-705.
[66] Moller, J., et al., Work related stressful life events and the risk of myocardial infarction. Case-control and case-crossover analyses within the Stockholm heart epidemiology programme (SHEEP). *J Epidemiol Community Health,* 2005. 59(1): p. 23-30.
[67] Uchiyama, S., et al., [Risk factors of cerebro-cardiovascular events in treated hypertensive male workers in the fifth decade]. *Sangyo Igaku,* 1992. 34(4): p. 318-25.
[68] Uchiyama, S., et al., Job strain and risk of cardiovascular events in treated hypertensive Japanese workers: hypertension follow-up group study. *J Occup Health,* 2005. 47(2): p. 102-11.
[69] Xu, W., et al., When job stress threatens Chinese workers: combination of job stress models can improve the risk estimation for coronary heart disease--the BADCAR study. *J Occup Environ Med,* 2011. 53(7): p. 771-5.
[70] Holt-Lunstad, J., T.B. Smith, and J.B. Layton, Social relationships and mortality risk: a meta-analytic review. *PLoS Med,* 2010. 7(7): p. e1000316.
[71] Barth, J., S. Schneider, and R. von Kanel, Lack of social support in the etiology and the prognosis of coronary heart disease: a systematic review and meta-analysis. *Psychosom Med,* 2010. 72(3): p. 229-38.
[72] Williams, R.B., J.C. Barefoot, and N. Schneiderman, Psychosocial risk factors for cardiovascular disease: more than one culprit at work. *JAMA,* 2003. 290(16): p. 2190-2.
[73] Friberg, J., et al., Sex-specific increase in the prevalence of atrial fibrillation (The Copenhagen City Heart Study). *Am J Cardiol,* 2003. 92(12): p. 1419-23.
[74] Colquhoun, D.M., et al., Screening, referral and treatment for depression in patients with coronary heart disease. *Med J Aust,* 2013. 198(9): p. 483-4.
[75] Gulliksson, M., et al., Randomized controlled trial of cognitive behavioral therapy vs standard treatment to prevent recurrent cardiovascular events in patients with coronary heart disease: Secondary Prevention in Uppsala Primary Health Care project (SUPRIM). *Arch Intern Med,* 2011. 171(2): p. 134-40.
[76] Yan, L.L., et al., Psychosocial factors and risk of hypertension: the Coronary Artery Risk Development in Young Adults (CARDIA) study. *JAMA,* 2003. 290(16): p. 2138-48.
[77] Poitras, V.J. and K.E. Pyke, The impact of acute mental stress on vascular endothelial function: evidence, mechanisms and importance. *Int J Psychophysiol,* 2013. 88(2): p. 124-35.
[78] Rozanski, A., et al., Mental stress and the induction of silent myocardial ischemia in patients with coronary artery disease. *N Engl J Med,* 1988. 318(16): p. 1005-12.

[79] Chen, H., et al., Relationship of depression, stress and endothelial function in stable angina patients. *Physiol Behav,* 2013. 118: p. 152-8.

[80] Eriksson, M., et al., Mental stress impairs endothelial vasodilatory function by a beta-adrenergic mechanism. *Endothelium,* 2007. 14(3): p. 151-6.

[81] Park, J.H., S.J. Tahk, and S.H. Bae, Depression and Anxiety as Predictors of Recurrent Cardiac Events 12 Months After Percutaneous Coronary Interventions. *J Cardiovasc Nurs,* 2014.

[82] Jespersen, L., et al., Persistent angina: highly prevalent and associated with long-term anxiety, depression, low physical functioning, and quality of life in stable angina pectoris. *Clin Res Cardiol,* 2013. 102(8): p. 571-81.

[83] Geovanini, G.R., et al., Obstructive Sleep Apnea and Depression are common and independently associated with refractory angina in patients with coronary artery disease. *Chest,* 2014.

[84] Vukovic, O., et al., Type D personality in patients with coronary artery disease. *Psychiatr Danub,* 2014. 26(1): p. 46-51.

[85] Jamil, G., et al., "Personality traits and heart disease in the Middle East". Is there a link? *Am J Cardiovasc Dis,* 2013. 3(3): p. 163-9.

[86] Ahmadi, N., et al., Post-traumatic stress disorder, coronary atherosclerosis, and mortality. *Am J Cardiol,* 2011. 108(1): p. 29-33.

[87] Lazzarino, A.I., et al., The combined association of psychological distress and socioeconomic status with all-cause mortality: a national cohort study. *JAMA Intern Med,* 2013. 173(1): p. 22-7.

[88] Rajagopalan, S., et al., Abnormal brachial artery flow-mediated vasodilation in young adults with major depression. *Am J Cardiol,* 2001. 88(2): p. 196-8, A7.

[89] Broadley, A.J., et al., Arterial endothelial function is impaired in treated depression. *Heart,* 2002. 88(5): p. 521-3.

[90] Suarez, E.C., R.R. Krishnan, and J.G. Lewis, The relation of severity of depressive symptoms to monocyte-associated proinflammatory cytokines and chemokines in apparently healthy men. *Psychosom Med,* 2003. 65(3): p. 362-8.

[91] Skantze, H.B., et al., Psychosocial stress causes endothelial injury in cynomolgus monkeys via beta1-adrenoceptor activation. *Atherosclerosis,* 1998. 136(1): p. 153-61.

[92] Nemeroff, C.B. and D.L. Musselman, Are platelets the link between depression and ischemic heart disease? *Am Heart J,* 2000. 140(4 Suppl): p. 57-62.

[93] Frimerman, A., et al., Changes in hemostatic function at times of cyclic variation in occupational stress. *Am J Cardiol,* 1997. 79(1): p. 72-5.

[94] Kittel, F., et al., Job conditions and fibrinogen in 14226 Belgian workers: the Belstress study. *Eur Heart J,* 2002. 23(23): p. 1841-8.

[95] Vrijkotte, T.G., L.J. van Doornen, and E.J. de Geus, Work stress and metabolic and hemostatic risk factors. *Psychosom Med,* 1999. 61(6): p. 796-805.

[96] Emeny, R., et al., Job strain associated CRP is mediated by leisure time physical activity: results from the MONICA/KORA study. *Brain Behav Immun,* 2012. 26(7): p. 1077-84.

[97] Emeny, R.T., et al., Job strain-associated inflammatory burden and long-term risk of coronary events: findings from the MONICA/KORA Augsburg case-cohort study. *Psychosom Med,* 2013. 75(3): p. 317-25.

[98] Strike, P.C. and A. Steptoe, Psychosocial factors in the development of coronary artery disease. *Prog Cardiovasc Dis,* 2004. 46(4): p. 337-47.

[99] Nemeroff, C.B., et al., Elevated concentrations of CSF corticotropin-releasing factor-like immunoreactivity in depressed patients. *Science,* 1984. 226(4680): p. 1342-4.

[100] Kemper, J.W., A.H. Baggenstoss, and C.H. Slocumb, The relationship of therapy with cortisone to the incidence of vascular lesions in rheumatoid arthritis. *Ann Intern Med,* 1957. 46(5): p. 831-51.

[101] Raadsheer, F.C., et al., Increased numbers of corticotropin-releasing hormone expressing neurons in the hypothalamic paraventricular nucleus of depressed patients. *Neuroendocrinology,* 1994. 60(4): p. 436-44.

[102] Troxler, R.G., et al., The association of elevated plasma cortisol and early atherosclerosis as demonstrated by coronary angiography. *Atherosclerosis,* 1977. 26(2): p. 151-62.

[103] Theorell, T., et al., Employee effects of an educational program for managers at an insurance company. *Psychosom Med,* 2001. 63(5): p. 724-33.

[104] Merchenthaler, I., et al., Immunocytochemical localization of corticotropin-releasing factor (CRF) in the rat brain. *Am J Anat,* 1982. 165(4): p. 385-96.

[105] Anfossi, G. and M. Trovati, Role of catecholamines in platelet function: pathophysiological and clinical significance. Eur J Clin Invest, 1996. 26(5): p. 353-70.

[106] Borchini, R. and M.M. Ferrario, [Job strain and heart rate variability. New evidence and new prospects]. *G Ital Med Lav Ergon,* 2012. 34(3 Suppl): p. 174-6.

[107] Thayer, J.F., et al., A meta-analysis of heart rate variability and neuroimaging studies: implications for heart rate variability as a marker of stress and health. *Neurosci Biobehav Rev,* 2012. 36(2): p. 747-56.

[108] Thayer, J.F. and J.E. Fischer, Heart rate variability, overnight urinary norepinephrine and C-reactive protein: evidence for the cholinergic anti-inflammatory pathway in healthy human adults. *J Intern Med,* 2009. 265(4): p. 439-47.

[109] Thayer, J.F., S.S. Yamamoto, and J.F. Brosschot, The relationship of autonomic imbalance, heart rate variability and cardiovascular disease risk factors. *Int J Cardiol,* 2010. 141(2): p. 122-31.

[110] de Groot, M., et al., Association of depression and diabetes complications: a meta-analysis. *Psychosom Med,* 2001. 63(4): p. 619-30.

[111] Choksy, P., et al., Brain Natriuretic Hormone Predicts Stress-Induced Alterations in Diastolic Function. *Am J Med Sci,* 2014.

[112] Manzoni, G.M., et al., Short-term effects of a multi-disciplinary cardiac rehabilitation programme on psychological well-being, exercise capacity and weight in a sample of obese in-patients with coronary heart disease: a practice-level study. *Psychology, health & medicine,* 2011. 16: p. 178-89.

[113] Geneva1993, W.G.W.H.O., *Needs and action priorities in cardiac rehabilitation and secondary prevention in patients with CHD.*

[114] Neubeck, L., et al., Participating in cardiac rehabilitation: a systematic review and meta-synthesis of qualitative data. *Eur J Prev Cardiol,* 2012. 19(3): p. 494-503.

[115] Grande, G. and B. Badura, *Cardiac rehabilitation from a health systems analysis perspective, in Contributions toward evidence-based psychocardiology: A systematic review of the literature.*, J. Jordan, B. Bardé, and A.M. Zeiher, Editors. 2007, American Psychological Association: Washington. p. 255-277.

[116] Balady, G.J., B.J. Fletcher, and E.F. Froelicher, Cardiac rehabilitation programs: a statement for healthcare professionals from the American Heart Association. *Circulation,* 1994. 90: p. 1602-1610.

[117] Greco, C., et al., [Selection criteria for patient admission to cardiac rehabilitation centers]. G Ital Cardiol (Rome), 2011. 12(3): p. 219-29.

[118] [Guidelines for psychology activities in cardiologic rehabilitation and prevention]. *Monaldi Arch Chest Dis,* 2003. 60(3): p. 184-234.

[119] Humphrey, R., M. Guazzi, and J. Niebauer, Cardiac rehabilitation in Europe. *Prog Cardiovasc Dis,* 2014. 56(5): p. 551-6.

[120] Child, A., et al., Meeting the psychological needs of cardiac patients: an integrated stepped-care approach within a cardiac rehabilitation setting. *Br J Cardiol,* 2010. 17(4): p. 175-9.

[121] Castelnuovo, G., Empirically supported treatments in psychotherapy: towards an evidence-based or evidence-biased psychology in clinical settings? *Front Psychol,* 2010. 1: p. 27.

[122] Spatola, C.A., et al., The ACTonHEART study: rationale and design of a randomized controlled clinical trial comparing a brief intervention based on Acceptance and Commitment Therapy to usual secondary prevention care of coronary heart disease. *Health Qual Life Outcomes,* 2014. 12: p. 22.

[123] Capodaglio, P., et al., Rationale for hospital-based rehabilitation in obesity with comorbidities. *Eur J Phys Rehabil Med,* 2013. 49(3): p. 399-417.

[124] Pietrabissa, G., G.M. Manzoni, and G. Castelnuovo, Motivation in psychocardiological rehabilitation. *Front Psychol,* 2013. 4.

[125] Pietrabissa, G., et al., Addressing motivation in globesity treatment: a new challenge for clinical psychology. *Front Psychol,* 2012. 3: p. 317.

[126] Beckie, T.M. and J.W. Beckstead, The effects of a cardiac rehabilitation program tailored for women on their perceptions of health: a randomized clinical trial. *J Cardiopulm Rehabil Prev,* 2011. 31(1): p. 25-34.

[127] Bellg, A.J., Maintenance of health behavior change in preventive cardiology. Internalization and self-regulation of new behaviors. *Behav Modif,* 2003. 27(1): p. 103-31.

[128] Bredie, S.J., et al., Effectiveness of Nurse Based Motivational Interviewing for smoking cessation in high risk cardiovascular outpatients: a randomized trial. *Eur J Cardiovasc Nurs,* 2011. 10(3): p. 174-9.

[129] Brennan, L., et al., Motivational interviewing and cognitive behaviour therapy in the treatment of adolescent overweight and obesity: study design and methodology. Contemp Clin Trials, 2008. 29(3): p. 359-75.

[130] Everett, B., et al., Pragmatic insights into a nurse-delivered motivational interviewing intervention in the outpatient cardiac rehabilitation setting. *J Cardiopulm Rehabil Prev,* 2008. 28(1): p. 61-4.

[131] Miller, N.H., Motivational interviewing as a prelude to coaching in healthcare settings. *J Cardiovasc Nurs,* 2010. 25(3): p. 247-51.

[132] Miller, N.H., Adherence behavior in the prevention and treatment of cardiovascular disease. *J Cardiopulm Rehabil Prev,* 2012. 32(2): p. 63-70.

[133] Burke, L.E., J.M. Dunbar-Jacob, and M.N. Hill, Compliance with cardiovascular disease prevention strategies: a review of the research. *Ann Behav Med,* 1997. 19(3): p. 239-63.
[134] Miller, N.H., et al., The multilevel compliance challenge: recommendations for a call to action. A statement for healthcare professionals. Circulation, 1997. 95(1085-1090).
[135] Castelnuovo, G., et al., The need of psychological motivational support for improving lifestyle change in cardiac rehabilitation. *Experimental & Clinical Cardiology*, 2014.
[136] Lambert, M.J. and A.E. Bergin, *The effectiveness of psychotherapy, in Issues in Psychotherapy Research,* A.E. Bergin and S.L. Bellack, Editors. 1994, Plenum Press: New York. p. 313-359.
[137] Castelnuovo, G., et al., The STRATOB study: design of a randomized controlled clinical trial of Cognitive Behavioral Therapy and Brief Strategic Therapy with telecare in patients with obesity and binge-eating disorder referred to residential nutritional rehabilitation. *Trials,* 2011. 12: p. 114.
[138] Castelnuovo, G. and S. Simpson, Ebesity - e-health for obesity - new technologies for the treatment of obesity in clinical psychology and medicine. *Clin Pract Epidemiol Ment Health,* 2011. 7: p. 5-8.
[139] Manzoni, G.M., et al., Internet-based behavioral interventions for obesity: an updated systematic review. *Clin Pract Epidemiol Ment Health,* 2011. 7: p. 19-28.
[140] Castelnuovo, G., et al., From psychotherapy to e-therapy: the integration of traditional techniques and new communication tools in clinical settings. *Cyberpsychol Behav,* 2003. 6(4): p. 375-82.

In: Myocardial Infarctions
Editor: Pattie Wilkonson

ISBN: 978-1-63321-726-3

Chapter 4

Risk of Myocardial Infarction in the Pathophysiology and Treatment of Prostatic Diseases

***Claudio de Lucia*[1*#], *Grazia Daniela Femminella*[1#], *Klara Komici*[1], *Giuseppe Rengo*[1,2] and *Nicola Ferrara*[1,2]**

[1]Department of Translational Medical Sciences,
University Federico II of Naples
[2]Salvatore Maugeri Foundation, IRCCS,
Scientific Institute of Telese Terme (BN), Italy

Abstract

Benign prostatic hyperplasia (BPH) and prostate cancer (PC) have shown an increased prevalence among elderly population in the last ten years leading to a significant deterioration in the quality of life and life span. BPH is a non-malignant adenofibromyomatous overgrowth of the periurethral portion of prostate gland that becomes clinically manifest through bladder outlet obstruction symptoms. PC is the most common malignancy in men and often shows an adenocarcinoma histology with symptoms such as hematuria and obstruct urine flow.

Pharmacological treatment of BPH includes α-adrenergic blockers and PDE-5 inhibitors though surgery is necessary if medical therapy fails or obstructive symptoms are impressive. Transurethral resection of the prostate (TURP) is the gold standard surgery for PBH; however open prostatectomy could also be considered as an option.

PC therapy is determined by PSA level, grade and stage of tumor, age and comorbidity. Generally, surgery or radiation therapy are preferred for localized cancer while hormonal therapy, radiation therapy or chemotherapy are utilized for symptomatic, advanced, and metastatic PC.

---

* Corresponding author: de Lucia Claudio, Department of Translational Medical Sciences, University Federico II of Naples, Via Sergio Pansini n.5, 80131 Naples, Italy. Phone: +390817463677. Fax: +390817462339. E-mail: claudiodelucia@libero.it.

# Contributed equally.

Particularly, in patients with a locally advanced tumor or metastases, androgen deprivation therapy (ADT) by bilateral orchiectomy or medical therapy with gonadotropin-releasing hormone (GnRH) agonists and antagonist are commonly utilized.

Recently, several studies exploring the relationship between cardiovascular (CV) risk and prostatic diseases have been published. In fact, there are some factors involved in the pathophysiology and treatment of prostatic diseases that may influence the establishment and progression of myocardial infarction (MI) in elderly patients with comorbidities.

First of all, perioperative and postoperative urological surgery are associated with cardiological complications as MI. Indeed, some studies showed an increase in MI-related mortality after TURP vs open prostatectomy. Furthermore, ADT (GnRH agonists and orchiectomy) induces a status of hypogonadism, which is related to adverse events as metabolic syndrome, diabetes and CV diseases. In fact, it has been demonstrated an increased risk of a CV events (coronary heart disease, MI and cardiac death) in PC patients treated with GnRH agonists. Besides, 6-months therapy with GnRH agonists is related to an earlier timing of fatal MI in elderly patients while GnRH antagonists administration decreases cardiac events (ischemic cerebrovascular diseases, MI, and other ischemic heart disease) in patients with preexisting CV disease during the first year of treatment compared to GnRH agonists.

Therefore, in this chapter we will analyze in detail the aforementioned data of the literature and we will discuss the CV, hormonal and metabolic factors involved in the development either of MI than prostatic disease. In particular, establishment of metabolic syndrome increases the estrogen-to-androgen ratio leading to sympathetic overactivity and influences the progression of BPH. Subsequently we will evaluate the surgical elements and the factors related to medical therapy for prostatic disease that are connected to myocardial damage.

Finally we will emphasize that in patients with prostatic disease is very important to evaluate pre-existing CV diseases and myocardial function and to strictly recommend a healthy lifestyle that includes a moderate and adequate exercise training associated to a balanced diet.

Abbreviations

Benign prostatic hyperplasia (BPH)
Prostate cancer (PC)
Transurethral resection of the prostate (TURP)
Androgen deprivation therapy (ADT)
Gonadotropin-releasing hormone (GnRH)
Cardiovascular (CV)
Myocardial Infarction (MI)
Prostate-Specific Antigen (PSA)
Metabolic Syndrome (MS)
Diabetes Mellitus (DM).

1. Background

Benign prostatic hyperplasia (BPH) and prostate cancer (PC) have shown an increased prevalence among elderly population in the last ten years leading to a significant deterioration in the quality of life and life span [1, 2]. BPH is a non-malignant adenofibromyomatous overgrowth of the periurethral portion of prostate gland that becomes clinically manifest through bladder outlet obstruction symptoms. Pharmacological treatment of BPH includes α-adrenergic blockers and PDE-5 inhibitors though surgery is necessary if medical therapy fails or obstructive symptoms are impressive. Transurethral resection of the prostate (TURP) is the gold standard surgery for PBH; however open prostatectomy could also be considered as an option [3].

PC is the most common noncutaneous malignancy in men worldwide, is second only to lung cancer in carcinoma-associated mortality. Half a million new cases occur each year, representing almost 10% of all cancers in men.

In most industrial countries, prostate cancer incidence rates are increasing, whereas mortality rates are declining. The reduction in mortality is largely due to the early detection of the disease (secondary prevention) [4]. PC often shows an adenocarcinoma histology that has been defined in two sub-groups. The first group includes histological variants of acinar adenocarcinoma and the second group non-acinar carcinoma variants or types with symptoms such as hematuria and obstruct urine flow.

The number of diagnosed PC is significantly increased because of a wide application of Prostate-Specific Antigen (PSA) screening and at the same time, the mortality was decreased thanks to earlier diagnosis and substantial therapeutic progresses. PC therapy is determined based on PSA level, grade and stage of tumor, age and comorbidity.

Generally, surgery or radiation therapy are preferred for localized cancer while hormonal therapy, radiation therapy or chemotherapy are utilized for symptomatic, advanced, and metastatic PC. Particularly, in patients with a locally advanced tumor or metastases, androgen deprivation therapy (ADT) by bilateral orchiectomy or medical therapies acting on gonadotropin-releasing hormone (GnRH) receptors are commonly utilized [5].

Recently, several studies exploring the relationship between cardiovascular (CV) risk and prostatic diseases have been published [6, 7]. In fact, there are some factors involved in the pathophysiology and treatment of prostatic diseases that may influence the establishment and progression of myocardial infarction (MI) in elderly patients with comorbidities. Therefore, in this chapter we will analyze in detail the aforementioned data of the literature and we will debate CV, hormonal and metabolic factors involved in the development either of MI than prostatic disease. Subsequently, we will discuss the urological factors (perioperative and postoperative) that can determinate CV complications as MI. Indeed, some studies showed an increase in MI-related mortality after TURP vs open prostatectomy [8]. After, we will argue some adverse events occurring during ADT as metabolic syndrome (MS), diabetes (DM) and CV diseases (MI, and stroke) that are dramatically connected to mortality of patients with PC [9].

Hence, we will emphasize that in patients with prostatic disease is fundamental to evaluate pre-existing CV diseases and cardiac function and to strictly recommend a healthy lifestyle. Prevention and therapeutic strategies are necessary to decrease morbidity and mortality in these elderly patients that usually die of conditions other than their prostatic disease [4].

2. Risk Factors for Prostatic Diseases and Cardiovascular Pathologies: Many Similarities

CV disease and BPH have been shown to share the same risk factors. These include obesity, diabetes, dyslipidemia and hypertension [10]. Obesity dramatically increases the risk of BPH, with an increases by 10% in BPH incidence for each 0.05-increase in the waist-to-hip ratio. Moreover, it has been demonstrated that abdominal adiposity increases the estrogen-to-androgen ratio and may lead to sympathetic overactivity, which can affect the development of BPH [11].

Different mechanisms have been proposed to explain the relationship between obesity and increased sympathetic tone. Pro-inflammatory cytokines might have a role, since elevated serum concentrations of IL-6 and TNF-a, and increased insulin and leptin levels result in sympathetic hyperactivation. Diabetes may also significantly influence the risk of BPH as the compensatory hyperinsulinemia observed in DM can, directly and/or indirectly, promote prostatic growth. Indeed, hyperinsulinemia stimulates the production of insulin-like growth factor (IGF) by the liver, a potent mitogen and an anti-apoptotic hormone which stimulates prostate growth. Moreover, it has been demonstrated that high circulating and prostatic levels of IGFs and IGF binding are associated with BPH risk [12].

Vice versa, a healthy lifestyle is not only cardio-protective, but can also prevent the development of BPH. A diet with high intake of proteins and polyunsaturated fatty acids results in a greater risk of BPH, while aerobic exercise and a low-fat, high-fiber diet can ameliorate metabolism [13, 14].

Hypercholesterolemia, a major risk factor for cardiovascular disease, is also a risk factor for BPH. Both preclinical and clinical findings indicate that the inhibition of cholesterol absorption from the intestine can reduce prostate gland size [15]. In addition to that, a significant association between BPH and hypertension exists, probably due to increased sympathetic activity as a common pathophysiological mechanism [16]. Elderly patients with BPH symptoms have higher blood pressure and higher serum catecholamine levels compared to age-matched healthy individuals.

Not only BPH, but also PC is related to the same lifestyle factors which constitute a risk for CV diseases. In particular, recent evidences have indicated in MS a significant risk factor for development and progression of PC.

The central feature of MS is insulin resistance, whose metabolic consequences are evident in adipose tissue where it stimulates hydrolysis of stored triglycerides and raised levels of circulating free fatty acids, in skeletal muscle where it reduces glucose uptake and in liver, where reduces glucose storage resulting in hyperglycemia [17]. According to current guidelines (The National Cholesterol Education Program Adult Treatment Panel III), MS is diagnosed when 3 or more of the following are present: central obesity, elevated triglycerides, reduced HDL cholesterol, raised blood pressure, or raised fasting plasma glucose [18]. All the individual components of MS have been related to increased risk of PC. A recent study showed that middle-aged men with MS had a 1.9-fold risk of PC than controls without MS. Similarly, in another prospective study a positive association between MS and PC has been identified. Other groups have shown a negative correlation between MS and PC, mainly evident in some ethnic groups (African-Americans) and less in others (White) [19]. These discrepancies in study results might be ascribed to the differences populations between

American and European cohorts, especially in terms of ethnicity, prevalence of obesity and MS.

Conflicting data also characterize the association between diabetes and PC. Recently, epidemiological studies have shown that diabetes might be a protective factor for PC, with a 20% lower risk of developing PC in diabetic compared to non-diabetic individuals. Moreover, diabetic patients had significantly lower levels of PSA compared to non-diabetic [20]. This could be ascribed at least in part to the fact that pancreas is not able to produce anymore insulin in long-term diabetes,. Thus, while transient hyperinsulinemia in early phases of diabetes might increase the risk of PC, the progressive reduction in insulin production in diabetic patients acts as a protective factor on PC risk.

Also, the possibility of an association between insulin/insulin resistance, diabetes, and cancer has become of increasing interest. A possible mechanistic explanation is that insulin is a growth factor for epithelial tumors and hyperinsulinemia produces a secondary increase in the availability of IGF-1, promoting survival and proliferation of early malignant cells [9].

In terms of prognostic significance, metabolic alterations related to PC might be associated with poor outcomes, in particular with a more advanced disease state and high-grade tumor at diagnosis. Evidence from cross-sectional studies identified an association between metabolic alterations with a more advanced PC. Stage T3 patients were more obese than stage T2 patients and, similarly, subjects with a G3 tumor were more dyslipidemic and had higher plasma insulin level than those with a G1 tumor [21].

Moreover, MS has also been associated with an increased mortality risk in PC. In a case-control study in PC patients, obese men at baseline had a higher mortality risk [22] while in a different cohort it has been demonstrated that higher serum insulin levels, lower HDL cholesterol, and higher prevalence of diabetes at the time of PC diagnosis were associated with a higher mortality risk [23].

3. Risk of Myocardial Infarction after Prostatectomy

Although prostatectomy is a well-established procedure that is used in clinical and the risk of severe complications is very low, surgical factors (perioperative and postoperative) can determinate CV complications as MI. Indeed, some studies showed an increase in MI-related mortality after TURP vs open prostatectomy [8]. During TURP procedure, one of the most recognized cardiac stressors can be identified in the excessive fluid absorption via blood vessels in the resection area. Small amounts of fluids are probably of little consequence, but the accidental transfer of more than 3L of fluid in the circulation results in symptoms originating from the CV system, as well as neurologic disturbance as confusion, aggressiveness and depressed consciousness. The so-called 'TURP syndrome' is a very rare systemic complication, caused by excessive absorption of electrolyte-free irrigation fluids, with an estimated incidence of less than 1% TURP, but milder forms are more common. This complication is very dangerous because it is characterized by symptoms ranging from an asymptomatic hyponatremic state to convulsions, CV symptoms, coma and death. The role of irrigation solution is to distend the bladder, clear the surgical site and wash away residual tissue and blood. Various irrigation fluids (glycine, sorbitol, mannitol and normal saline) have been used for TURP, and glycine solution is the most commonly used fluid in traditional urologic procedures. Several reports showed that glycine absorption causes neurologic symptoms, ECG changes such as T-wave depression or inversion (subacute effects on the myocardium), prolongation of the RR interval and QRS duration and acute MI (the latter in about 0.5% of patients) [8, 24, 25].

Measuring serum electrolytes during TURP is a simple and effective method for assessment of fluid absorption and early detection of TURP syndrome [26].

In addition to this, hemodynamic factors have been suggested as potential triggers of myocardial ischemia during TURP. In particular, it has been reported that the use of cold irrigating fluids resulting in body temperature lowering might also lead to "cardiac stress" as demonstrated by increased peripheral resistance and arterial pressure, as well as reduced stroke volume and cardiac output after TURP compared to control procedures [27].

The hypothesis of TURP-related cardiac stress is also supported by data deriving from studies evaluating cardiac enzyme levels after this surgical procedure. A slight increase in creatinine kinase-B subunit and lactate dehydrogenase 1 has been reported in patients undergoing TURP, but the criteria for MI were never fulfilled [24]. Recently, it has been demonstrated that Troponin T is not increased in patients undergoing TURP, without previous cardiac comorbidity. Pro-brain natriuretic peptide is slightly increased, but without any significant clinical dysfunction [28].

Thus, the relevance of these increases is still unknown and it can be hypothesized that patients with a history of cardiac disease are at a higher risk of myocardial damage during TURP. Moreover, in elderly patients without cardiovascular disease undergoing TURP, continuous ECG monitoring during the pre-, intra- and post-operative phases was not able to detect any significant variations in electrocardiographical features indicative for ischemic disease [29]. However, it is mandatory in old patients undergoing to prostatectomy (both TURP and open prostatectomy) to evaluate CV risk factors and previous CV events with the purpose to identify the most appropriate surgery or evaluate alternative treatments.

4. Cardiovascular Risk of Androgen Deprivation Therapy in Prostate Cancer: Myocardial Infarction and Other Cardio-Metabolic Complications

The effectiveness of ADT in patients with PC is well known from 1941 when Huggins and Hodges described for the first time the relationship between testosterone levels and PC and demonstrated that castration produced dramatic therapeutic responses [30]. ADT includes bilateral orchiectomy, estrogens, anti-androgens, GnRH agonists and GnRH antagonists and plays an important role in the therapy of PC, improving considerably overall survival. Over the years, GnRH agonists (leuprolide, goserelin and triptorelin are the most common) have become a valid alternative to surgical castration or anti-androgens and are actually a cornerstone of the treatment of local and metastatic PC [31]. GnRH is a key regulator of the hypothalamus-pitiuitary-gonad axis in the gonadotropin release. GnRH agonists bind with a long half-life to the GnRH receptor. Initially, there is an increase in FSH and LH secretion FSH (so-called "flare effect"). GnRH agonists, also known as LHRH, agonist prevent the pulsatile stimulation of the LHRH receptor due to a longer half-life and receptor binding time, this leads to receptors down regulation and to a profound hypogonadal effect. GnRH are useful in locally advanced PC by suppressing PSA, stabilizing disease, alleviating symptoms and determining an enhance in disease-free and overall survival either in association with external radiation than post-prostatectomy and pelvic lymphadenectomy (adjuvant therapy). In addition, GnRH agonists are a palliative therapy in metastatic PC improving pain and quality of life and, despite no overall survival advantage, they should be considered the first-line treatment. Although ADT is helpful in these patient populations, it is frequently used as primary therapy in men with localized disease and with biochemical recurrence, despite no evidence of advantage in survival [5]. The extensive long-term use of GnRH derivative in last years, especially in elderly patients with comorbidity and polypharmacy, has led to a better understanding of their side effects. Recently, in addition to well established adverse effects (such as flare phenomenon, anemia, osteoporosis, flushing, sexual dysfunction, impotence, reduction of functional performance, fatigue, gynecomastia/mastodynia), cardio-metabolic alterations seems to be at least equally impressive. Indeed, insulin-resistance/DM, dyslipidemia, hypertension and MS are emerging as fundamental complications of ADT, particularly due to their role in establishment and progression of CV disease [32].

Presently, standard duration of GnRH agonist therapy is not established (from few months to 3 years) and the correlation between this length and side effects is still uncertain. It seems fairly clear that longer duration of treatment is associated with elevated osteoporosis and fracture but there is no accordance with risk of cardiac events.

In last ten year, the development of GnRH antagonists has offered an effective alternative to GnRH agonist treatment. GnRH antagonists (degarelix seems to be the most promising drug for PC therapy) competitively bind to GnRH receptors and determine a rapid suppression of testosterone levels. Hence, GnRH antagonists lead to an equivalent testosterone reduction without transient testosterone surge and flare phenomenon compared to GnRH agonists.

In patients with advanced disease, the testosterone surge lead to a flare-up of the tumor characterized by typical symptoms such as bone pain, ureteral obstruction, and neurological problems, consequently it is common to associate anti-androgens to GnRH agonists. In addition to the positive effects in patients with metastatic disease, high baseline PSA (>20 ng/mL) and very symptomatic disease, GnRH antagonists reduce the number of cardiac events in PC patients with preexisting cardiovascular disease than GnRH agonists [33].

a) Cardio-Metabolic Effects of Androgen Deprivation Therapy

Over recent years, cardio-metabolic alterations related to ADT and particularly collected to GnRH treatment are gaining importance due to their potential cardiovascular consequence. Previous studies have clarify that low testosterone levels are associated with an augmented CV risk and a pro-thrombotic state [34, 35].

Some authors suggest a direct effect of GnRH agonists on cardiomyocytes in the heart. Indeed, Dong F. et al. have proven that in cardiomyocytes isolated from mice the stimulation of GnRH receptors determinate an activation of the PKA pathway (but not the PKC pathway) with important effects on contractility and intracellular Ca^{2+} response [36]. They hypothesize that a chronic stimulation with GnRH agonists in patient with PC should directly determinate a cardiac dysfunction.

Furthermore, since lymphocytes T-helper 1 are important determinant in the pathogenesis of the atherosclerotic plaque and GnRH receptors lead to the proliferation and differentiation of these lymphocytes, someone might speculate that GnRH agonists may partly endorse destabilization of atherosclerotic plaques [33].

However, indirect mechanism due to hypogonadism seems to play the prominent part in CV effects of ADT therapy through metabolic alterations leading to a faster evolution and potential rupture of the atherosclerotic plaque [37].

Therefore, these negative indirect effects should be understood considering the physiological role of androgens on cellular lipids and glucose metabolism of (remarkable influence on adipose tissue and muscle), on blood vessels dilatation, on arterial stiffness and on endothelial function.

Indeed, androgens control body composition enhancing the lean body mass/decreasing fat mass, stimulate mesenchymal pluripotent stem cells towards myogenic lineage instead of adipogenic lineage, determinate lipolysis in adipose tissues and mobilize lipids from the visceral fat deposit [38, 39]. Based on the above mentioned data, it is reasonable that GnRH agonist therapy cause detrimental changes in body composition that predispose to metabolic alterations such as increased waist circumference, reduced muscle mass and strength and increased fat mass (sarcopenic obesity); these alterations occur mostly during the first year of treatment but they can continue even after 2 years [40].

Moreover, rise of adipose tissue in hypogonadal patients determinates an increase in conversion of testosterone in estradiol by aromatase and an enhance in leptin levels that lead to a further hypogonadism (vicious circle) [9]. These modifications are often associated to hyperinsulinemia, insulin resistance, hyperglycemia, enhanced HbA1c levels, augmented levels of total cholesterol, low-density lipoprotein (LDL) cholesterol and triglycerides [9, 41]. Of note, during ADT it has been shown that insulin levels increased of 26–65% within 3 months from the start of treatment while fasting glucose levels increase after 6 months from the start of the therapy, probably indicating compensatory changes [42]. Lage et al. demonstrated an enhancement in prevalence of DM which correlate with duration of ADT and these authors estimated that the relative risk of incident diabetes associated with this treatment was 1.36 ($P = 0.01$) [43].

It is well known that pro-inflammatory cytokines (in particular IL-6 and tumor necrosis factor – TNF) are related to the development of DM and MS. Recently, it has been shown that testosterone determinates the reduction of IL-6 *in vivo* and an inhibition of TNF production on macrophages. Since in hypogonadal men with DM, testosterone replacement resulted in decreased TNF, and IL-6 levels (*ex-vivo* model), it could be hypostasize that in hypogonadism ADT-related lead to metabolic changes of MS via an inflammatory mechanism [42].

The severity of all these changes is directly related to the duration of ADT and lead to the development of DM and MS (MS has been shown in 50% of patients treated with long-term ADT) that are widely known to be among the most important CV risk factors [44].

MS in men is defined by three of the following five criteria: fasting plasma glucose level>100 mg/dl^{-1}, serum triglyceride level > 150 mg/dl^{-1}, serum high-density lipoprotein (HDL) cholesterol level < 40 mg/dl^{-1}, blood pressure $\geq$ 130/85mmHg and waist circumference >102 cm [32, 45, 46].

However, the MS due to GnRH treatment is partially different to the "classical" MS. In fact, ADT can determinate: increase in HDL, subcutaneous (rather than visceral abdominal fat), in adiponectin levels (rather than decreasing) and unchanged waist-to-hip ratio and C-reactive protein levels (than augmented) [42].

b) Risk of Myocardial Infarction and Other Cardiovascular Disease during Androgen Deprivation Therapy

In the last years, some studies have suggested that GnRH treatment in patients with PC should increase the risk of CV morbidity (MI, coronary heart disease, arrhythmia, QT interval prolongation, and stroke) and mortality [32]. However, although several authors have widely shown this relationship [47-50], other studies did not find a statistically significant association [51-53].

From the SEER (Surveillance, Epidemiology and End Results registry) database, Keating et al. proved that medical endocrine therapy determined increase in MI (Hazard Ratio [HR]:1.11; p<0.03), in coronary heart disease (adjusted HR:1.16; p<0.001) and in sudden cardiac death or life-threatening ventricular arrhythmia (HR:1.16, p<0.04)(49) while Saigal et al. have shown that in 22816 men with PC, CV events occurs in 24% of subjects with ADT and this treatment was associated with a 1.2 relative increased risk of CV accidents [35]. Subsequently the study group of Keating confirmed the previous data in an Observational study conducted on veterans with PC showing that GnRH agonists are associated with a statistically significant increased risk of MI (adjusted HR = 1.28), incident coronary heart disease (adjusted HR = 1.19) and sudden cardiac death (adjusted HR = 1.35) [50]. D'Amico and colleagues have evidenced that ADT is associated with significant cardiac events particularly in the elderly population: men ≥ 65 years who received 6 months of AST, underwent an earlier onset of fatal MI than men without hormonal treatment (P <0.017) and men younger than65 yea rs (P <0.016) [47].

Recently, Jespersen et al. have analyzed 31,571 subjects with PC and they have shown cardiac outcome for different kinds of ADT. Patients treated with GnRH agonists have showed an augmented risk of MI (HR of 1.31) compared to patients without hormonal therapy while orchiectomy was not associated to an increased risk of MI (HR: 0.90) [54].

Importantly, a Swedish study described an increased risk of developing arrhythmias after hormonal treatment in PC patients. In this study the authors have shown that men who underwent surveillance and curative treatment had an increased risk of CV pathologies but less severe than those who underwent ADT. This finding suggests that PC itself may enhance the risk of CV disease via a biologic mechanism linking PC and CV system or that there are some common causes such as neurohormonal (e.g. sympathetic nervous system) and inflammatory overactivation [55].

Moreover, in some papers was discussed the importance of a complete evaluation of pre-existing CV risk factors that can influence the mobility and mortality related to ADT. In a prospective randomized controlled trial published in JAMA, D'Amico et al. showed in patients with PC treated with Radiotherapy that addition of ADT increased risk of MI in the subgroup of patients with moderate to severe comorbidities [48]. Besides, Nanda et al. have found that neo adjuvant ADT use is significantly associated with an increased risk of all-cause mortality, in men with a history of coronary artery disease–induced congestive heart failure or MI, but not in those patients without comorbidities or at least a single coronary artery disease risk factor suggesting that in these patients, alternative strategies such as watching waiting or treatment with external beam radiation therapy or prostatectomy should be evaluated [56]. Furthermore, recently the same study group showed that coronary artery disease risk factors (DM and hypertension; no hypercholesterolemia) and sequelae (congestive heart failure or MI) are associated with an increased risk of all-cause of mortality in old men treated for PC and confirmed the preeminent importance of CV comorbidity, particularly in elderly [57].

Regarding the risk of CV mortality, Tsai et al. have indicated that ADT (GnRH agonists and/or an anti-androgen) (adjusted HR = 2.6) and aging (adjusted HR = 1.07) were associated with a statistically significant increase in the risk of CV death in patients treated with radical prostatectomy [7].

Of note, metabolic alterations connected to hormonal therapy in PC seem to predispose also to thromboembolic events and cerebrovascular events (increased risk of transient ischemic attacks or strokes) although data are conflicting [50, 54, 58-60]

On the other hand, several other studies have not confirmed the relationship between hormonal therapy and CV events in patients with PC.

Particularly, three large phase III randomized controlled trials of the Radiation Therapy Oncology Group (men randomized to radiotherapy and ADT vs radiotherapy alone) did not evidence a statistically significant increase of CV mortality risk with ADT use [51, 61, 62].

Furthermore, Alibhai et al. have shown that prolonged ADT (mean follow-up was 6.47 years) was associated with an increased risk of DM and fragility fractures but not MI (HR 0.91) or sudden cardiac death [53] while Punnen et al. using the Cancer of the Prostate Strategic Urologic Research Endeavor registry have shown that patients treated by watching waiting/active surveillance had a higher risk of CV death than patients treated with primary ADT, maybe due to unevaluated factors in treatment selection [52].

Of note, the first study could be biased since subjects had to receive an hormonal treatment for 6 months to be classified as ADT users and, the latter study received some critics for the not blinded determination, not rigorous definitions of cause of death and limited evaluation of CV risk factors (there was absence of CV family history, smoking, type of cardiac disease and body mass index; for 31% of patients resulted missing comorbidity data) [63].

Wherefore, the relationship between GnRH treatment and CV system remains unresolved mostly because none of the described studies was designed with CV morbidity or mortality as primary outcome and the conclusion are a result of secondary analyses of oncological trial. Furthermore, the above mentioned studies have shown a diverse follow-up period, a small number of events, a different type of ADT and potential confounding factors, such as comorbidities.

Recently, it has been shown that a GnRH antagonist (degarelix) was associated to lower cardiac events (6.5%) in PC patients with preexisting cardiovascular disease during the first year of ADT, when compared to GnRH agonists, leuprolide and goserelin (14.7%). However, since there was not a difference in patients without pre-existing CV disease, it could be hypostasize that GnRH antagonists should be most suitable and safe in patients with a CV history [33]. This interesting results derive from a post hoc analysis of data from six phase 3 randomized trials (2328 subjects) and thus need to be confirmed in further studies also because in a previous study Smith and colleagues suggest that degarelix and leuprolide have similar cardiovascular safety profiles (risk of arrhythmias) [64].

c) Management of Patients with Prostate Cancer Treated with Hormonal Therapy

Since a large part of elderly subject with an early-stage PC usually do not die of conditions strictly related to their tumor, it is mandatory to evaluate the side-effects of anti-cancer drugs. In last years, cardio-metabolic adverse events of ADT in PC patients have been widely studied and discussed due to their important impact on quality life and mortality. Furthermore old men that suffered from PC show an extensive amount of comorbidities that can influence therapeutic choice and outcomes [32]. In particular CV disease, such as MI, heart failure, atrial fibrillation and stroke have an impressive prevalence and incidence in the elderly population [65]. Hence, an accurate management of patients with PC has to include a deep evaluation of the most appropriate treatment, carefully weighting the potential benefits vs the possible risks (e.g. GnRH agonists vs GnRH antagonists).

Cardiotoxicity is emerging as one of the most frequent complication of antineoplastic drugs particularly in patient that are affected by malignancy, such as PC, that typically allow a long-term survival [66]. However the real impact of ADT and CV morbidity and mortality is controversial. Probably, these discordant data are justifiable by the nature of the studies. In fact, mostly of the above described analysis derive from an evaluation of oncologic and radiologic trial and have not CV events as the primary outcome. Moreover, the common association of hormonal therapy with radiological treatment could collaborate to enhance the risk of CV side effects. Therefore, there is a real need for further clinical investigations that can explain the relation between hormonal therapy and cardio-metabolic adverse effects, that may identify potential prevention and management strategies to reduce morbidity and mortality in patients with PC. Particularly, it is important to screen the pre-existing CV risk factors and pathologies with the purpose to find the most suitable treatment for each patient. For example, recent studies suggest that degarelix (a GnRH antagonist)is associated to lower cardiac events in PC patients with preexisting cardiovascular disease during the first year of ADT when compared to GnRH agonists, (leuprolide and goserelin) [33].

Moreover, given the metabolic effects of ADT in patients with PC, it is indicated a periodic (every three or six months) cardiac follow-up, as suggested by the Science Advisory from the American Heart Association, American Cancer Society, the American Urological Association and the American Society for Radiation Oncology [67]. This evaluation should include a measurement of body weight, body mass index, blood pressure, lipid profile (total cholesterol, LDL cholesterol, HDL cholesterol, triglycerides), fasting glucose and insulin level with the purpose of an early diagnosis of MS. In our opinion, it should be also suggested a periodic cardiologic assessment including physical examination, ECG and echocardiography, particularly in elderly patients with pre-existing CV risk factor and cardiac disease. Additionally, in the recent years cardiac magnetic resonance is emerging as a successful method to recognize cardiac dysfunction (myocardial injury and ventricular alterations) related to anti-cancer treatment. In fact, this diagnostic method allows to identify preclinical manifestations of cardiac diseases [68].

Presently, there are not standardized strategies to control and treat ADT-related cardio-metabolic effects and consequently it is necessary to utilize the guidelines and the recommendations for MS, DM and CV disease (hypertension and dyslipidemia) for the general population. Hence, it is strongly suggested an healthy lifestyle that include a balanced diet, regular-moderate physical activity and smoking cessation.

Recent studies confirmed the beneficial effect of physical activity during ADT treatment in patients with PC: a resistance exercise intervention (for at least 3 months) reduced significantly fatigue, improved quality of life and muscular fitness, whereas a combined program, including aerobic and resistance exercise, ameliorated cardiovascular fitness, muscular strength, total cholesterol-to-HDL cholesterol ratio, fatigue and mental health [69, 70].

Moreover, in a more advanced stage of each disease, it could be required a specific pharmacological treatment: antihypertensive drugs (beta-blockers, ACE-inhibitors or angiotensin II receptor blocker), oral hypoglycemic agents (e.g. metformin) or insulin analogs and statins.

The European Society of Hypertension/European Society of Cardiology (ESH/ESC) guidelines recommend BP ≥140/90 mmHg as a reference values to start antihypertensive therapy. In addition, in the elderly it is important to avoid rapid reduction in blood pressure, while there is not a general consensus regarding the best glycemic goals in this population [71].

Recently, a working group including the International Association of Gerontology and Geriatrics, the European Diabetes Working Party for Older People and the International Task Force of Experts in Diabetes have suggested some advice:

1) The clinician must consider individual comorbidities, cognitive and functional status; glucose goals should be agreed with the patient and/or caregiver;
2) HbA1c target range should be between 7.0% and 7.5 %;
3) Glucose-lowering therapy should be started if fasting glucose levels are ≥ 7 mmol/L [72].

Regarding the management of dyslipidemias, statins are recommended only for elderly patients with established CV disease [73, 74]. In addition, Nobes et colleagues published an interesting randomized pilot study estimating the efficacy of 6-months intervention including metformin and lifestyle changes in patients with PC treated with ADT. They evidenced a significant increase in abdominal circumference, body weight, body mass index and systolic blood pressure [75]. Interestingly, another trial ('MVENT' trial - ClinicalTrials.gov Identifier: NCT01077479) is currently ongoing to assess the efficacy of metformin in contrasting ADT-induced insulin resistance, as measured by homeostasis model assessment (HOMAIR) in men with non-metastatic prostate cancer. The results of this trial will open new interesting scenarios and will inspire other studies with the aim to determine whether this drug should influence CV morbidity and mortality. Further researches are necessary to produce more extensive evidence-based guidelines that could lead to an appropriate and complete management of PC patients treated with long-term ADT.

Conclusion

Prostatic diseases (BPH and PC) have shown an increased prevalence among elderly population in the last ten years, leading to a significant deterioration in the quality of life and life span [1, 2].

It is now well-established that cardio-metabolic factors are involved in the pathophysiology of both prostatic diseases and cardiovascular diseases; moreover, surgical factors related to prostatectomy are associated to CV complications such as MI (Figure 1). Indeed, the presence of MS in men with PC is associated with worse prognosis (higher tumor grade and stage) and increased mortality. However, this latter association seems even more important, since MS and diabetes can often represent a complication for PC patients, as a consequence of ADT, leading to further alterations, mainly of the cardiovascular system (Figure 1). Thus, it is extremely important to assess and monitor CV and metabolic function in patients with prostatic diseases, as it is equally important to prevent cardiac disease in subjects with established cardiovascular risk factors.

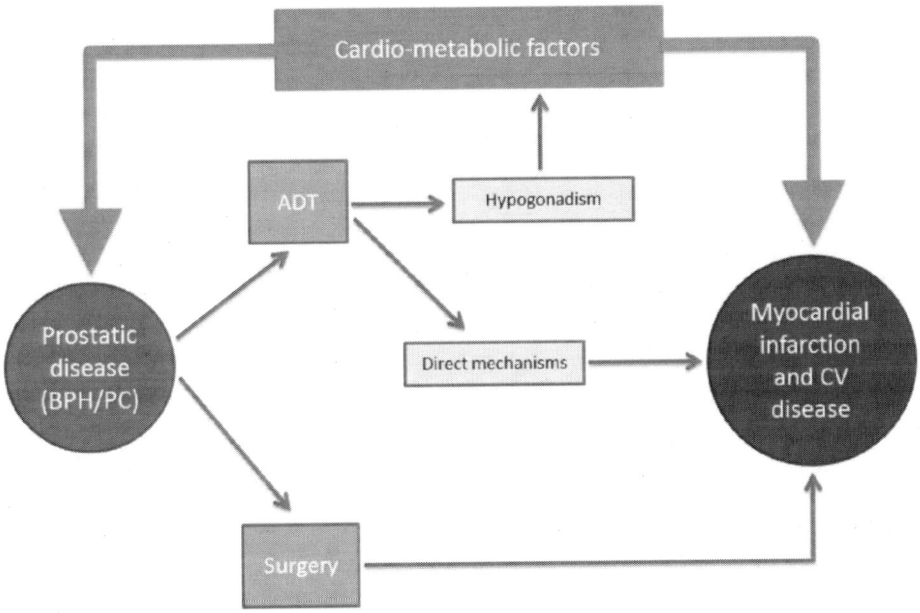

Figure 1. Abbreviations: BPH: benign prostatic hyperplasia; PC: prostatic cancer; ADT: androgen deprivation therapy; CV: cardiovascular.

Schematic representation of the close relationship between Prostatic disease and Myocardial infarction/CV disease. Cardio-metabolic factors are involved in the pathophysiology of both prostatic diseases (BPH and PC) and CV disease (including myocardial infarction, heart failure, stroke and arrhythmias). Furthermore, surgical factors (perioperative and postoperative) can lead to CV complications such as myocardial infarction and ADT could determinate cardiac dysfunction through direct mechanism (cardiomyocyte stimulation and destabilization of atherosclerotic plaques). However, indirect mechanism due to hypogonadism, seems to play the prominent part in CV effects of ADT by metabolic alterations (changes in body composition, metabolic syndrome, diabetes). For more information, refer to the main text.

Future longitudinal studies elucidating the relationship between cardiac, metabolic and prostatic risk factors are needed in order to provide better diagnostic, prognostic and therapeutic tools in the management of these frequently associated conditions.

References

[1] Siegel R, Ma J, Zou Z, Jemal A. Cancer statistics, 2014. *CA: a cancer journal for clinicians.* 2014;64(1):9-29.

[2] Patel ND, Parsons JK. Epidemiology and etiology of benign prostatic hyperplasia and bladder outlet obstruction. Indian journal of urology: *IJU: journal of the Urological Society of India.* 2014;30(2):170-6.

[3] Biester K, Skipka G, Jahn R, Buchberger B, Rohde V, Lange S. Systematic review of surgical treatments for benign prostatic hyperplasia and presentation of an approach to investigate therapeutic equivalence (non-inferiority). *BJU international.* 2012;109(5):722-30.

[4] DeSantis CE, Lin CC, Mariotto AB, Siegel RL, Stein KD, Kramer JL, et al. Cancer treatment and survivorship statistics, 2014. *CA: a cancer journal for clinicians.* 2014.

[5] Horwich A, Parker C, de Reijke T, Kataja V, Group EGW. Prostate cancer: ESMO Clinical Practice Guidelines for diagnosis, treatment and follow-up. *Annals of oncology: official journal of the European Society for Medical Oncology / ESMO.* 2013;24 Suppl 6:vi106-14.

[6] Weaver KE, Foraker RE, Alfano CM, Rowland JH, Arora NK, Bellizzi KM, et al. Cardiovascular risk factors among long-term survivors of breast, prostate, colorectal, and gynecologic cancers: a gap in survivorship care? *Journal of cancer survivorship: research and practice.* 2013;7(2):253-61.

[7] Tsai HK, D'Amico AV, Sadetsky N, Chen MH, Carroll PR. Androgen deprivation therapy for localized prostate cancer and the risk of cardiovascular mortality. *Journal of the National Cancer Institute.* 2007;99(20):1516-24.

[8] de Lucia C, Femminella GD, Rengo G, Ruffo A, Parisi V, Pagano G, et al. Risk of acute myocardial infarction after transurethral resection of prostate in elderly. *BMC surgery.* 2013;13 Suppl 2:S35.

[9] Collier A, Ghosh S, McGlynn B, Hollins G. Prostate cancer, androgen deprivation therapy, obesity, the metabolic syndrome, type 2 diabetes, and cardiovascular disease: a review. *American journal of clinical oncology.* 2012;35(5):504-9.

[10] Parsons JK. Modifiable risk factors for benign prostatic hyperplasia and lower urinary tract symptoms: new approaches to old problems. *The Journal of Urology.* 2007;178(2):395-401.

[11] Parsons JK, Sarma AV, McVary K, Wei JT. Obesity and benign prostatic hyperplasia: clinical connections, emerging etiological paradigms and future directions. *The Journal of urology.* 2013;189(1 Suppl):S102-6.

[12] Wang Z, Olumi AF. Diabetes, growth hormone-insulin-like growth factor pathways and association to benign prostatic hyperplasia. *Differentiation; research in biological diversity.* 2011;82(4-5):261-71.

[13] Suzuki S, Platz EA, Kawachi I, Willett WC, Giovannucci E. Intakes of energy and macronutrients and the risk of benign prostatic hyperplasia. *The American journal of clinical nutrition.* 2002;75(4):689-97.

[14] Parsons JK. Lifestyle factors, benign prostatic hyperplasia, and lower urinary tract symptoms. *Current opinion in urology.* 2011;21(1):1-4.

[15] Freeman MR, Solomon KR. Cholesterol and benign prostate disease. *Differentiation; research in biological diversity*. 2011;82(4-5):244-52.

[16] Michel MC, Heemann U, Schumacher H, Mehlburger L, Goepel M. Association of hypertension with symptoms of benign prostatic hyperplasia. *The Journal of urology*. 2004;172(4 Pt 1):1390-3.

[17] Conteduca V, Di Lorenzo G, Bozza G, Ardito R, Aieta M. Metabolic syndrome as a peculiar target for management of prostate cancer patients. *Clinical genitourinary cancer*. 2013;11(3):211-20.

[18] Stone NJ, Bilek S, Rosenbaum S. Recent National Cholesterol Education Program Adult Treatment Panel III update: adjustments and options. *The American journal of cardiology*. 2005;96(4A):53E-9E.

[19] Beebe-Dimmer JL, Nock NL, Neslund-Dudas C, Rundle A, Bock CH, Tang D, et al. Racial differences in risk of prostate cancer associated with metabolic syndrome. *Urology*. 2009;74(1):185-90.

[20] Pierce BL, Plymate S, Ostrander EA, Stanford JL. Diabetes mellitus and prostate cancer risk. *The Prostate*. 2008;68(10):1126-32.

[21] Hammarsten J, Hogstedt B. Clinical, haemodynamic, anthropometric, metabolic and insulin profile of men with high-stage and high-grade clinical prostate cancer. *Blood pressure*. 2004;13(1):47-55.

[22] Gong Z, Agalliu I, Lin DW, Stanford JL, Kristal AR. Obesity is associated with increased risks of prostate cancer metastasis and death after initial cancer diagnosis in middle-aged men. *Cancer*. 2007;109(6):1192-202.

[23] Hammarsten J, Hogstedt B. Hyperinsulinaemia: a prospective risk factor for lethal clinical prostate cancer. *European journal of cancer*. 2005;41(18):2887-95.

[24] Hahn RG, Essen P. ECG and cardiac enzymes after glycine absorption in transurethral prostatic resection. *Acta anaesthesiologica Scandinavica*. 1994;38(6):550-6.

[25] Ashton CM, Lahart CJ, Wray NP. The incidence of perioperative myocardial infarction with transurethral resection of the prostate. *Journal of the American Geriatrics Society*. 1989;37(7):614-8.

[26] Gupta K, Rastogi B, Jain M, Gupta PK, Sharma D. Electrolyte changes: An indirect method to assess irrigation fluid absorption complications during transurethral resection of prostate: A prospective study. *Saudi journal of anaesthesia*. 2010;4(3):142-6.

[27] Evans JW, Singer M, Chapple CR, Macartney N, Walker JM, Milroy EJ. Haemodynamic evidence for cardiac stress during transurethral prostatectomy. *BMJ*. 1992;304(6828):666-71.

[28] Manikandan R, Nathaniel C, Lewis P, Brough RJ, Adeyoju A, Brown SC, et al. Troponin T and N-terminal pro-brain natriuretic peptide changes in patients undergoing transurethral resection of the prostate. *The Journal of urology*. 2005;174(5):1892-5; discussion 5.

[29] Cancado TO, Leitao FB, Torres ML, Brito FS. Peri-operative evaluation by holter in elderly patients submitted to prostatectomy. *Arquivos brasileiros de cardiologia*. 2009;93(4):409-17, 1-9.

[30] Huggins C, Hodges CV. Studies on prostatic cancer. I. The effect of castration, of estrogen and androgen injection on serum phosphatases in metastatic carcinoma of the prostate. *CA: a cancer journal for clinicians*. 1972;22(4):232-40.

[31] Schroder F, Crawford ED, Axcrona K, Payne H, Keane TE. Androgen deprivation therapy: past, present and future. *BJU international*. 2012;109 Suppl 6:1-12.

[32] Conteduca V, Di Lorenzo G, Tartarone A, Aieta M. The cardiovascular risk of gonadotropin releasing hormone agonists in men with prostate cancer: an unresolved controversy. *Critical reviews in oncology/hematology*. 2013;86(1):42-51.

[33] Albertsen PC, Klotz L, Tombal B, Grady J, Olesen TK, Nilsson J. Cardiovascular morbidity associated with gonadotropin releasing hormone agonists and an antagonist. *European urology*. 2014;65(3):565-73.

[34] Corona G, Rastrelli G, Monami M, Guay A, Buvat J, Sforza A, et al. Hypogonadism as a risk factor for cardiovascular mortality in men: a meta-analytic study. European *journal of endocrinology / European Federation of Endocrine Societies*. 2011;165(5):687-701.

[35] Saigal CS, Gore JL, Krupski TL, Hanley J, Schonlau M, Litwin MS, et al. Androgen deprivation therapy increases cardiovascular morbidity in men with prostate cancer. Cancer. 2007;110(7):1493-500.

[36] Dong F, Skinner DC, Wu TJ, Ren J. The heart: a novel gonadotrophin-releasing hormone target. *Journal of neuroendocrinology*. 2011;23(5):456-63.

[37] Fahed AC, Gholmieh JM, Azar ST. Connecting the Lines between Hypogonadism and Atherosclerosis. *International journal of endocrinology*. 2012;2012:793953.

[38] Saylor PJ, Smith MR. Metabolic complications of androgen deprivation therapy for prostate cancer. *The Journal of urology*. 2013;189(1 Suppl):S34-42; discussion S3-4.

[39] Bhasin S, Taylor WE, Singh R, Artaza J, Sinha-Hikim I, Jasuja R, et al. The mechanisms of androgen effects on body composition: mesenchymal pluripotent cell as the target of androgen action. *The journals of gerontology Series A, Biological sciences and medical sciences*. 2003;58(12):M1103-10.

[40] van Londen GJ, Levy ME, Perera S, Nelson JB, Greenspan SL. Body composition changes during androgen deprivation therapy for prostate cancer: a 2-year prospective study. *Critical reviews in oncology/hematology*. 2008;68(2):172-7.

[41] Basaria S, Muller DC, Carducci MA, Egan J, Dobs AS. Hyperglycemia and insulin resistance in men with prostate carcinoma who receive androgen-deprivation therapy. *Cancer*. 2006;106(3):581-8.

[42] Trost LW, Serefoglu E, Gokce A, Linder BJ, Sartor AO, Hellstrom WJ. Androgen deprivation therapy impact on quality of life and cardiovascular health, monitoring therapeutic replacement. *The journal of sexual medicine*. 2013;10 Suppl 1:84-101.

[43] Lage MJ, Barber BL, Markus RA. Association between androgen-deprivation therapy and incidence of diabetes among males with prostate cancer. *Urology*. 2007;70(6):1104-8.

[44] Nobes JP, Langley SE, Laing RW. Metabolic syndrome and prostate cancer: a review. *Clinical oncology*. 2009;21(3):183-91.

[45] Berwick ZC, Dick GM, Tune JD. Heart of the matter: coronary dysfunction in metabolic syndrome. *Journal of molecular and cellular cardiology*. 2012;52(4):848-56.

[46] Collins L, Basaria S. Adverse effects of androgen deprivation therapy in men with prostate cancer: a focus on metabolic and cardiovascular complications. *Asian journal of andrology*. 2012;14(2):222-5.

[47] D'Amico AV, Denham JW, Crook J, Chen MH, Goldhaber SZ, Lamb DS, et al. Influence of androgen suppression therapy for prostate cancer on the frequency and

timing of fatal myocardial infarctions. *Journal of clinical oncology: official journal of the American Society of Clinical Oncology*. 2007;25(17):2420-5.

[48] D'Amico AV, Chen MH, Renshaw AA, Loffredo M, Kantoff PW. Androgen suppression and radiation vs radiation alone for prostate cancer: a randomized trial. *JAMA : the journal of the American Medical Association*. 2008;299(3):289-95.

[49] Keating NL, O'Malley AJ, Smith MR. Diabetes and cardiovascular disease during androgen deprivation therapy for prostate cancer. *Journal of clinical oncology: official journal of the American Society of Clinical Oncology*. 2006;24(27):4448-56.

[50] Keating NL, O'Malley AJ, Freedland SJ, Smith MR. Diabetes and cardiovascular disease during androgen deprivation therapy: observational study of veterans with prostate cancer. *Journal of the National Cancer Institute*. 2010;102(1):39-46.

[51] Efstathiou JA, Bae K, Shipley WU, Hanks GE, Pilepich MV, Sandler HM, et al. Cardiovascular mortality and duration of androgen deprivation for locally advanced prostate cancer: analysis of RTOG 92-02. *European urology*. 2008;54(4):816-23.

[52] Punnen S, Cooperberg MR, Sadetsky N, Carroll PR. Androgen deprivation therapy and cardiovascular risk. *Journal of clinical oncology: official journal of the American Society of Clinical Oncology*. 2011;29(26):3510-6.

[53] Alibhai SM, Duong-Hua M, Sutradhar R, Fleshner NE, Warde P, Cheung AM, et al. Impact of androgen deprivation therapy on cardiovascular disease and diabetes. *Journal of clinical oncology: official journal of the American Society of Clinical Oncology*. 2009;27(21):3452-8.

[54] Jespersen CG, Norgaard M, Borre M. Androgen-deprivation therapy in treatment of prostate cancer and risk of myocardial infarction and stroke: a nationwide Danish population-based cohort study. *European urology*. 2014;65(4):704-9.

[55] Van Hemelrijck M, Garmo H, Holmberg L, Ingelsson E, Bratt O, Bill-Axelson A, et al. Absolute and relative risk of cardiovascular disease in men with prostate cancer: results from the Population-Based PCBaSe Sweden. *Journal of clinical oncology: official journal of the American Society of Clinical Oncology*. 2010;28(21):3448-56.

[56] Nanda A, Chen MH, Braccioforte MH, Moran BJ, D'Amico AV. Hormonal therapy use for prostate cancer and mortality in men with coronary artery disease-induced congestive heart failure or myocardial infarction. *JAMA: the journal of the American Medical Association*. 2009;302(8):866-73.

[57] Nanda A, Chen MH, Moran BJ, Braccioforte MH, D'Amico AV. Cardiovascular comorbidity and mortality in men with prostate cancer treated with brachytherapy-based radiation with or without hormonal therapy. *International journal of radiation oncology, biology, physics*. 2013;85(5):e209-15.

[58] Azoulay L, Yin H, Benayoun S, Renoux C, Boivin JF, Suissa S. Androgen-deprivation therapy and the risk of stroke in patients with prostate cancer. *European urology*. 2011;60(6):1244-50.

[59] Ehdaie B, Atoria CL, Gupta A, Feifer A, Lowrance WT, Morris MJ, et al. Androgen deprivation and thromboembolic events in men with prostate cancer. *Cancer*. 2012;118(13):3397-406.

[60] Chung SD, Chen YK, Wu FJ, Lin HC. Hormone therapy for prostate cancer and the risk of stroke: a 5-year follow-up study. *BJU international*. 2012;109(7):1001-5.

[61] Efstathiou JA, Bae K, Shipley WU, Hanks GE, Pilepich MV, Sandler HM, et al. Cardiovascular mortality after androgen deprivation therapy for locally advanced

prostate cancer: RTOG 85-31. *Journal of clinical oncology: official journal of the American Society of Clinical Oncology*. 2009;27(1):92-9.

[62] Roach M, 3rd, Bae K, Speight J, Wolkov HB, Rubin P, Lee RJ, et al. Short-term neoadjuvant androgen deprivation therapy and external-beam radiotherapy for locally advanced prostate cancer: long-term results of RTOG 8610. *Journal of clinical oncology : official journal of the American Society of Clinical Oncology*. 2008;26(4):585-91.

[63] Alibhai SM. Cardiovascular toxicity of androgen deprivation therapy: a new door opens. *Journal of clinical oncology: official journal of the American Society of Clinical Oncology*. 2011;29(26):3500-2.

[64] Smith MR, Klotz L, Persson BE, Olesen TK, Wilde AA. Cardiovascular safety of degarelix: results from a 12-month, comparative, randomized, open label, parallel group phase III trial in patients with prostate cancer. *The Journal of urology*. 2010;184(6):2313-9.

[65] Go AS, Mozaffarian D, Roger VL, Benjamin EJ, Berry JD, Blaha MJ, et al. Heart disease and stroke statistics--2014 update: *a report from the American Heart Association. Circulation*. 2014;129(3):e28-e292.

[66] Albini A, Pennesi G, Donatelli F, Cammarota R, De Flora S, Noonan DM. Cardiotoxicity of anticancer drugs: the need for cardio-oncology and cardio-oncological prevention. *Journal of the National Cancer Institute*. 2010;102(1):14-25.

[67] Levine GN, D'Amico AV, Berger P, Clark PE, Eckel RH, Keating NL, et al. Androgen-deprivation therapy in prostate cancer and cardiovascular risk: a science advisory from the American Heart Association, American Cancer Society, and American Urological Association: endorsed by the American Society for Radiation Oncology. *Circulation*. 2010;121(6):833-40.

[68] Vasu S, Hundley WG. Understanding cardiovascular injury after treatment for cancer: an overview of current uses and future directions of cardiovascular magnetic resonance. *Journal of cardiovascular magnetic resonance: official journal of the Society for Cardiovascular Magnetic Resonance*. 2013;15(1):66.

[69] Segal RJ, Reid RD, Courneya KS, Sigal RJ, Kenny GP, Prud'Homme DG, et al. Randomized controlled trial of resistance or aerobic exercise in men receiving radiation therapy for prostate cancer. *Journal of clinical oncology: official journal of the American Society of Clinical Oncology*. 2009;27(3):344-51.

[70] Cormie P, Galvao DA, Spry N, Joseph D, Chee R, Taaffe DR, et al. Can Supervised Exercise Prevent Treatment Toxicity in Prostate Cancer Patients Initiating Androgen Deprivation Therapy: A Randomised Controlled Trial. *BJU international*. 2014.

[71] Mancia G, Fagard R, Narkiewicz K, Redon J, Zanchetti A, Bohm M, et al. 2013 ESH/ESC guidelines for the management of arterial hypertension: the Task Force for the Management of Arterial Hypertension of the European Society of Hypertension (ESH) and of the European Society of Cardiology (ESC). *European heart journal*. 2013;34(28):2159-219.

[72] Sinclair A, Morley JE, Rodriguez-Manas L, Paolisso G, Bayer T, Zeyfang A, et al. Diabetes mellitus in older people: position statement on behalf of the International Association of Gerontology and Geriatrics (IAGG), the European Diabetes Working Party for Older People (EDWPOP), and the International Task Force of Experts in Diabetes. *Journal of the American Medical Directors Association*. 2012;13(6):497-502.

[73] European Association for Cardiovascular P, Rehabilitation, Reiner Z, Catapano AL, De Backer G, Graham I, et al. ESC/EAS Guidelines for the management of dyslipidaemias: the Task Force for the management of dyslipidaemias of the European Society of Cardiology (ESC) and the European Atherosclerosis Society (EAS). *European heart journal.* 2011;32(14):1769-818.
[74] Tsigos C, Bitzur R, Kleinman Y, Cohen H, Cahn A, Brambilla G, et al. Targets for body fat, blood pressure, lipids, and glucose-lowering interventions in healthy older people. *Diabetes care*. 2013;36 Suppl 2:S292-300.
[75] Nobes JP, Langley SE, Klopper T, Russell-Jones D, Laing RW. A prospective, randomized pilot study evaluating the effects of metformin and lifestyle intervention on patients with prostate cancer receiving androgen deprivation therapy. *BJU international.* 2012;109(10):1495-502.

In: Myocardial Infarctions
Editor: Pattie Wilkonson

ISBN: 978-1-63321-726-3

Chapter 5

Albuminuria: Marker or Maker of Atrial Fibrillation and Mortality in Patients with Acute Myocardial Infarction

Rafel Sanjuan, [*] ***PhD and Maria L. Blasco*** [†]***, PhD***
Coronary Care Unit, University Clinic Hospital of Valencia, Valencia, Spain

Abstract

Background/Aims: Albuminuria is a marker of a cardiovascular morbimortality. We assessed the relationship between albuminuria, atrial fibrillation and mortality in a cohort of patients with acute myocardial infarction.

Methods: In the observational prospective study, we examined 636 consecutive patients with a diagnosis of acute myocardial infarction. Urine specimens were analyzed for albuminuria and were corrected with urinary creatinine to obtain a reliable estimate of Albumin/Creatinine rate. Albumin/Creatinine ≥ 30 mg/g^{-1} was considered abnormal. Association between Albumin/Creatinine, atrial fibrillation and mortality was assessed by multivariate analysis.

Results: The incidence of atrial fibrillation was 7.5% when Albumin/Creatinine was normal. When the albuminuria ranged from 30 to 300 mg.Cr^{-1}, the incidence of atrial fibrillation was 17.8%. Macroproteinuria (>300 mg.Cr^{-1}) was detected in 48 patients and the incidence of atrial fibrillation was 27%. In-hospital mortality was 42 (6.6%) and increased to 16.7% when macroalbuminuria was present. In a multivariate adjusted risk, Albumin/Creatinine ≥ 30 mg.Cr^{-1} (OR=1.8;1.1-2.9), previous coronary artery by-pass (OR=2;1.1-4) and chronic renal disease (OR=1.6;1-2.6) were independent prognostic factors for the incidence of atrial fibrillation. Albuminuria increased the model prediction (C-statistic analysis) for atrial fibrillation in 0.026. Neither albuminuria nor atrial fibrillation increased the model prediction for mortality. In a multivariate analysis for mortality, the most important prognostic factors were a Killip class>1 (OR=6;2.8-15) and

[*] sanjuan_raf@gva.es. AV Blasco Ibañez 17, Valencia. 46010. Spain; Tel: +34963862627. Fax number: +34963868830.
[†] blasco_luicor@gva.es.

initial or complicate Bundle Brunch Block (OR=3;1.5-6) on admission meanwhile a previous history of hypertension had a protective factor (OR=0.22; 011-0.45)(<0.001)

Conclusions: An early increase of albuminuria was associated with atrial instability but was not a marker for a poor in-hospital prognosis in patients with acute myocardial infarction.

Introduction

Microalbuminuria, a subclinical rise in the urinary albumin excretion (30–300 mg/day), has been proposed as an independent prognostic factor of cardiovascular morbidity and mortality in the fields of diabetes mellitus, metabolic syndrome and arterial hypertension [1-3]. Microalbuminuria may result from a glomerular overfiltration or a tubular reabsorption or a combination of both. Persistent albuminuria suggests progression of chronic renal disease at all levels of estimated glomerular filtration rate [4] and has been linked to abnormalities of the vasculature, such as endothelial dysfunction and reduced vascular dilatation. The changes in urinary albumin excretion may therefore reflect underlying microvascular abnormalities.

It has been 22 years since Gosling et al. [5] observed a transient increase in albumin excretion rate during acute myocardial infarction (AMI) attributed to a systemic increase in vascular permeability as part of the early acute inflammatory process accompanying AMI, independent of blood pressure, diabetes, renal disease and thrombolytic treatment [6-9].

Some reports, which included both diabetic and non-diabetic patients, have shown that increased urinary protein excretion appears to be an early and proportional response to AMI and it yields prognostic information about early [10-12] and late mortality [13, 14].

On the other hand, atrial fibrillation (AF) is common in end-stage renal disease, but the relation between more modest decrements in kidney function or albuminuria with AF is uncertain. An association between resting heart rate, AF and albuminuria has been recently described to occur in chronic kidney disease and hypertensive patients [15, 16] with or without a history of AF. Regardless of severity, chronic kidney disease is associated with an increased prevalence of AF among a population-based cohort of US adults [17]. The precise pathological mechanisms that link AF and albuminuria or chronic renal disease, are those due to direct effects (ischemic burden and/or ventricular hypertrophy or dysfunction), but also, indirect mechanisms related to autonomic deregulation could be responsible.

None of these studies explored whether the association of albuminuria and AF could be done in patients with acute coronary syndromes. Therefore, we examined the relationship between albumin excretion and atrial instability in patients with AMI. Also, we hypothesized that individuals with more severe albuminuria would have increased risk of dying during hospitalization independently of classical cardiovascular risk factors.

Materials and Methods

Patients

This was a single-centre observational prospective study. Six-hundred and thirty six consecutive and unselected patients admitted to our Coronary Care Unit for AMI were prospectively studied. The entry criteria for the study were: chest pain with ST segment changes elevation (STEMI) or depression (NSTEMI) or acute bundle branch block with specific biomarkers increased according to the criteria established by current guidelines [18].

Subjects were excluded from the study if they had acute inflammatory diseases (n=12), hepatic failure (n=3), autoimmunity or cancer (n=4) and patients with chronic renal failure in haemodialysis programme (n=5). Moreover eleven patients with a permanent history of atrial fibrillation also were excluded. After echocardiography was performed, six patients were ruled out because significant aortic stenosis was observed. Fifteen additional patients were excluded because of insufficient data collection.

Cardiovascular Risk Factor

The presence of hypertension, type II diabetes, dyslipidemia, smoking habits and body mass index were considered. Patients with a fasting glucose level <110 mg/dl and without a history of diabetes were classified as normoglycemic. We defined Chronic Kidney Disease based on the recommendations of the National Kidney Foundation [19]. Estimated Glomerular Filtration Rate (eGFR) was calculated using the modification of diet in renal disease (MDRD) equation, which includes serum creatinine, age, race, and gender.

Measurements

The project design included a medical examination, biochemical analyses and instrumental exams as echocardiography and coronary angiography results. The presence and degree of heart failure was assessed on admission at the emergency department, following the Killip classification [20].

Coronary angiography was performed as soon as possible, and the number of damaged coronary arteries evaluated. Patients with STEMI and having contraindication for thrombolytic therapy were referred for urgent invasive angiography with the intention of performing primary percutaneous coronary interventions (PCI). Moreover, patients after unsuccessful fibrinolytic therapy were treated with rescue PCI. Left ventricular ejection fraction (LVEF) was assessed by two-dimensional echocardiography within 2 days after admission. Once the presence of valvular cardiopathy was ruled out, LVEF was calculated by the Simpson method.

All analyses were measured by conventional laboratory methods. Urine specimens was collected on admission and processed immediately or the next morning after admission. Albuminuria was corrected for urinary creatinine to obtain a reliable estimate of Albumin/ Creatinine Rate (ACR) [21]. In statistical analysis presented in this paper the ACR was used because it showed slightly better predictive power than the albumin excretion rate. Urinary albumin excretion up 30 mg.g Cr^{-1} was considered normal.

Continuous monitoring was performed in all patients during stay at the Coronary Care Unit in order to determine any type of significant arrhythmia. After discharge from Coronary Care Unit an electrocardiogram was performed every day and when patients had symptoms.

The study was closed on October 2013. All patients gave their informed consent and the study was carried out according to the principles of the Declaration of Helsinki.

Statistical Analysis

Continuous variables with abnormal distribution (Kolmogorov–Smirnov test) were transformed by neperian logarithm before analysis. Continuous variables were expressed as mean ± standard deviation or standard error mean, determining the differences between groups by Student's t-test. The categorical variables were compared by chi-square analysis, contingency coefficient risk for asymptotic methods. The following dichotomous categorical indicator variables were classified such that being, gender, age, smoking, site of myocardial infarction, previous myocardial infarction, chronic renal disease, Killip class on admission, the most important cardiovascular risk factor, etc. scored 1 and the opposite scored 2. The cut-offs were chosen on information obtained through ROC curve analysis. The significant variables in the univariate analysis and no significant but important clinical cardiovascular risk factors, were introduced (Forward:Conditional) in a multivariate logistical regression model to obtain the predictive variables of adverse outcomes (in-hospital AF and mortality). The ACR was utilized in some analysis as a continuous (logged) variable and in the others as dichotomous variable. The model's discriminative ability was assessed with Harrell's C statistic. The probability of concordance between observed and predicted AF and mortality on the basis of pairs of individuals was calculated for baseline clinical variables, hemodynamic and metabolic parameters, chronic renal failure and ACR the first day after admission. A value of $p < 0.05$ was considered statistically significant. Data were analyzed using SPSS version 11.0 (SPSS Inc., Chicago, Ill, USA).

Results

Baseline Characteristics

The median age of our sample (636 consecutive AMI patients) was 65 (30-95) years old 76% were males and Body Mass Index>30 were present in 24% of patients. Median time from onset of chest pain to admission was 3 h (range 1–48 h), and patients were discharged from hospital after an average of 8 days (range 1–48 days) (mean 10±8 days). STEMI was observed in 406 (64%) and reperfusion therapy (primary angioplasty vs thrombolysis) was performed in 66% (268/406) of STEMI patients. In 566/636 (89%) of patients percutaneous coronary interventions was carried out and a significant lesion of left coronary artery trunk was observed in 51 patients (8%).

Patients were divided into two groups according to ACR value: 1°) Patients with abnormal ACR ≥ 30 (262 patients; 42%) and 2°). Patients with normal ACR <30 (374 patients) (control group).Unadjusted relative risks for clinical, hemodynamic, metabolic characteristics and in-hospital follow-up are given in Table 1 according to ACR. In-hospital mortality was 6.6% (42/636) and atrial fibrillation was present in 79 patients (12%). Initial or new bundle branch block was observed in 54 patients (8.5%). An association between abnormal ACR and severity of coronary artery disease, NSTEMI myocardial infarction and lower left ventricular ejection fraction were observed. All patients with no specific contraindications received the recommended drugs in the acute phase.

Table 1. Acute myocardial infarction: Clinical, hemodynamic and metabolic characteristics of the study population according to albuminuria/creatinine rate

Variable	ACR≥30 (262 patients) (41%)	ACR<30 (374 patients (59%)	OR (CI)	P
Anthropometric Parameters				
Male	77%	77%	0.99(0.89-1.2)	0.83
Aged (m ± sd)	67±12	62±13		<0.001
Aged>70years	49%	34%	1.4(1.19-1.72)	<0.001
BMI (kg/m^2)	28±4	27.8±4		0,57
Previous Disorders				
NYHA>2	6.7%	2.5%	1.6 (1.2-2.2)	<0.01
Diabetes	49%	28%	1.6 (1.4-1,9)	<0.001
Hypertension	74%	59%	1.5(1.21-1..9)	<0.001
Previous Myocardial Infarction	32%	23%	1.28 (1-1.5)	0.015
Current smoker	36%	43%	0.8 (0.7-1.1)	0.79
Dyslipemia	47%	50%	0.9 (0.7-1.1)	0.52
Chronic Renal Disease	14%	29%	2(1.6-2.4)	<0.001
Previous Coronary Artery By-pass	5%	4.5%	1(0.69-1.6)	0.8
ACUTE MYOCARDIAL INFARCTION				
GRACE risk score	179±44	155±41		<0.001
NSTEMI (230 patients)	38%	31%	1.22 (1-1.4)	0.04
Killip>1 (admission)	45%	17%	2 (1.7-2.4)	<0.001
Heart Rate (admission)(bpm)	89±21	77±19		<0.001
Left Ventricular EF (440 patients)	47±13	53±11		<0.001
N° of Coronary Artery Disease (m±sd)	1.7±0.9	1.4±0.8		0.003
N° of Coronary Artery Disease>1	53%	35%	1.5 (1.2-1.9)	<0.001
Creatine Kinase MB (ng/ml)(m±SEM).	128±10	130±9		0.9
Reperfusion therapy (STEMI)				
Fibrinolisys agents (STEMI)	31.4%	36.4%	0.8 (0.59-1)	0.19
Primary Angioplasty (STEMI)	37%	31%	1.15 (0,9-1,5)	0.28
In-Hospital Follow-up				
GRACE risk score (mortality)	9.8%	3.9%	2 (1.3-2.5)	<0.001
In-Hospital Mortality	9.9%	4.3%	1.5 (1.2-2)	0.005
Atrial fibrillation	19%	7%	1.7 (1.4-2.2)	<0.001
Initial or complicated BBB	15.6%	3.5%	1.99 (1.6-2.4)	<0.001
Primary Ventricular Fibrillation	6.5%	4.8%	1.19 (0.8-1.6)	0.36
AV Block ≥2°	6.5%	5.3%	1.12 (0.7-1.6)	0.54
In-Coronary Care Unit (m±sd)	3.5±2	3.18±1.6		0.04
In-Hospital Stay (days) (m±sd)	11±3	9±3		0.003

Table 1. (Continued)

Variable	ACR≥30 (262 patients) (41%)	ACR<30 (374 patients (59%)	OR (CI)	P
Metabolic and Inflammatoryparameters				
Glycemia (mg/dL) (admission)	202±999	158±70		<0.001
Glycemia >140 mg/dL	66%	46%	1.6(1.3-1.9)	<0.001
HbA1c (%)	6.6±1.5	6.1±1.3		<0.001
Insulin (μU/ml)	16±15	12±9		0.002
Triglyceride (mg/dL)	139±68	146±80		0.3
Cholesterol (mg/dL)	172±49	181±47		0.022
High Density Lipoprotein (mg/dL)	42±12	42±12		0.8
Low Density Lipoprotein (mg/dL)	107±42	117±43		0.005
Creatine (mg/dl)(admission)	1.47±1.3	1±0.3		<0.001
eGFR<60 ml/min	26%	9.4%	1.8(1.46-2.18)	<0.001
C-Reactive Protein (mg/dl)	64±5	37±3		0.002
White blood cell counts (109/L)	11994±436	11000±359		0.079
BNP (ng/mL) (m±SEM)	683±66	264±25		<0.001
Concomitant hospital therapies				
Aspirin	97%	97%	0.9(0.58-1.3)	0.87
Clopidogrel	89%	92%	0.8 (0.6-1.1)	0.29
Heparin	84%	84%	0.97 (0.7-1.3)	0.95
B-Blockers	31%	42%	0.7(0.5-0.9)	0.005
ACE inhibitors	62%	62%	1 (0.8 -1.2)	0.76
Statin	91%	94%	0.8(0.6-1.1)	0.07
Diuretics	46%	18%	2(1.6-2.3)	<0.001
Inotropic agents	18%	6%	1.7(1.4-2)	0.001
Insulin (214patients)(34%)	50%	25%	1.8(1.5-2.1)	<0.001

ACR: Albuminuria/creatinine rate, BMI: Body Mass Index; NYHA: New York Heart Association; GRACE: Global Registry of Acute Coronary Events; NSTEMI: non ST elevation myocardial infarction; EF: ejection fraction; M: mean; SD: standard deviation; SEM: standard error mean; STEMI: ST elevation myocardial infarction; BBB: Bundle Branch Block; AV: atrioventricular; eGFR: estimates glomerular filtration rate; BNP: brain natriuretic peptide; ACE: angiotensin-converting enzyme; CI: confidence interval; OR: odds ratio.

Albuminuria and Atrial Fibrillation

The following urinary ACR measurement on the first day after admission were observed: normal ACR (9±7 mg.g.Cr^{-1}) was present in 374 patients (59%); microalbuminuria (30-300 mg.g.Cr^{-1})(100±64 mg.g.Cr^{-1}) was detected in 214 patients (34%) and macroproteinuria (>300 mg.g.Cr^{-1}) (491±194 mg.g.Cr^{-1}) in 48 patients (7%).

AF was observed in 79 patients (12%), 96% of them during the immediate post-infarction period in the Coronary Care Unit stay: 10 patients suffer AF in the first 24h; 38 patients presented AF during 24h-48h; 12 patients suffer an episodic of AF between 48h-72 h. In 4% of patients (three patients) AF were observed after discharge from coronary care unit.

The incidence of atrial fibrillation was 7.5% when Albumin/Creatinine was normal. When the albuminuria ranged from 30-300 mg.Cr^{-1}, the incidence of atrial fibrillation reaches 17.8%. Macroproteinuria (>300 mg.Cr^{-1}) was detected in 48 patients and the incidence of atrial fibrillation was 27% (Figure 1). The arrhythmia was self-limited in 35 patients. Pharmacological therapy (amiodarone, bolus followed by a continuous infusion) was necessary to terminate auricular tachyarrhythmia in 19 patients. A direct-current cardioversion was done in seven patients because the arrhythmic episode was symptomatic. In 12 patients, several episodes (recurrent) of paroxysmal AF were observed.

The significant variables in the univariate analysis associated with AF were older (>70 year old) 2.5 (1.6-3.8)($p<0.001$), chronic renal disease (2.6;1.6-4.3)($p<0.001$), previous coronary artery by-pass (2.9;1.6-3.8)($p<0.001$), hypertension (2.4;1.3-4.2)($p=0.001$), chronic myocardial infarction (1.78;1.17-2.7)($p=0.006$), NSTEMI (1.08;1.01-1.16)($p=0.01$), number of coronary artery disease>1 (2.4;1.4-4)($p<0.001$), Killip Class >1 (3.2 (2.1-4.9)($p<0.001$), Left Ventricular ejection fraction<45% (2;1.2-3.3)($p=0.005$) and ACR>30 mg.Cr^{-1} (1.7;1.4-2.2)($p<0.001$) . In a multivariate adjusted risk Albumin/Creatinine ≥30 mg.Cr^{-1} (OR=1.7), previous coronary artery by-pass (OR=2.5) and chronic renal disease (creatinine>1.4 or e-GFR<60% on admission) (OR=1.7) were independent predictive factors for the incidence of atrial fibrillation (Table 2). Albuminuria significantly increased the model prediction (C-statistic analysis) for atrial fibrillation in 0.026 (0.741-0.715=0.026) regardless chronic renal disease (Table 3). (Figure 2).

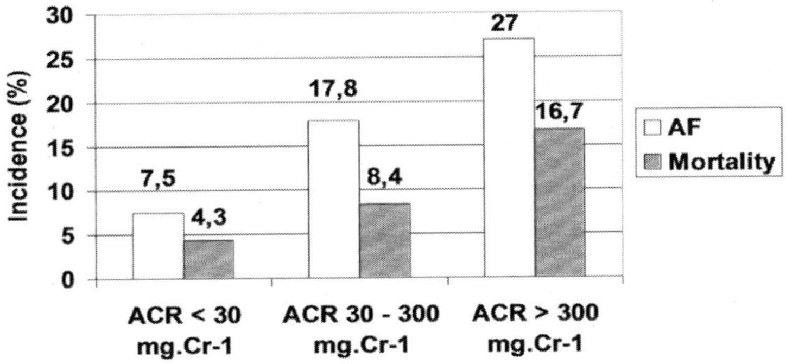

Figure 1. Mortality (dark bar) and atrial fibrillation (AF) in patients with acute myocardial infarction according to albumin/creatinuria ratio (ACR). The patients with normal albuminuria (ACR<30 mg.Cr^{-1}) presented a lower incidence as AF as mortality. In the microalbuminuria range (30-300 mg.g.Cr^{-1}), the incidence of AF and mortality was 17.8% and 8,4% respectively. Patients with macroalbuminuria suffer a higher incidence of AF (27%) and mortality (16.7%).

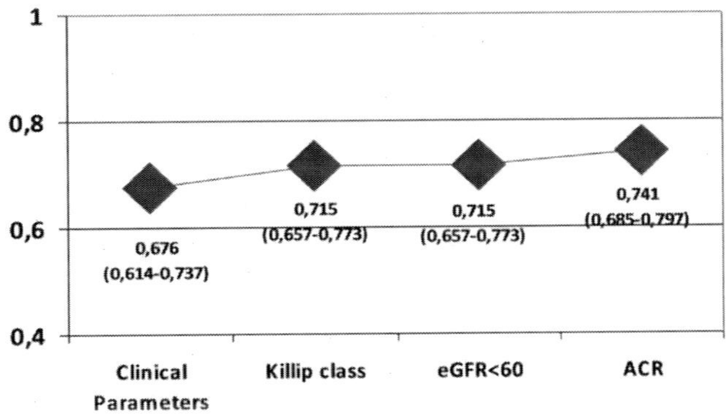

Figure 2. Predictive models for atrial fibrillation tested with C-statistic method. Albuminuria significantly increased the model prediction (slightly) for atrial fibrillation in 0.026 (0.741-0.715=0.026), regardless chronic renal disease.

Table 2. Multivariate adjusted risk for the incidence of Atrial Fibrillation (AF)

	OR	CI 95%	P value
Albumin/Creatinine Ratio ≥30 mg.g.Cr^{-1}	1.7	1.1-2.8	0.01
Creatinine>1.4 or e-GFR<60%	1.7	1-2.8	0.03
Previous Coronary Artery By-pass	2.5	1.2-5	0.012

CI: Confidence Intervals. OR: Odds Ratio; eGFR: estimated glomerular filtration rate.

Table 3. Predictive models (logistic regression model) for atrial fibrillation tested with C-statistic analysis

Predictive models	C-statistic	Asymptotic 95% CI	P
Clinical parameters (admission)	0.676	0.614-0.737	0.001
Hemodynamic (Killip Class) and acute reactants parameters (Glycemia; CRP; WBC)	0.715	0.657-0.773	0.001
Chronic Renal Disease (Creatinine>1.4;eGFR<60%)	0.715	0.657-0.773	0.001
ACR ≥30 mg.g.Cr^{-1}	0.741	0.685-0.797	0.001

CRP: C-reactive protein, WBC: White blood cell count, eGFR: estimated glomerular filtration rate, ACR: Albumin/Creatinine ratio, CI: confidence intervals.

In-Hospital Mortality, Albuminuria and Atrial Fibrillation

In-hospital mortality was 6.6%. A higher in-hospital mortality (9.9%) was documented in patients with ACR≥30 mg.g.Cr^{-1} (OR=1.5). It was an association between ACR and mortality (OR=1.5;1.2-2)(p=0.005). The risk increases progressively with albuminuria. Mortality was 4.3% when albuminuria was normal (<30 mg.g.Cr^{-1}) and increased to 16.7% when macroalbuminuria was present (Figure 1). Table 4 shows the predictive models for mortality tested with C-statistic analysis. Albuminuria did not increase the model prediction for mortality (from C-statistic 0.904 to 0.904) (Figure 3). In a multivariate adjusted risk initial or new bundle branch block (OR=2.8), eGFR<60% (OR=4.8), WBC count>10400 (2.68), glycemia>140 mg/ml, (OR=3.4) and Killip class>1 (OR=2.7) on admission were independent predictive factors for in-hospital mortality, meanwhile a previous history of hypertension was a protective factor (OR=0.22). Albuminuria did not increase risk for dying during hospitalization (OR=1.2; 0.58-2.5) (p=0.6) (Table 5).

Table 4. Predictive models (logistic regression model) for mortality, tested with C-statistic analysis

Predictive models	C-statistic	Asymptotic 95% CI	P
Clinical parameters (admission)	0.747	0.671-0.824	0.001
Number of diseased vessels>1	0.834	(0.772-0.896	0.001
Killip Class>1	0.904	0.863-0.944	0.001
Atrial Fibrillation	0.904	0.863-0.944	
ACR ≥30 mg.g.Cr^{-1}	0.904	0.863-0.944	

ACR: Albumin/Creatinine ratio. CI: confidence intervals.

Table 5. Multivariate adjusted risk for in-hospital mortality

	OR	CI 95%	P value
Albumin/Creatinine Ratio ≥30 mg.g.Cr^{-1}	1.2	0.58-2.5	0.6
BBB (initial or complicated)	2.8	1.3-6	0.005
Chronic Renal Disease	4.8	2.4-9	<0.001
WBC>10400 (admission)	2.68	1.1-5	0.019
Glycemia>140 mg/ml (admission)	3.4	1.2-9	0.014
Killip>1 (admission)	2.7	1.9-6	<0.001
Previous History of Hypertension	0.22	0.11-0.45	<0.001

CI: Confidence Intervals. OR: Odds Ratio;BBB: Bundle Brunch Block, WBC: white blood cells.

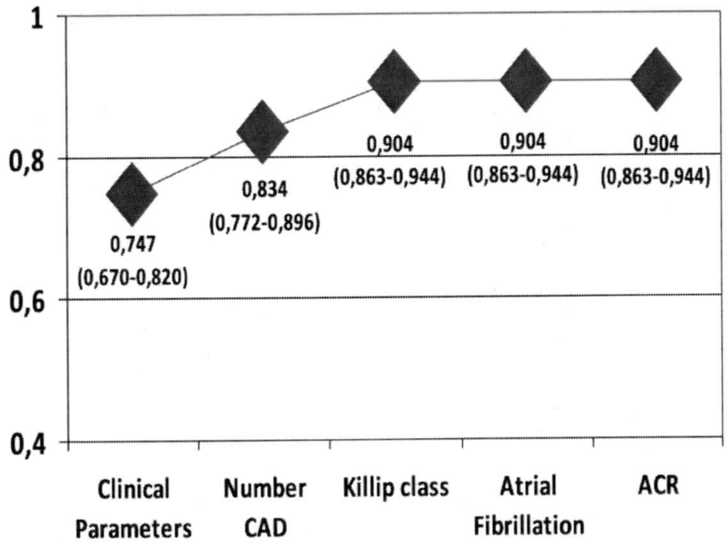

Figure 3. Predictive models for mortality (C-statistic analysis). Albuminuria did not increase risk for dying during hospitalization (0.904-0,904=0).

Discussion

This prospective study demonstrates that: 1) microalbuminuria is a common finding during AMI; 2) in the present analysis, it was shown that a history of AF is associated with an increased prevalence of albuminuria; 3) urinary albumin improved the predictive power of the model for the presence of atrial fibrillation when it was added to the baseline of traditional risk factors; 4) however, the high incidence of abnormal albuminuria limits its prognostic usefulness and the model prediction for in-hospital mortality was not modified when albuminuria is added.

Albuminuria increases with age and has been proposed as a marker or maker of chronic kidney disease and coronary heart disease [19]. Persistent albuminuria suggests progression of chronic renal disease at all levels of estimated glomerular filtration rate [4]. In addition to its function as a marker of kidney damage, microalbuminuria represents an indirect window to monitor the status of the whole vasculature [21]. Microalbuminuria may, in fact, indicate endothelial cell dysfunction and increase permeability not just in the kidney but throughout the vascular system [6-8].

Some reports have shown that increased urinary protein excretion in acute myocardial yields prognostic information about early [10, 12] and late mortality [13, 14] additional to that provided by clinical or hemodynamic evaluation of left ventricular performance. The finding of Lekatsas et al., [9] that microalbuminuria remained a powerful prognostic indicator even if we excluded AMI patients with Killip class>1 from the analysis, may suggest that albuminuria is related to the adverse prognosis of AMI with a mechanism different from the development of congestive heart failure. Bandyopadhayay et al., [12] observed in 80 non-diabetic patients with AMI, that microalbuminuria had a positive correlation with deteriorating Killip's class and short-term mortality. We have observed only an association between in-hospital mortality and albuminuria with similar to GRACE risk scores in univariate analyses. But in our experience, albuminuria was not an independent predictive factor for in-hospital mortality. Potential explanations for the discrepancy could be explained by methodological analysis. Lekatsas et al., [9] included only a subgroup of non-diabetic patients; moreover they excluded all the events that happened in the first two hospital days because albuminuria was measured at third day after admission. According to Berton et al., [22], the incidence of albuminuria in AMI appeared to be a dynamic process with the highest values on the first day and decreases on the third and seventh day; the ACR measured on the third day never should be used as a predictive in-hospital mortality factor. Also to obtain a reliable estimate of albumin excretion independent of urine flow rate, albuminuria should be corrected for urinary creatinine because it is closely associated to the real albumin loos than only albuminuria.

Although the pathogenesis of albuminuria in acute coronary syndromes is not clear, we suggest that microalbuminuria, chronic kidney disease, and coronary heart disease share common pathways involving inflammation and oxidative stress. The main pathophysiological mechanism is the development of endothelial dysfunction, leading to widespread vascular damage. Neurohumoral changes [23], inflammation [24] and ischemia seem to be others determinants factors which are associated with albuminuria. An association between abnormal albuminuria, number of significant coronary artery disease and NSTEMI myocardial infarction was observed in our patients. Urinary albumin and renal failure, has been related to extent and severity of angiography estimated coronary artery damage, independent of blood pressure, diabetes mellitus and renal disease [9, 25, 26]

Atrial fibrillation is the most frequently supraventricular arrhythmia and increases the risk of cardiovascular mortality by approximately two-fold. The presence of hypertension accompanied by left ventricular hypertrophy, poor ventricular compliance and left atrial chamber dilatation and fibrosis are regarded as a cardiac risk factor for the development of AF [27].

The pathogenesis of AF in acute myocardial infarction is likely multifactorial. Overall incidence rate of AF (9.8%) observed in the present analysis is within the range of the most recently published studies [27, 28] (5%-23%)..Data presented herein suggests that early vascular and *renal end organ damage* might be associated. Albuminuria (the main marker of renal dysfunction) and atrial fibrillation share many cardiovascular risk factors. Multivariable analysis, including other factors contributing to AF, revealed that abnormal albuminuria and chronic renal disease are independently associated with higher odds for AF. Moreover, the cardiovascular effects of myocardial ischemia in ventricular infarction/dysfunction, increased atrial stretch, pericarditis, and autonomic nervous system changes are potentially important in contributing to a heterogeneous electrical and structural milieu and, thereby, resulting in AF [29]. Atrial fibrillation could be considered the consequence of the *end organ damage* (cardiomyopathy) or the result from prolonged vascular damage, albuminuria being the marker in both situations.

Limitations

Some study limitations should be noted and some potential problems probably need further validation. The study population is relatively small and a large number of predictors for only 79 patients with atrial fibrillation may give unstable estimations. The possibility of bias selection and/or residual confounding from unknown or unmeasured covariates cannot be excluded resulting in attenuation or inflation of the odds ratios (type 1 or type 2 errors). Such issues are inherent limitations of observational cohort studies.

A 24-hour urine collection is the gold standard for the detection of albuminuria. However, screening can be more simply achieved by a timed urine collection. A value above 30 $mg.g.Cr^{-1}$ suggests that albumin is above 30 mg/day. The standardized procedure for determining albuminuria might allow interpreting the results with some confidence.

In our analysis, incident AF was identified mostly before coronary care unit discharges; so, the incidence of AF in the albuminuria group may have been over-estimated because these patients spent more time under continuous monitoring in the Coronary Care Unit (3.5±2 vs 3.18±1.6 days). Moreover, episodic, transient and asymptomatic atrial fibrillation could not be detected in patients without continuous monitoring after discharge from the coronary care unit.

No further information on type or duration of AF was collected.

Conclusion

Our observation suggests that albuminuria itself is a predictor of atrial instability in patients with acute myocardial infarction. The practical consequences of these data are that screening measurement of urinary albumin-to-creatinine ratio using spot urine sample can help predict the presence of atrial fibrillation but in our experience it is not a marker for in-hospital mortality. Nevertheless, further studies will need to determine whether albuminuria remains a good intermediate variable to predict in-hospital cardiovascular outcomes patients with AMI.

Statement of Conflict of Interest

All authors declare that there are no conflicts of interest.

We wish to thank Miss Chris Guevara from Mercé V. Electromedicina S.L, who was involved in translation support.

References

[1] Gomal F, Deshmukh A, Shah S, Mehta JL. Triad of metabolic syndrome, chronic kidney disease and coronary heart disease with a focus on miocroalbuminuria. *J Am Coll Cardiol* 2011; 57: 2303-8.

[2] Afonso L, Hari P, Kondur A, Veeranna V, Manickam P, Simegn M et al. Usefulness of Microalbuminuria in Patients With the Metabolic Syndrome to Predict Subclinical Atherosclerosis and Cardiovascular Disease Outcomes. *Am J Cardiol* 2010; 106: 976-83.

[3] Danziger J. Importance of low-grade albuminuria. *Mayo Clin Proc* 2008; 83: 806-12.

[4] Chronic Kidney Disease Prognosis Consortium: Association of estimated glomerular filtration rate and albuminuria with all cause and cardiovascular in general population cohort: a collaborative meta-analysis. *Lancet* 2010; 375: 2073-81.

[5] Gosling P, Hughes EA, Reynolds TM, Fox JP. Microalbuminuria is an early response following acute myocardial infarction. *Eur Heart J* 1991; 12:/508-13.

[6] Deckert T, Feldt-Rasmussen B, Borch-Johnsen K, Jensen T, Kofoed-Enevoldsen A. Albuminuria reflects widespread vascular damage. The Steno hypothesis. *Diabetologia* 1989; 32: 219–226.

[7] Pedrinelli R, Giampietro O, Carmassi F, Melillo E, Dell'Omo G, Catapano G, et al. Microalbuminuria and endotelial dysfunction in essential hypertension. *Lancet* 1994; 344: 14–18.

[8] Stehouwer CD, Henry RM, Dekker JM, Nijpels G, Heine RJ, Bouter LM. Microalbuminuria is associated with impaired brachial artery, flow-mediated vasodilation in elderly individuals without and with diabetes: further evidence for a link between microalbuminuria and endothelial dysfunction–the Hoorn Study. *Kidney Int Suppl* 2004; S42–S44.

[9] Lekatsas I, Kranidis A, Ioannidis G, Kalofoustis Ch, Tavernarakis A, Thalassinos N et al. Comparison of the extent and severity of coronary artery disease in patients with acute myocardial infarction with and without microalbuminuria. *Am J Cardiol* 2004; 94: 334-37.

[10] Taskiran M, Feldt-Rasmussen B, Jensen GB, Jensen JS.Urinary albumin excretion in hospitalized patients with acute myocardial infarction. *Scand Cardiovasc J* 1998; 32:/163-6.

[11] Berton G, Citro T, Palmieri R, Petucco S, De Toni R, Palatini P. Albumin excretion rate increases during acute myocardial infarction and strongly predicts early mortality. *Circulation* 1997;/96:/3338-45.

[12] Bandyopadhyay SK, Ghosh S, Bandyopadhyay R, Ghosh S, Sarkar N. Micro-albuminuria: a predictor of 7-day mortality in acute myocardial infarction. *J Indian Med Assoc* 2010; 108: 826-8.

[13] Berton G, Cordiano R, Mazzuco S, Katz E, De Toni R, Palatini P. Albumin excretion in acute myocardial infarction: a guide for long-term prognosis. *Am Heart J* 2008; 156: 760-8.

[14] Koulouris S, Lekatsas I, Karabinos I, Ioannidis G, Katostaras T, Kranidis A, et al. Microalbuminuria: A strong predictor of 3-year adverse prognosis in nondiabetic patients with acute myocardial infarction *Am Heart J* 2005; 149: 840- 5.

[15] Alonso A, Lopez FL, Matsushita K, Loehr LR, Agarwal SK, Chen LY, et al. Chronic Kidney Disease Is Associated With the Incidence of Atrial Fibrillation .The Atherosclerosis Risk in Communities (ARIC) Study. *Circulation* 2011; 123: 2946-53.

[16] Böhm M, Thoenes M, Neuberger HR, Gräber S, Reil JC, Bramlage P, Volpe M. Atrial fibrillation and heart rate independently correlate to microalbuminuria in hypertensive patients. *Eur Heart J;* 2009: 30, 1364–1371.

[17] Baber U, Howard VJ, Halperin JL, Soliman EZ, Zhang X, McClellan W et al. Association of Chronic Kidney Disease With Atrial Fibrillation Among Adults in the United States: REasons for Geographic and Racial Differences in Stroke (REGARDS) Study. *Circ Arrhythm Electrophysiol* 2011; 4: 26-32.

[18] Kristian Thygesen, Joseph S. Alpert, Allan S. Jaffe, Maarten L. Simoons, Bernard R. Chaitman and Harvey D. White: the Writing Group on behalf of the Joint ESC/ACCF/AHA/WHF Task Force for the Universal Definition of Myocardial Infarction. Third Universal Definition of Myocardial Infarction. *JACC* 2012; 60: 1581-1588.

[19] Levey AS, Coresh J. Chronic kidney disease. *Lancet* 2012; 14; 379(9811): 165-80.

[20] Killip T and Kimball JT. Treatment of myocardial infarction in a coronary care unit. A two year experience with 250 patients. *Am J Cardiol* 1967; 20: 457-64.

[21] Abdelhafiz AH, Ahmed Sh, El Nahas M. Microalbuminuria: marker or maker of cardiovascular disease. *Nephron Exp Nephrol* 2011; 119 (suppl 1): e6-e10.

[22] Berton G. Measurement of albuminuria during acute myocardial infarction and its relation with prognosis. Letter to editor. *Eur Heart J* 2005; 26: 1242-44

[23] Foy SG, Crozier IG, Richards AM et al. Neurohumoral changes after acute myocardial infarction. Relationships with haemodynamic indices and effects of ACE inhibition. *Eur Heart J* 1995; 16: 770-9.

[24] Lagrand WK, Niessen HW, Wolbink GJ, Jaspars LH, Visser CA, Verheugt FW, et al. C-reactive protein colocalizes with complements in human hearts during acute myocardial infarction. *Circulation* 1997; 95: 97-103.

[25] Young JH, Myung HJ, Yun HCh, Jin AS, Khurshid A, Dong HK, et al. Relationship between microalbuminuria and vulnerable plaque components in patients with acute coronary syndrome and with diabetes mellitus *Circ J* 2011; 75: 2893 – 2901.

[26] Blasco L, Sanjuan R, Carbonell N, Miguel A, Puchades MJ, Torregrosa I et al.Estimated Glomerular Filtration Rate in Short-Risk Stratification in Acute Myocardial infarction. *Cardiorenal Med* 2011;1:131–138.

[27] Savelieva I, Camm J. Update on atrial fibrillation. Clin Cardiol 2008; 31: 55-62.

[28] Saczynski JS, Mcanus D, Zhou Z, Spencer F, Yarzebski J, Lessard D, et al. Trends in atrial fibrillation complicating acute myocardial infarction. *Am J Cardiol* 2009; 104: 169-174.

[29] Schmitt J, Duray G, Gersh BJ, Hohnloser SH. Atrial fibrillation in acute myocardial infarction: a systematic review of the incidence, clinical features and prognostic implications. *Eur Heart J* 2008; 30, 1038–1045.

In: Myocardial Infarctions
Editor: Pattie Wilkonson
ISBN: 978-1-63321-726-3

Chapter 6

Effect and Mechanism of Luteolin on Cardiac Protection and Anti-Apoptosis in Rat Cardiomyocytes with Ischemia-Reperfusion Injury

Dongye Li[1,2,•] ***and Haochen Xuan***[1]
[1]Institution of cardiovascular disease, Xuzhou Medical College, Xuzhou, Jiangsu, China
[2]Department of Cardiology, The Affiliated Hospital of Xuzhou Medical College, Xuzhou, Jiangsu, China

Abstract

Acute myocardial infarction (AMI) is one of the leading causes of death in the adult population. Myocardial ischemia/reperfusion (I/R) injury is an important complication of acute coronary arterial occlusion and subsequent recanalization, whether it is spontaneous or therapeutic. Following AMI, therapeutic coronary artery recanalization by thrombolytic therapy or percutaneous coronary intervention (PCI) is used to minimize infarct size. In most cases, the damaged structure can be repaired, and heart function can be restored to its basal level through reperfusion. However, in some instances, I/R exerts the opposite effect, not only failing to improve heart function but instead exacerbating cardiac function and worsening structural damage. Cellular damage after reperfusion of previously viable ischemic tissue is defined as I/R injury (IRI).

There is growing evidence that apoptosis plays a key role during myocardial I/R and much discussion has been undertaken to elucidate the detailed mechanisms, relevant gene expression, and signaling transduction pathways. Protection of cardiomyocytes from I/R induced cell death would in principle increase the viable myocardium, thus providing acute and chronic benefits after AMI. Therefore, cardiomyocyte apoptosis may be an

• E-mail: dongyeli@medmail.com.cn.

excellent target for therapeutic modulation in the context of AMI and IRI. Drug pretreatment has been one of the main focus for ameliorating IRI.

Luteolin is a common flavonoid that exists in many types of plants, including fruits, vegetables and medicinal herbs. Preclinical studies have revealed the diverse beneficial effects of luteolin, such as cardiovascular protection, antioxidant, anti-inflammatory, antimicrobial, anticancer effects and other biological activities. Recent studies have suggested that administration of luteolin yields cardioprotective effects during I/R in rats. Pretreatment with luteolin can improve cardiomyocyte shortening amplitude, decrease the apoptosis rate, upregulate Bcl-2/Bax ratio under a simulated I/R condition. Moreover, luteolin pretreatment can activate multiple endogenous signaling pathways such as PI3K/Akt, JAK/STAT and MAPKs, which further protect the myocardium against IRI through different mechanisms. The aim of this chapter is to summarize luteolin's anti-apoptotic roles and mechanisms following I/R in rats, and luteolin may be a potential candidate for preventing and treating cardiovascular diseases.

Introduction

Myocardial ischemia refers to a clinical state characterized by low coronary blood flow triggered by various causes. It results in the lack of myocardial oxygen supply that can damage myocardial structure and heart function. In recent years, with the increasing routine utilization of coronary artery bypass grafts and PCI, it is now feasible to restore blood flow and oxygen supply to the ischemic myocardium in a short period of time. However, reperfusion itself can induce ventricular contractile dysfunction, microvascular impairment and lethal reperfusion arrhythmia beyond that caused by the original myocardial ischemia insult alone. Because of the resultant aggravation of myocardial ischemic tissue damage after blood flow is increased, this phenomenon is known as myocardial IRI. Therefore, it is very important to develop cardioprotective agents that can improve myocardial function, decrease the incidence of cardiovascular events and reduce the total extent of infarction during I/R.

In recent years, emerging evidence has shown remarkable progress in tackling IRI [1]. Ischemic preconditioning (IP) is used to induce the production of endogenous myocardial protective substances as powerful agents against IRI by repeated transient I/R. This is a well-described adaptive response to I/R, markedly enhancing the ability of the heart to tolerate a subsequent IRI. Drug pretreatment has been designed based on the signaling pathways activated by IP, with the end goal of using the drugs to stimulate or simulate endogenous substances to inhibit IRI [2]. Some of the drugs have already tested positive for cardioprotective effects through inducing the release of endogenous substances or by directly stimulating endogenous mechanisms to inhibit IRI. The discovery of these major cardioprotective mechanisms has prompted the exploration of new drugs to protect ischemic myocardium against IRI. However, previous pharmacological approaches to attenuate the deleterious effects of IRI either showed limited experimental efficacy or failed to be translated into clinical practice. It is pivotal to keep in mind that a clinical trial is always based on a specific treatment strategy, which may lead to the failure of a drug to achieve its desired effects despite its inherent efficacy. Meanwhile, it is an urgent need to acquire additional insight into the molecular events during I/R, and that could be exploited therapeutically. In addition, such preconditioning effects can occur at relatively low concentrations, while higher levels, which may be difficult to achieve through diet, are needed for direct antioxidant effects.

Luteolin (Figure 1) is a widely distributed flavonoid, a member of a group of naturally occurring polyphenolic compounds found in many plants, fruits, vegetables and medicinal herbs. Plants rich in luteolin have been used for treating various diseases, such as hypertension, infection diseases and cancer. Furthermore, preclinical studies have shown that luteolin possesses a variety of biological and pharmacological activities, including antioxidant, anti-inflammatory, antimicrobial and anticancer activities [3], which could be against IRI, which is mainly dependent on its antioxidant and anti-inflammatory properties [4]. Some research has indicated that apoptosis is involved in myocardial IRI, and that luteolin plays an important anti-apoptotic role during IRI. However, the underlying mechanism regarding the involvement of luteolin in the apoptosis pathway that contributes to the cardioprotection against IRI has not been elucidated. Recently, it has been reported that luteolin plays an important role in the cardioprotection against anti-inflammatory and antioxidant activities of luteolin affect its role in cardioprotection against IRI in vivo [4], the aim of this chapter is not to summarize the existing cardioprotective therapies in IRI animal models but to illustrate the potential mechanisms for cardioprotection against IRI through anti-apoptosis by luteolin pretreatment in a rat model. Understanding the mechanisms by which luteolin regulates apoptosis has revealed new therapeutic targets that could potentially improve heart function during myocardial IRI.

Evidence Supporting that Cell Apoptosis Occurs in Myocardial IRI

Up to date, some experiments and clinical studies have suggested that cell apoptosis may be an important link between the pathogenesis of myocardial IRI. In 1994, Gottlieb [5] first found that apoptosis was apparent after reperfusion injury in rabbit hearts. Later, Fliss [6] observed a typical apoptotic morphological phenotype, changes in DNA ladder electrophoresis and reperfusion injury after I/R, indicating that I/R could lead to cardiomyocyte apoptosis in rats.

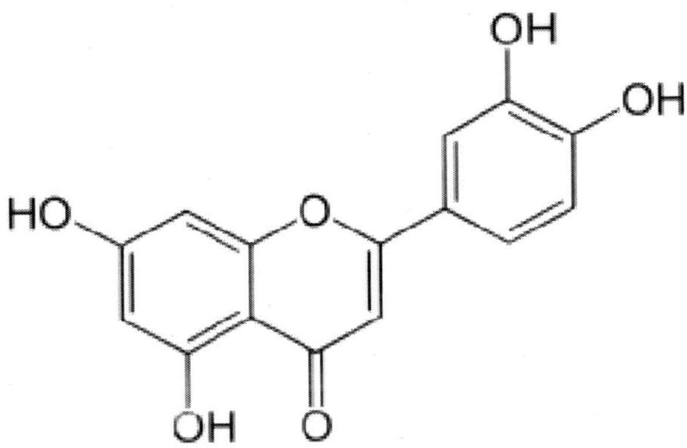

Figure 1. Chemical structure of luteolin.

Chakrabarti found evidence that supported the occurrence of cell apoptosis after 10min of myocardial ischemia in rat hearts [7], which peaked after 30min of ischemia. In clinical studies, myocardial apoptosis was also observed in ACS patients even after PCI treatment [8]. These results further confirmed that ischemia could cause myocardial apoptosis, indicating that cell apoptosis is closely correlated to myocardial IRI.

Mechanism of Cell Apoptosis in Myocardial IRI

1. Oxygen Free Radical

A large quantity of oxygen free radicals are generated during myocardial IRI and promote the occurrence and development of IRI by lipid and nucleic acid destructive molecular chain reactions (Figure 2). Mitochondria are an important source for oxygen free radical production, in which a large number of oxygen free radicals selectively impair ion permeability or change mitochondrial membrane permeability. The change in mitochondrial membrane potential causes the release of apoptosis-inducing factor or apoptotic protease-activating factor 1 from mitochondria, which in turn activates cysteinyl aspartate-specific proteases (caspases) to induce apoptosis.

2. Calcium Overload

The cellular Ca^{2+} content increases significantly, after the blood flow in ischemic tissues is restored, which causes cellular damage.

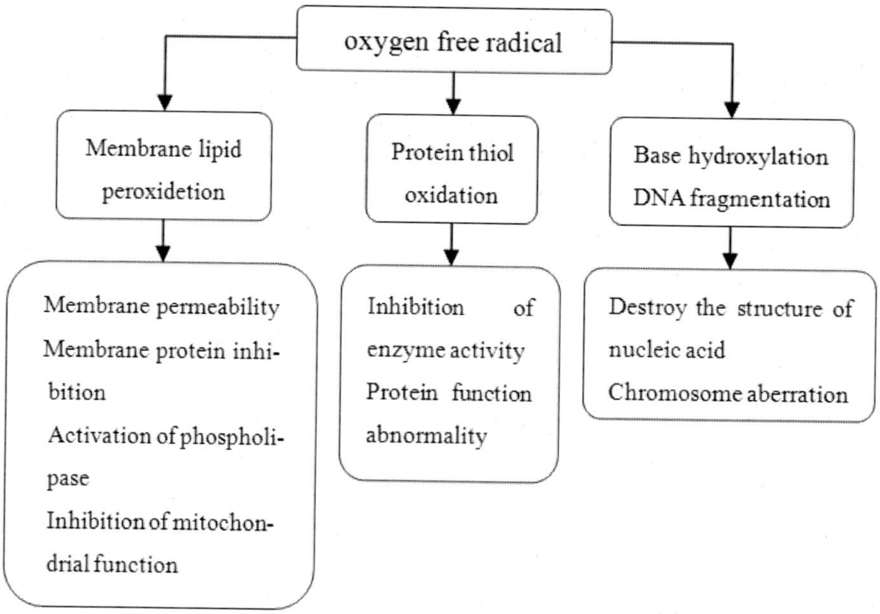

Figure 2. Damage effects of oxygen free radicals.

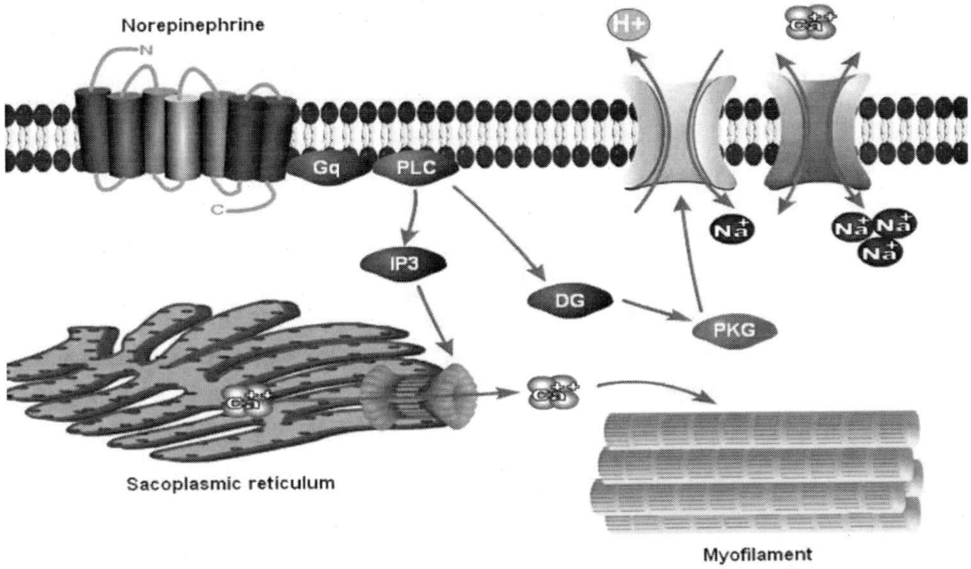

Figure 3. The mechanism of calcium overload during ischemia reperfusion.

This process is known as calcium overload (Figure 3). Calcium overload and a series of following harmful metabolic events are the "last common access". During myocardial IRI, Ca^{2+} are mostly accumulated in the mitochondria, which causes the mitochondrial membrane permeability transition pore (mPTP) to open and facilitates the release of cytochrome C into the cytoplasm, therefore activating caspases to induce apoptosis. Overproduction of oxygen free radicals can directly damage cell membranes and increase cell membrane permeability, resulting in calcium overload. Calcium overload can also activate the Ca^{2+}-dependent protease, triggering the catalytic conversion of xanthine dehydrogenase into xanthine oxidase. Xanthine oxidase can simultaneously promote xanthine decomposition into uric acid and induce the overproduction of oxygen free radicals in the presence of oxygen.

3. Neutrophils

It has been shown that during the evolution of AMI, neutrophils are recruited to the ischemic myocardium and become activated in response to the IRI. Because the neutrophil reaction is most intense during reperfusion and the neutrophils are rich sources of toxic oxidants and proteolytic enzymes, it has become a widely held view that activation of neutrophils is an important mechanism of myocardial injury during reperfusion. In the IRI process, activated neutrophils can adhere to endothelium and cause a no-reflow phenomenon. Furthermore, the neutrophils infiltrated into the ischemic myocardium can release oxygen free radicals, proteases, pro-inflammatory cytokines and other inflammatory mediators, which increase the infiltration of neutrophils into the jeopardized myocardium and lead to further myocardial injury. Studies have found that the content of neutrophils with determinant pulp peroxidase activity is three times higher in rats with apoptotic cardiomyocytes induced by 45min of ischemia and 4h of reperfusion, compared to that in normal rats, indicating an increase in the number of neutrophils in ischemic myocardium.

4. Mitochondrial Damage

Some researchers have proposed that cell apoptosis correlates with mitochondrial damage. During periods of apoptosis, mitochondria may still maintain its normal ultrastructure. However, its function has been significantly changed, including increased mitochondrial membrane permeability, decreased mitochondrial membrane potential and significantly reduced energy synthesis. Some current evidence has shown that these functional changes in mitochondria play a key role in cell apoptosis. Such evidence shows that apoptosis can result from the perturbation of mitochondrial cycle or the inhibition of its respiratory chain function. Usually, before apoptosis is apparent in the nucleus, the mitochondrial membrane potential has already been decreased. In vivo experiments have demonstrated that reversing the changes on mitochondrial permeability can prevent apoptosis. In addition, as a key component of the mitochondrial respiratory chain, cytochrome C is necessary to activate the protease caspases-3 to cause DNA fragmentation.

Gene Regulation in Apoptotic Cardiomyocytes

Myocardial regulatory genes involved in cell apoptosis are divided into three groups: pro-apoptosis genes (Fas, Bax and Caspases), anti-apoptosis genes (Bcl-2 and heat shock proteins) and two-way regulatory genes (p53, c-myc and NF-κB) (Chart 1).

Chart 1. Gene Regulation in apoptotic cardiomyocytes

Gene names	*Type*	Function	References
Fas/Apo-1/ CD95	cell membrane antigen	pro-apoptosis	9
p53	cancer gene	anti-apoptosis: mutation p53 pro-apoptosis:wild p53	10
Bcl-2	Bcl-2 family	anti-apoptosis:Bcl-2, Bcl-X_L, Mcl-1, Bcl-W ; pro-apoptosis:Bax, Bad, Bak, Bid	11
HSP	molecular partner of eukaryotic cells	anti-apoptosis: HSP10, HSP60, HSP70	12
caspase	Caspase family protease	pro-apoptosis: caspase-3, caspase-8,	13
NF-κB	Rel protein family members	pro-apoptosis:long-term activation anti-apoptosis:short-term activation	14
C-myc	Translocation and regulatory gene	anti-apoptosis: presence of growth factors; pro-apoptosis: absence of growth factors	15

1. *Fas.* Fas, a cell membrane antigen that belongs to the tumor necrosis factor (TNF)/nerve growth factor receptor family, is also called Apo-1 or CD95. It is widely expressed in many cell types. Fas ligand (FasL) is a cell surface membrane protein that is abundant in myocardial cells, whose expression increases in the

presence of pathological stimuli. An anti-Fas antibody, membrane-bound FasL and plasma sFasL may be targeted for Fas binding, which ultimately induces apoptosis through signal transduction. Some experiments showed that a large amount of Fas receptor protein was located near the infarction area after myocardial I/R. They also found that cell apoptosis in this area was inhibited by 77%, and that the expression of Fas receptors was significantly reduced following the pretreatment of carvedilol or antioxidants combined with beta blockers prior to IRI [9]. Compared to that in wild-type mice, heart IRI was significantly reduced in global Fas knockout mice, further indicating that Fas could promote cell apoptosis. Overexpression of FasL led to cardiomyocyte apoptosis in vitro, whereas in FasL knockout mice, the size of I/R-induced myocardial infarct was smaller, and apoptosis was inhibited, compared to the control.

2. *p53.* The cancer gene p53 is present in two types: wild-type and mutant. The former contributes to cell apoptosis, whereas the latter inhibits apoptosis. Wild-type p53 is a transcription factor that can regulate the expression of many genes related to cell cycle and apoptosis (such as p21 and Bax) [10]. It plays an important role in apoptosis by directly or indirectly regulating the apoptosis pathways, such as the death receptor pathway and the mitochondrial pathway. It is well known that p53 mediates cell cycle arrest and apoptosis; however, its role in IRI in myocardial cells remains unclear.
3. *Bcl-2 family.* The Bcl-2 protein family can be divided into anti-apoptotic proteins and pro -apoptotic proteins, based on their structure and function. The former mainly includes Bcl-2, Bcl-X_L, Mcl-1 and Bcl-W, whereas the latter includes Bax, Bad, Bak, Bid etc. Bax and Bcl-2 also function as p53 regulatory genes. Previous studies have demonstrated the role of Bcl-2 family members in the apoptosis pathway and the importance of the Bax/Bcl-2 ratio in determining cell behavior [11]. The anti-apoptotic members, such as Bcl-2 and Bcl-X_L, are important for cell survival and for protecting cardiomyocytes against various harmful stressors. For example, overexpression of Bcl-X_L can protect H9c2 cardiac cells against doxorubicin and hypoxia-mediated apoptosis by maintaining mitochondrial integrity. Bcl-2 has also been shown to prevent p53-mediated apoptosis in cardiomyocytes. Moreover, transgenic mice overexpressing Bcl-2 in the heart presented reduced IRI and fewer apoptotic cells, compared to wild-type mice, indicating that the cardioprotective role of Bcl-2 is via the inhibition of the mitochondrial death pathway.

   In conclusion, the interaction between pro-apoptotic proteins and anti-apoptotic proteins play a key role in myocardial cell survival in I/R.
4. *Heat shock protein (HSP).* The HSP family is one of the most well characterized protein families with the function of myocardial protection. HSP70 belongs to a group of protective proteins that maintain cellular homeostasis upon stimulation. As one of the most important molecular chaperons in eukaryotic cells, it plays an important role in regulating protein folding, assembling, translocation and degradation. Previous research showed that the number of apoptotic cells in transgenic mice transfected with HSP70 was significantly reduced, compared to the control. However, clinical studies have reported a significant increase of HSP70, C-reactive protein and interleukin-6 (IL-6) in AMI patient blood. The extent of left ventricular ejection fraction has been shown to negatively correlate with HSP70

concentration after 1 day of AMI, suggesting that HSP70 concentration may be related to the infarct size. Other studies found that in cardiomyocytes of newborn rats, transfected with HSP10 and (or) HSP60 and treated with I/R, the extent of myocardial apoptosis was decreased, accompanied with reduced caspase-3 activity and the low content of cytochrome C in the cytoplasm [12].

5. *Cysteinyl aspartate-specific proteases (Caspases).* Caspases play an important role in apoptosis. Propagation and execution of apoptotic signals in cells is largely dependent upon active caspases. Caspase family proteases share similar characteristics with cysteine protein enzymes and specific enzymes that digest proteins at the Asp amino acid. Caspase proteins normally exist in an inactive form and are regarded as key regulators in apoptosis through induced activation, which, however, is not their only function. After the application of zVAD-fmk (pan-caspase inhibitor) in a myocardial I/R model in both rats and rabbits, it was found that the number of apoptotic cells identified by the in situ nick-end labeling method was reduced, and that the size of the myocardial infarction area was smaller. Excessive expression of the heart-specific caspase-3 in the transgenic mice impaired heart function, increased the size of the myocardial infarction area and exacerbated ultrastructural changes in the nucleus, mitochondria and cardiomyocytes. However, typical apoptotic characteristics, such as the "apoptotic body", were not observed [13]. These results suggest that the occurrence of apoptosis may result from the activation of multiple caspase cascades.
6. *Nuclear factor (NF)-κB.* NF-κB is a Rel protein family member. During I/R, it can be activated by cytokines such as TNF-α, interleukin-1 (IL-l) and IL-17. NF-κB activation can be elevated by peroxide, and it regulates the expression of a variety of cytokines, such as IL-6 and IL-8, as well as adhesion molecules. NF-κB can exert pro-apoptotic functions due to its role in the up-regulation of harmful cytokines. In cardiomyocytes, recent studies have shown that NF-κB can be cardioprotective during acute hypoxia and IRI. However, prolonged NF-κB activation appears to be detrimental and promotes apoptosis in cardiomyocytes after I/R, by eliciting signals that promote chronic inflammation through inducing the production of cytokines such as IL-1, TNF and IL-6, resulting in endoplasmic reticulum (ER) stress responses and cell apoptosis. The underlying multifaceted mechanisms and differential impact of NF-κB activation on cardiac cell fate warrant further investigation [14].
7. *C-myc.* The cellular homologue of avian myelocytomatosis virus oncogene (C-myc) is not only a translocation gene but also a regulatory gene that can be induced by a variety of stimuli. C-myc has a dual nature, both anti-apoptotic and pro-apoptotic. Its role in apoptosis depends on the presence or absence of growth factors. When growth factors are insufficient, it induces apoptosis. Otherwise, it promotes cell proliferation [15].

Many basic and clinical studies have investigated the mechanisms of apoptosis in I/R, including the inducers, second messengers, effectors and links among them. Most of these studies focused on the inducers and effectors. Little addressed second messengers and intracellular signaling pathways.

Myocardial IRI involves a complex network of signaling transduction, regulation of a number of intracellular signaling pathways and interactions at multiple levels, as well as many other aspects.

Luteolin and Signaling Pathways Involved Cell Apoptosis during I/R

To date, detailed mechanisms regulating apoptosis in myocardial IRI remain unclear. It has been proposed that myocardial apoptosis is mainly mediated through the following pathways: caspase, mitogen-activated protein kinases (MAPKs), phosphatidylinositol-3-kinase/Akt (PI3K/Akt), janus kinase/signal transduction and activator of transcription (JAK/STAT), small G protein and lectin-like oxidized low-density lipoprotein receptor-1 (LOX-1). Furthermore, crosstalk among these pathways is also involved. Elucidating the cardioprotective mechanism and identifying the drug targets in I/R myocardial cells can provide a theoretical basis for clinical application.

Here, we present the most recent progress and current perspectives regarding the role of luteolin in apoptosis during IRI. Mounting evidence has indicated that apoptosis is involved in myocardial I/R, and that luteolin plays an important anti-apoptotic role during IRI.

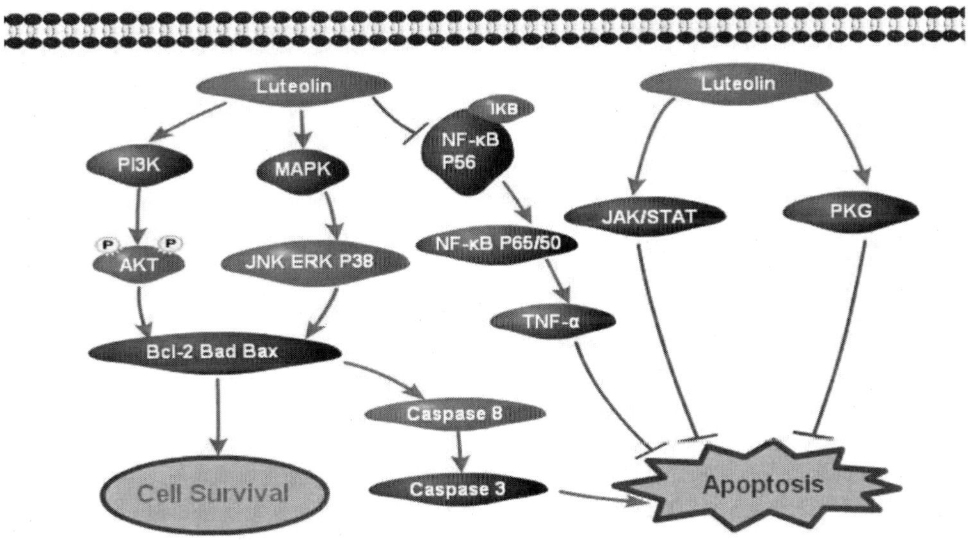

Figure 4. Possible mechanisms for luteolin exerting its protective effects on cardiomyocytes following I/R.

Although the underlying mechanisms of luteolin-induced cardioprotection are complex, they can be summarized as enhancing cell survival by either inhibiting apoptosis or inducing survival signaling in myocardial I/R (Figure 4).

1. Luteolin and the Caspase Signaling Pathway Mediating Cell Apoptosis during I/R

Apoptosis is a highly regulated program of cell death and can be mediated by death receptors in the plasma membrane, mitochondria and ER. Caspase signaling pathways includes:

(1) Death receptor pathway: Death receptor belongs to the TNF family. TNF and Fas are pro-apoptotic factors that have been intensively studied. FasL binds Fas to interact with procaspase-8. Together, they form the death induction signal compounds (DISC) and trigger the caspase cascade, leading to caspase-3 activation and eventually the induction of apoptosis [16]. TNF can bind tumor necrosis factor receptor (TNFR) to induce caspase cascade activation and apoptosis. Researches have shown that calcium-sensing receptors (CaSR) can maintain Ca^{2+} homeostasis in a myocardial IRI model. CaSR activation induces calcium overload and activates the death receptor signaling pathway mediated by Fas/FasL, which inhibits Bcl-2.

(2) Mitochondria involvement in caspase-induced apoptosis: As stated above, mPTP opening is the key event leading to IRI. Therefore, inhibiting mPTP opening is the common mechanism of many cardioprotective substances against IRI. In cardiac physiology and pathology, mitochondria serve as an integrator of signal transduction and energy production [17]. When apoptotic signals are present, a series of events occur in mitochondria, including mPTP opening, after which the outer membrane ruptures. Therefore, the contents of the intima, such as cytochrome C and apoptotic peptidase-activating factor 1 (Apaf-1), are released, and the caspase-activating complex, namely the apoptosis body, forms. Activated caspase-9 in the apoptosis body can activate caspase-3 and caspase-7, initiating the caspase cascade to activate a series of hydrolytic enzymes in the cell, which eventually results in apoptosis. In the model of experimental stress-induced cardiopathology, the action of luteolin was studied. In this model, Mesaton injection disturbed the blood flow in the coronary circulation, inducing cardiopathology and heart function decompensation in rats. Moreover, administration of luteolin preparations exerted cardioprotection. Changes in some metabolic parameters and the endocrinal status of the animals also supported the therapeutic effect of luteolin. These findings suggested that luteolin might protect cardiomyocytes by stimulating mitochondrial biogenesis. Thus, preserving mitochondrial integrity is essential for therapeutic efficacy.

(3) ER approach: ER plays pivotal roles in maintaining Ca^{2+} homeostasis in cells and membrane protein synthesis, modification and folding. ER stress not only induces caspase-12 expression but also leads to the translocation of cytoplasmic caspases to the ER surface, where the latter activates the former. For example, activated caspase-12 can further cleave caspase-3 to induce apoptosis. The stress condition of myocardial IRI triggers an unfolded protein response (UPR) in the ER, which eases ER stress by inducing changes in transcription and translation, thereby, maintaining cell function. However, prolonged UPR in cardiomyocytes causes evident cardiac dysfunction by inducing myocardial apoptosis.

2. Luteolin and Calcium Signaling Pathways Mediating Cell Apoptosis during I/R

For the calcium signaling pathways, after the binding of ligands to their respective surface receptors, G-protein-coupled receptor ligands (GPCRs), ion channels and other channels can activate various phospholipase C (PLC) isoenzymes, generating two second messengers, diacylglycerol (DAG) and inositol 1, 4, 5-triphosphate (IP_3). DAG can activate protein kinase C (PKC), while IP_3 can induce Ca^{2+} release from intracellular storage pools to the cytoplasm, Once PKC activated, PKC can also catalyze plasma membrane calcium channel phosphorylation, and promote calcium ions influx into cytoplasm, both of which can increase the myocardial intracellular Ca^{2+} concentration. The imbalance of energy metabolism causes an increase of the myocardial cytoplasm Ca^{2+} concentration in early ischemia/hypoxia and then changes in myocardial cell membrane and sarcoplasmic reticulum permeability, which induce Ca^{2+} overload, further leading to irreversible damages. Apparently, Ca^{2+} accumulation is the key event in myocardial IRI. Increased myocardial calcium concentration impairs myocardial systolic and diastolic function by damaging the excitation-contraction coupling, and activates intracellular calcium-sensitive signaling pathways, such as PKC, MAPKs, calcium/calmodulin-dependent protein kinase and calcineurin. In the intracellular calcium-sensitive signaling transduction cascade, calmodulin is the most important adapter. Calcium-calmodulin complex may directly act on the target enzyme and activate Ca^{2+}/CaMK, prior to the phosphorylation of the target enzyme. Studies have shown that elevated Ca^{2+} concentration can change the activity of transcription factors, such as c-fos, c-jun and CREB, to initiate apoptosis in myocardial IRI. Ca^{2+} chelators, calcium channel blockers and calmodulin antagonists can alleviate or inhibit apoptosis. However, whether luteolin exerts the protection against apoptosis directly or indirectly through calcium signaling pathways has not been well defined.

3. Luteolin and the Calcium-dependent Mitochondrial Signaling Pathway Mediating Cell Apoptosis during I/R

Lysophosphatidylcholine (LPC)-induced apoptosis is characterized by a calcium-dependent mitochondrial pathway, involving calcium influx, calpain activation, cytochrome C release and caspase activation. Luteolin can reduce calcium influx. Junna et al. have found that luteolin also inhibits calpain activation and prevents cytochrome C release from the mitochondria. Inhibiting cytochrome C release by luteolin blocks the activation of caspase-3 and, thus, prevents subsequent endothelial apoptosis. These results suggested that luteolin might inhibit LPC-induced apoptosis in endothelial cells by blocking the calcium-dependent mitochondrial pathway [18] (Figure 5). However, whether luteolin inhibits apoptosis in myocardial I/R by blocking the caspase pathway remains unclear.

Choi et al. have found that luteolin can inhibit endothelial apoptosis, increase the protein expression of Bcl-2 and inhibit both the protein expression of Bax and the cleavage and activation of caspase-3 in endothelial cells. This study suggested that luteolin might exert anti-apoptotic effects through multiple mechanisms. The anti-apoptotic activity of luteolin appears to be mediated through the mitochondrial pathway. However, whether luteolin inhibits apoptosis in cardiomyocytes during I/R by this mechanism has not been elucidated. Kim et al. [2] have investigated whether ER stress and the Bcl-2 protein are associated with the protective effect of luteolin on I/R-induced cardiac damage. In the experiment, H9c2 cardiac muscle cells were exposed to luteolin prior to ischemia (12h)/reperfusion (4h). They observed that luteolin protected the cells against I/R-induced cell death. The results also showed that luteolin pretreatment significantly increased the expression of the anti-apoptotic protein Bcl-2, while decreasing the expression of the pro-apoptotic protein Bax. Additionally, luteolin down-regulated the expression of ER stress proteins, suggesting that cardiac I/R might be related to the ER stress response, in which mitochondrial Bcl-2 protein might also be involved.

In summary, luteolin regulates the ER stress response and is most likely associated with the mitochondrial apoptosis pathway to exert cardiac cell protection.

4. Luteolin and the PI3K/Akt Signaling Pathway Mediating Cell Apoptosis during I/R

Akt or protein kinase B (PKB) is a serine/threonine protein kinase. Activated Akt can inhibit cardiomyocyte apoptosis during myocardial I/R.

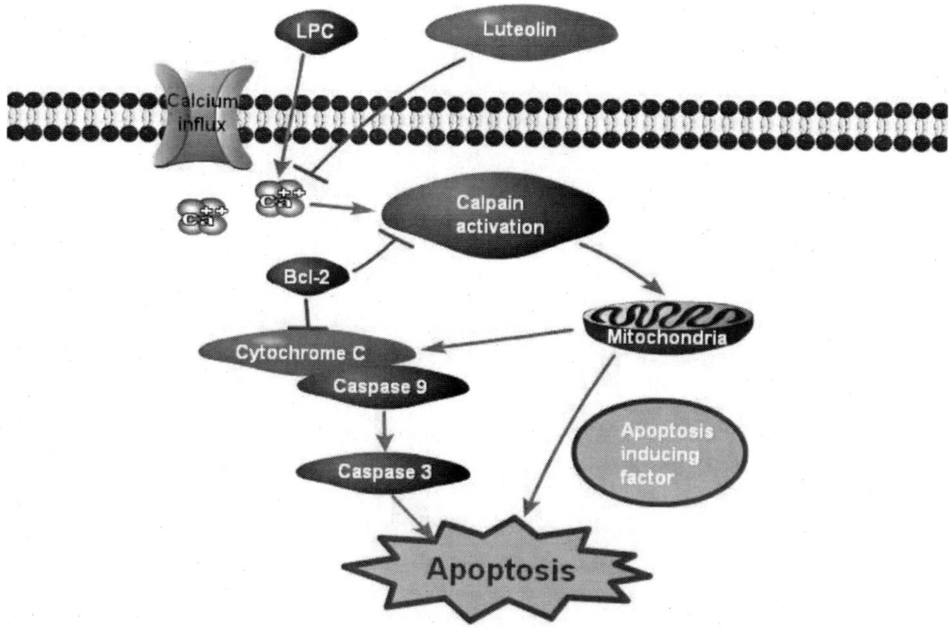

Figure 5. Possible mechanisms of luteolin inhibiting LPC-induced apoptosis in endothelial cells through the blockage of the calcium-dependent mitochondrial pathway.

Akt inhibits apoptosis mainly through the PI3K signaling pathway, and the possible mechanism is as follows: activated Akt inhibits cardiomyocyte apoptosis through the PI3K/Akt/NF-κB signaling pathway. Akt can regulate pro-apoptotic proteins (such as Bad and caspase) by phosphorylation or inactivation, thereby suppressing apoptosis. Akt is a critical regulator of PI3K-mediated cell survival. Constitutive activation of Akt signaling is sufficient to block cell death induced by a variety of apoptotic stimuli. Several downstream targets of Akt have been identified as apoptosis regulatory molecules, including the Bcl-2 family member Bad and procaspase-9. Activation of Akt also directly or indirectly regulates multiple transcription factor families, including Foxhead, NF-κB and p53. Akt can also inhibit the mitochondrial release of cytochrome C.

Recent studies have confirmed the cardioprotective role of this pathway in IRI [19-21]. In an in vitro experiment in rabbit hearts, by comparing 30min ischemia to 6 cycles of 30s ischemia and 30s reperfusion, Yang [21] showed that the area of infarct (33.3±2.2)% was reduced to (10.4±3.4)%. After 5min reperfusion, the specific PI3K inhibitor Wortmannin was administrated, and the area of infarction returned to 31.2±4.2%. The protective effect of the reperfusion treatment disappeared. These results suggested that the protective effect of luteolin might be exerted through the PI3K pathway. Although the downstream transduction pathways of some myocardial protective factors may be very complicated, in many cases, Akt activation is a characteristic event. It plays an important role in regulating various growth factors required for cardiomyocyte survival, growth, proliferation and nutrient metabolism. The Akt signaling pathway is considered the most important pathway involved in regulating cell survival. It can transduce the anti-apoptotic signals in cells [22]. In vitro, PI3K/Akt activation reduced hypoxia-induced myocardial apoptosis [23]. In vivo, exogenous expression of activated Akt in the heart, using adenoviral vectors, appeared to inhibit myocardial apoptosis after short periods of ischemia and shrank the infarction area [24].

The anti-apoptotic effect of Akt is exerted through the phosphorylation of its downstream targets. The expression of various anti-apoptotic molecular markers downstream of Akt has been confirmed in cardiomyocytes. The overall effects of Akt activation is likely the collective results of regulating many signaling pathways. We found that Akt activation not only reduced mortality in the I/R model of cardiomyocytes in vivo but also improved regional and global cardiac function [19, 20]. As the control, we also showed that endogenous Akt activation was inhibited, and that cardiomyocyte function was impaired during hypoxia, when expressing a dominant negative Akt [24].

These findings indicate that Akt regulates the survival and function of cardiomyocytes; however, the exact pathway through which this occurs has yet to be elucidated. Communal et al. have found that caspase-3 activation directly targets three components of cardiac myofilament: a-actin, a-actinin and troponin T, which severely affects cardiomyocyte function. Further investigation has proposed another possible mechanism: Akt activation may increase Ca^{2+} circulation to maintain heart contractile function. In recent studies [19, 20], we have also demonstrated that luteolin ameliorates I/R-induced cardiomyocyte contractile dysfunction, evidenced by the significant dose-dependent increase in single cardiomyocyte shortening amplitude. In these experiments, we tested the contractile function of left ventricular cardiomyocytes with the administration of different concentrations of luteolin after simulation. Our results demonstrated that the PI3K/Akt pathway is one of the most important intracellular survival signaling pathways. We utilized the PI3K inhibitor LY294002 to examine whether the cardioprotective effect of luteolin treatment was indeed mediated by the PI3K/Akt pathway. Inhibition of the Akt activity abolished the luteolin-induced positive contraction and the inhibition of apoptosis in cardiomyocytes during I/R. These results indicate that luteolin inhibits apoptosis and improves cardiomyocyte contractile function in I/R, at least partly through the PI3K/Akt pathway.

5. Luteolin and the MAPK Signaling Pathway Mediating Cell Apoptosis during I/R

The pro-apoptosis effect of the MAPK pathway in cardiomyocytes is an increasing concern. MAPKs mediate the effects of double-phosphorylated serine and tyrosine protein kinase family members, including extracellular regulation kinases (ERKs), c-jun N end kinase/stress-activated protein kinases (JNK/SAPKs) and the protein kinase p38. Several laboratories [25] have found that p38 and ERKs are activated during myocardial I/R in rats. Other studies have shown that the JNK/SAPK pathway is also involved in cell apoptosis.

Accumulating evidence suggests the involvement of MAPKs in the regulation of mitochondrial translocation and activation of pro-apoptotic Bax and Bim via phosphorylation of Bcl-2 family members. Researchers tested the exact role of the interaction between MAPKs and mitochondrial signaling pathways. In the experiment, Kang observed the activation of JNK, p38 and ERK within 10min after luteolin treatment, reduced mitochondrial translocation of Bax after the treatment of each specific MAPK inhibitor, as well as cytochrome C release induced by luteolin. Therefore, Kang suggested that MAPKs might play a role in luteolin-induced Bax translocation, matrix metallopeptidase (MMP) reduction, cytochrome C release and subsequent cell death in Neuro-2a cells [26]. They hypothesized that crosstalk may occur among the three MAPK signaling pathways to regulate Bax activity and mitochondrial function.

In recent years, studies have suggested that luteolin inhibits lipoteichoic acid -induced ERK 1/2, p38, and JNK phosphorylation in H9c2 cells, the phenomenon has also been found in human gingival fibroblasts [27]. However, the myocardial protective effects of luteolin against IRI and the mechanisms by which it affects the ERK1/2 and JNK family have not been clarified. In recent studies [28], we have demonstrated that I/R mainly activates JNK, rather than the ERK1/2 pathway. JNK is a key factor in the signal transduction leading to myocardial injury after I/R; in contrast, ERK1/2 is not activated during I/R. However, several recent studies have found that ERK is activated during the I/R stages, and was shown to be required for survival signaling. This difference observed between our study and the aforementioned reports may be due to differences in the cell types and experimental protocols employed. Our results showed that I/R led to the apoptosis of cardiomyocytes, the release of LDH in coronary effluent, and decrease of contractile function and infarction of myocardial tissue. Pretreatment with luteolin or SP600125 significantly attenuated I/R-induced cardiomyocyte death, LDH leakage and infarct size. Further, it also improved the systolic/diastolic function of single cardiomyocytes and whole heart, with a concomitant increase in p-ERK1/2 and decrease in p-JNK expression. All these effects of luteolin were abolished by ERK1/2 inhibitor. Moreover, luteolin effectively improved the degeneration of cell shortening amplitude and cell death induced by I/R, with a maximal effect observed at a dose of 8mmol/l. This result [28] suggests that luteolin may actually exert anti-IRI effects in myocytes at this concentration.

Recently, we performed related experiments to further investigate the luteolin-induced protection against simulated I/R and its underlying mechanism. In this study, we examined the levels of p38 MAPK and phosphorylated p38 after 3h simulated ischemia and 2h simulated reperfusion in cardiomyocytes [unpublished data]. Pretreatment with luteolin substantially increased cell viability and shortening amplitude and repressed p38 phosphorylation. Furthermore, we observed contractile function in isolated hearts after they were subjected to 30min global ischemia followed by 120min reperfusion. Compared to the control, Bcl-2 expression was decreased, while Bax expression was increased during I/R. Luteolin treatment increased the Bcl-2 expression level while significantly decreased the Bax expression level, resulting in an increase in the Bcl-2/Bax ratio in cardiomyocytes subjected to I/R.

6. Luteolin and the JAK/STAT Signaling Pathway Mediating Cell Apoptosis during I/R

In recent years, many studies have found that the JAK/STAT pathway is involved in I/R-mediated apoptosis in cardiomyocytes [29]. STAT3 activation exerts cardioprotective effects, whereas STAT1 activation is associated with apoptosis. Using the JAK-2 specific inhibitor AG490 in a myocardial IRI rat model, it was observed that caspase-3 activity was greatly enhanced, while the Bax level was elevated, and the number of apoptotic cells increased, upon the treatment. On the contrary, the number of apoptotic cardiomyocytes in rat hearts decreased upon AG490 treatment in vitro. The JAK/STAT pathway may have a dual nature in regulating myocardial apoptosis, potentially through crosstalk with another pathway, which means the balance between protective and apoptotic mechanisms is determined by a network of signaling pathways that can interact with the JAK/STAT pathway to regulate the expression of either anti-apoptotic or pro-apoptotic genes [30]. Constitutive activation of the related pathways may be achieved by benefiting from the cross activation of the STATs by serine/threonine kinases in collateral signaling pathways. These pathways are activated by cytokines, such as TNF, FasL and G-protein-coupled receptor (GPCR) ligands released by ischemic myocardium. The interaction between these ligands and their respective signaling pathways, as well as their crosstalk with the JAK/STAT pathway, can affect the behavior of stressed cardiomyocytes [31]. However, whether luteolin inhibits apoptosis in cardiomyocytes during IRI via the JAK/STAT pathway has not been experimentally confirmed.

7. Luteolin and the cGMP/PKG Signaling Pathway Mediating Cell Apoptosis during I/R

In all forms of cardioprotection, cGMP production and protein kinase G (PKG) activation are key steps in the signal transduction pathway. Burley et al. have highlighted the roles of cGMP and PKG in their comprehensive review, which involve transactivation of a growth factor receptor, activation of membrane enzymes and lipid metabolism, activation of Akt, stimulation of nitric oxide (NO) production and subsequent activation of PKG, opening of mitochondrial ATP-dependent K^+ channels and release of reactive oxygen species.

As an important intracellular messenger substance, cGMP has three main targets: cGMP-dependent protein kinase or PKG, cAMP phosphodiesterase and cGMP-regulated ion channels, among which PKG is considered the most important target. PKG belongs to the serine/threonine protein kinase family. In mammals, PKG is present in two forms, namely pKG-I and pKG-II. PKG-I mainly functions in the cardiovascular system under physiological conditions, causing vasodilation, inhibition of endothelial cell permeability and platelet activation. It can also exert a negative inotropic effect on myocardial cells. In addition to these physiological functions, PKG is also involved in anti-apoptotic responses. In nerve cells, NO-cGMP-PKG exerts anti-apoptotic effects or activates the survival signaling pathway. Activating PKG or increasing cGMP prevents apoptosis, while decreasing the cGMP basal level is pro-apoptotic. For PC12 nerve cells, PKG activation by NO prevents mitochondrial cytochrome C release and inhibits apoptosis. In the liver mitochondria, NO prevents mPTP opening and cytochrome C release. A recent study also showed that through the activation of PKG, cGMP could reduce HZO, through the reduction of mitochondrial membrane potential, cytochrome C release and mPTP opening in astrocytes. It has been reported that by activating ATP-sensitive potassium (KATP) channels in myocardial cells, PKG is involved in the mechanism of preconditioning to protect myocardial cells. These findings indicate that PKG plays an important role in the regulation of mitochondrial function under a variety of pathophysiological conditions. However, the exact mechanism is unclear. Moreover, whether luteolin inhibits apoptosis in cardiomyocytes during IRI via the cGMP-PKG pathway remains to be elucidated.

8. Luteolin and the PKC Signaling Pathway Mediating Cell Apoptosis during I/R

The current view is that drug preconditioning, which activates intracellular signal transduction pathways to promote the release or synthesis of a variety of endogenous protective substances, may prime cells to produce adaptive responses. It is generally acknowledged that the G-coupled protein/PKC/ATP-sensitive potassium channel axis in the intracellular pathway and the activation of PKC in this pathway are the central link among all inherent cell protection pathways, while mitochondrial membrane potassium channels are involved in cell protection during I/R.

A large number of studies have shown that PKC plays a very important role in IP. There are many subtypes of PKC, among which PKC£ and PKCe are the main subtypes expressed in adult rat cardiomyocytes. Many clinical studies have directly proved that PKC activation is the central link of inherent cell protection pathways. Moreover, both ischemia and drug preconditioning lead to increased PKC activity in cells. The heart tissue-specific PKC knockout mice do not produce IP. However, the expression of PKC£ agonists in transgenic mice induces production against cardiac IRI, indicating that PKC also plays a role in regulating the apoptosis pathway. As a Ca^{2+} and phospholipid-dependent protein kinase, PKC is involved in maintaining cellular calcium homeostasis. These signaling molecules can increase the release and activation of PKC via the GPCR pathway during myocardial IR. GPCRs, such as adenosine, bradykinin and opioids, can activate phospholipase C to generate a diglyceride pool. Afterwards, PKC activation induces phosphorylation of the mPTP component porin, directly inhibiting the mPTP opening-mediated cardiac IP. The PKC pathway, which depends on Ca^{2+}, diacylglycerol and phosphatidylserine, plays a key role in cell survival. Application of PKC agonists can reduce the cardiomyocyte Ca^{2+} uptake and decrease the concentration of free Ca^{2+}. ROS and lipid peroxidation can also stimulate the phosphorylation of L-type calcium channels in the membrane via PKC activation, accompanied by the activation of ion channels, such as Na^{+}, H^{+} and Ca^{2+}, and the calcium pump, thereby regulating myocardial calcium homeostasis. However, whether the anti-apoptotic effect of luteolin in cardiomyocytes during IRI is exerted through PKC requires further investigation.

9. Luteolin and the LOX-1 Signaling Pathway Mediating Cell Apoptosis during I/R

Recent studies in this field has been mainly focusing on the role of LOX-1 in myocardial apoptosis during IRI. In I/R, low-density lipoprotein oxidation releases ROS. Both low-density lipoprotein oxidation and ROS can increase LOX-1 receptor expression. The work of Kataoka has shown that myocardial I/R can induce LOX-1 expression. With the administration of a LOX-1 monoclonal antibody prior to I/R, the area of myocardial injury was significantly reduced. Additionally, it was reported that during myocardial I/R, LOX-1 gene expression was upregulated, while cardiac injury was significantly reduced. The SOD activity was obviously enhanced in LOX-1 knockout mice during myocardial IRI, suggesting that LOX-1 might play an important role in IRI-mediated myocardial apoptosis.

In addition, researchers found that mice with luteolin supplemented in their drinking water exhibited decreased levels of plasma IL-6 and reduced IL-6 expression in their hippocampus. The enzymes cyclooxygenase (COX), LOX and inducible NO synthase (iNOS) are known to play an important role in inflammation and in the production of reactive species. Some reports have shown that luteolin can inhibit LOX [32]. However, whether luteolin exerts protection against IRI in rat hearts via the LOX pathway has not yet been elucidated.

10. Luteolin and other Signaling Pathways Mediating Cell Apoptosis during I/R

(1) *NF-κB:* Activation of the transcription factor on oxidative stress may directly or indirectly activate transcription factors, regulating the redox reaction on the transcription of target genes, such as the AP-1 transcription factor complex and NF-κB, to antagonize ROS toxicity. NF-κB can be activated by a variety of stimuli. Cooperated with the corresponding gene enhancer, it can initiates gene transcription. Upon activation, NF-κB undergoes nuclear translocation. In combination with other partners, the κB motif plays a transcriptional regulatory role. The downstream targets of NF-κB include molecules involved in the regulation of apoptosis, such as Bcl-2 family proteins. As a classical transcription factor, NF-κB plays a critical role in LPS-induced TNF-α production in cardiomyocytes [33]. Based on the function of NF-κB in cardiomyocytes, previous research has investigated whether luteolin can prevent LPS-induced TNF-α expression in cardiomyocytes through inhibiting the NF-κB signaling pathway. In the experiment, neonatal rat cardiomyocytes were pretreated with luteolin for 24h, prior to LPS stimulation. The result showed that luteolin inhibited LPS-induced TNF-α expression in a dose dependent manner in cultured cardiomyocytes. Further experiment showed that luteolin significantly inhibited the activation of the NF-κB signaling pathway and decreased the expression of myocardial TNF-α, in response to LPS stimulation. Taken together, these results indicate that luteolin inhibits LPS-induced NF-κB activation and subsequently down-regulates TNF-α synthesis to prevent cardiac dysfunction.

(2) *small G proteins:* In recent years, increasing studies have investigated the roles of small G proteins, such as Rac1, Rho kinase (Rho-kinase, ROCK) and ADP-ribose polymerase (poly(ADP-ribose)Polymerase PARP), in myocardial apoptosis during

I/R. Some studies have reported that Rho-kinase plays an important role in the pathogenesis of heart IRI, and that Rho-kinase activation can be reversed by ischemic preconditioning (IPC). Zhang et al. have studied the mechanisms of the role of Rho-kinase in I/R. In the experiment, they induced I/R by ligating the left anterior descending branch of the coronary artery (LAD) for 30min and releasing the ligature for 180min in Wistar rats. In the IPC rat model, two cycles of 5min ligation of the LAD and 5min reflow were conducted before I/R. They observed increased ERK1/2 activity and decreased Rho-kinase activity, as well as decreased cardiomyocyte apoptosis, in the IPC group. Administration of PD 98059 increased Rho-kinase activity. These results indicate that the ERK-MAPK signaling pathway inhibits Rho-kinase to reduce cardiomyocyte apoptosis in heart IPC, therefore implying that the crosstalk between the ERK-MAPK signaling pathway and Rho-kinase activity plays a role in regulating cardiomyocyte apoptosis in vivo [34].

Previous reports have shown that ROCK and PARP play an important role in the I/R rat heart. More specifically, both the ROCK/JNK/AIF signaling pathway and the PARP/JNK/AIF signal pathway are activated in I/R rat heart [35]. Furthermore, they identified the ROCK/Akt/caspase-3/PARP signaling pathway as a novel important signaling pathway in I/R rat cardiomyocytes. To explore whether small G proteins are involved in the effects of luteolin on apoptosis and its mechanism of action, both the heart capillary endothelial cell line H5V and human umbilical vein endothelial cells (HUVEC) were treated with pyrogallol in the experiment, and the induced apoptosis was studied. The result showed that luteolin could inhibit the poly (ADP-ribose) polymerase activation, caspase-8 cleavage and p38 MAPK activation, indicating that luteolin is an effective agent to protect endothelial cells, partly via inhibiting the poly (ADP-ribose) polymerase activation.

The function of Rac1 is mediated through NADPH oxidase activation and is associated with mitochondrial ROS production, suggesting that Rac1 may promote cardiomyocyte apoptosis. Studies have shown that Rac1 activation may promote the production of oxidase/reactive oxygen species in cardiomyocytes during I/R [36]. Moreover, Rac1 is required for cardiomyocyte apoptosis during hyperglycemia. Rac1 plays a critical role in hyperglycemia-induced apoptosis in cardiomyocytes through NADPH oxidase and ROS production, leading to myocardial dysfunction in diabetes. Meanwhile, disruption of Rac1 signaling reduces IRI in the diabetic heart by inhibiting calpain. Further, in endotoxemia, Rac1 activation induces TNF-α expression and cardiac dysfunction. In summary, Rac1 exacerbates apoptosis in cardiomyocytes during I/R, partly through inducing excess ROS production. However, RhoA was reported to protect the mouse heart against IRI [37]. Nevertheless, whether luteolin functions via small G proteins to exert protection against IRI in rat hearts has not yet been elucidated.

(3) *Focal adhesion kinase (FAK):* FAK is a non-receptor tyrosine kinase that regulates adhesion-dependent survival signals. In some cell types, FAK stimulates the activation of pro-survival kinases, such as ERK and Akt. Inactivation of FAK leads to apoptosis. Prolonged transverse aortic constriction in mice with cardiac-specific FAK deletion leads to dilated cardiomyopathy and heart failure. FAK deficiency enhances I/R-induced apoptosis. Previous research has investigated the function of FAK and found that it can inhibit stress-induced cardiomyocyte apoptosis. The

experiments showed that depletion of FAK markedly exacerbated hypoxia/re-oxygenation-induced cardiomyocyte cell death in vitro. Deletion of FAK in the adult myocardium resulted in a significant increase in the size of I/R-induced infarct and in cardiomyocyte apoptosis, with a concomitant reduction in left ventricular function. The results suggest that NF-κB signaling may play a key role in regulating FAK-dependent cardioprotection, because FAK inactivation inhibits NF-κB activation and reduces the expression of the NF-κB target genes, including Bcl-2 and Bcl-xl. Taken together, FAK may regulate cardiomyocyte survival during I/R [38].

11. The Crosstalk of Luteolin and other Signaling Pathways Mediating Cell Apoptosis during I/R

Signal transduction may involve several signaling pathways, interactions among which form the signal network. Therefore, one inducer can activate several signaling pathways. Signaling crosstalk means that different signals can be integrated at different joints of the signaling pathways, resulting in the same or similar biological effects.

Pharmacologic preconditioning involves multiple salvage signal transduction pathways, mainly including PI3K/Akt and ERK. As important therapeutic targets, drug-induced anti-apoptotic effects have been certificated for improving the tolerance to IRI. We hypothesized that drug treatment might activate several pro-survival signaling pathways, the crosstalk among which could be essential to coordinate a variety of biological and pharmacological activities. Therefore, after determining the involvement of luteolin and many signaling pathways in mediating cell apoptosis during IRI individually, we need to explore the role of the crosstalk among multiple signaling pathways related to luteolin in cardioprotection during I/R.

Since apoptosis is a highly regulated process, it is a good potential target for therapeutic intervention. Inhibition of cardiomyocyte apoptosis using novel research tools, including transgenic mice, gene deletion, recombinant proteins and pharmacological inhibitors, results in cardioprotection [39]. Although several potential therapeutic agents have been tested in animal models of IRI, showing promising results, almost none of the specific anti-apoptotic agents have reached the stage of clinical application. This is partly due to the fact that multiple signaling pathways are activated in response to IRI. In addition, it is not clear how much crosstalk occurs among those pathways during IR.

The complex signal transduction mechanisms during myocardial IRI involves extracellular signaling molecules on the cell membrane, a wide range of changes in intracellular signal transduction pathways and the downstream effects, which further interact at several levels and crosstalk with their canonical roles. Many myocardial protection approaches by activating anti-apoptotic or pro-survival signaling pathways ultimately reduce cardiac injury. Some studies have suggested that, other than the Akt, PKC, PKG, Ca^{2+} and NF-κB pathways, JAK/STAT and MAPK signaling pathways are also involved. However, which pathway plays the major role in reducing the injury is not determined [40].

Many experimental studies have shown that IP can activate certain pro-survival signaling pathways, such as Akt and GPCR. IP can activate tyrosine kinases, triggering PI3K activation, which in turn results in Akt phosphorylation through activation of phosphoinositide-dependent kinase 1 (PDK-1). It has been reported that IP induces Akt phosphorylation, and that inhibitors of Akt or PI3K can block IP. Moreover, Akt can increase eNOS phosphorylation, resulting in protective effect against NO through the PKG signaling pathway. Drug pretreatment mimics IP via activating certain pro-survival signaling pathways. The pathways involved in drug pretreatment and those activated by IP may be similar. Whether drug treatment induces multiple pro-survival signaling pathways and how the crosstalk occurs are of increasing concern.

For the calcium signaling pathways, after the binding between surface receptors and their ligands, GPCRs, ion channels and other channels can activate various PLC isoenzymes, generating two second messengers, DG and IP_3. DG can activate PKC, while IP_3 can induce Ca^{2+} release from intracellular storage pools to the cytoplasm, both of which can increase the myocardial intracellular Ca^{2+} concentration. The imbalance of energy metabolism causes an increase of the myocardial cytoplasmic Ca^{2+} concentration in early ischemia/hypoxia and then changes in myocardial cell membrane and sarcoplasmic reticulum permeability, which induce Ca^{2+} overload, further leading to irreversible damages. Apparently, Ca^{2+} accumulation is the key event in myocardial IRI. Increased myocardial calcium concentration impairs myocardial systolic and diastole function by damaging the excitation-contraction couple and by activating intracellular calcium-sensitive signaling pathways, such as PKC, MAPKs, calcium/calmodulin-dependent protein kinase (Ca^{2+}/CaMK) and calcineurin phosphatase (CaN). In the intracellular signaling transduction cascade, calmodulin (CaM) is the most important adapter. Ca^{2+}/CaM complexes may act directly on the target enzyme and activate Ca^{2+}/CaMK, prior to the phosphorylation of the target enzyme. Ca^{2+}/CaMK regulates L-type calcium channel current, as well as calcium release and uptake by sarcoplasmic reticulum. Ras expression is upregulated in myocardial I/R. Once forming a complex with p21-Ras, GPT can activate PLC, promote the metabolism of phosphorylation inositol, mobilize intracellular Ca^{2+} storages and activate PKC, therefore increasing Na^+/H^+ exchange and the intracellular pH value, which in turn activates the transcription of c-fos. The complex of p21-Ras-GPT can also translocate into the nucleus to regulate gene transcription involved in myocardial IRI. Studies have shown that elevated Ca^{2+} concentration can change the activity of transcription factors, such as c-fos, c-jun and CREB, to initiate apoptosis in myocardial IRI. Ca^{2+} chelators, calcium channel blockers and calcium calmodulin antagonists can alleviate or completely inhibit apoptosis. However, whether luteolin exerts the protection against apoptosis directly or indirectly through calcium signaling pathways has not been well defined.

Due to the complexity of signaling pathways involved in regulating apoptosis in cardiomyocytes during I/R, it is essential to develop multi-targeted drugs for cardioprotection. We and others have reported that the anti-apoptosis effect of luteolin on cardiac protection in I/R rat cardiomyocytes [18, 41-42]. Previous studies have shown that luteolin protects against ROS-mediated apoptotic cell death induced by zinc, partly via the PI3K/Akt/NF-κB/ERK1/2 pathways [43]. However, whether the crosstalk among these pathways mediates the cardioprotective role of luteolin is merely examined. Most researchers have been focusing on the apoptosis phenotype in I/R, and many drugs for cardioprotective effect lay particular emphasis on treating the phenotypic damage as well. In contrast, drugs with protective effects and targeting signaling cascades are rare. Given that luteolin induces apoptosis in cancer cells that are resistant to multiple drugs without affecting the drug transporter function [44], it is possible that the anti-apoptotic effect of luteolin in cardiomyocytes during I/R may involve multiply target signaling pathways. In another study [45], H9c2 cells were pretreated with 10μM biochanin A, 1μM daidzein, 25μM genistein, 10μM luteolin, 50μM quercetin or 50μM rutin for 30min and were then exposed to I/R for 12 h/4h, which did not affect cell viability. It was observed that I/R increased the Bcl-2 level and decreased the Bax level. In this experiment, the authors investigated the effect of flavonoids on the activation of MAPK family members, Akt and IL-1β expression in rat heart embryonic (H9c2) cells upon LTA stimulation. Pretreatment with four flavonoids, including quercetin, genistein, quercetagetin and luteolin, diminished LTA-induced phosphorylation of ERK1/2, JNK, p38 and Akt, as well as IL-1β gene expression, indicating that flavonoids interfere with LTA signal transduction. This finding suggests that both Akt and MAPKs may be involved in the role of luteolin during I/R.

Previous studies have shown that PI3K/Akt interplays with MAPKs. In the myocardium of obese animals, the activity of p38 and JNK was increased, accompanied by the downregulation of PI3K/Akt expression. By examining changes of Akt in I/R, Crozier et al. have found that SD rat myocardial I/R can activate p38 MAPK and ERK1/2, indicating a close relationship between PI3K/AKT and MAPK pathways in myocardial IRI. The upstream activators of MAPK family members partially overlap, and other important molecules in Erk1/2, Erk5, p38 and PI3K/Akt signaling pathways are closely related. Our preliminary results have shown that inhibition of p38 MAPK phosphorylation exerts antioxidant effects via the PI3K/Akt pathway in luteolin pretreatment, further suggesting that PI3K/Akt and MAPKs cooperate closely in myocardial IRI. We hypothesize that in myocardial IRI, luteolin pretreatment may exert anti-apoptotic effects via the PI3K/Akt and MAPK pathways. Confirming the collaboration between PI3K/Akt and MAPKs on regulating anti-apoptosis is our next research objective.

Luteolin and Signaling Pathways Mediating Cell Apoptosis in Diabetic Rats during I/R

We have discussed the effect and mechanism of luteolin on cardiac protection and anti-apoptosis in non-diabetic rats with myocardial IRI. Diabetes mellitus (DM) has been known to exacerbate ischemic or pharmacologic preconditioning in IRI. Diabetes is associated with significantly increased cardiomyocyte apoptosis. Due to the effect of PPARγ activation in HCEC by luteolin, as a PPARγ partial agonist, luteolin exerts a protective effect against diabetic complications in streptozotocin(STZ)-induced diabetic rats [46]. Luteolin reduces cardiac dysfunctions in STZ-induced diabetic rats. Kwak has reported that diabetes affect remifentanil preconditioning-induced cardioprotection in rat hearts during I/R through anti-apoptotic pathways [47]. In the experiment, STZ-induced diabetic rats and Sprague-Dawley(SD) rats were exposed to 30min ischemia followed by 1h of reperfusion. They examined the myocardial infarct size, the activity of ERK1/2, Bcl-2, and Bax, the release of cytochrome C and the expression of genes regulating Ca^{2+} homeostasis. The results showed that myocardial protective effects induced by remifentanil preconditioning were attenuated in the diabetic rat heart, compared to those in the wild-type rat heart. Given that diabetes minimized the remifentanil-induced correction of abnormal changes in sarcoplasmic reticulum genes and proteins in I/R rat hearts, they concluded that diabetes could mitigate remifentanil-induced cardioprotection against I/R.

The next question is that whether the effect of luteolin in DM and Non-DM is equivalent. In recent study, luteolin has been shown to improve cardiac function after myocardial IRI in diabetic rats. Sun evaluated whether diabetes affect luteolin preconditioning-induced cardioprotection in I/R rat hearts in respect of cardiac function and cardiomyocyte apoptosis [48]. In this study, STZ-induced diabetic rats and matched wild-type SD rats were subjected to 30min ischemia/3h reperfusion. They then examined the severity of myocardial I/R-induced LDH release, arrhythmia, infarct size, cardiac function impairment and cardiomyocyte apoptosis. The results indicated that luteolin could protect diabetic rats from cardiac IRI and cardiomyocytes apoptosis. Moreover, they observed that the PI3K inhibitor Wortmannin abolished the cardiac protective effects of luteolin, suggesting that luteolin might exert the anti-apoptotic effects by activating the PI3K/Akt pathway while increasing the Bcl-2/Bax ratio. The phenotype of STZ-induced diabetic rats mimics that of type I DM. In future studies, we will focus on the anti-apoptosis effects of luteolin and the potential mechanism through the PI3k/Akt and MAPK pathways in cardiomyocytes during I/R using Goto-Kakizaki (G-K) and Wistar rats.

Conclusion and Perspective

Up to now, a large number of studies have shown that cell apoptosis plays an important role during myocardial IRI, and that much work has been conducted to identify the detailed mechanisms and transduction pathways involved, aiming to elucidate the relationship between cardiomyocyte apoptosis and myocardial IRI. Many experiments have confirmed that multiple signaling pathways can be activated during myocardial I/R in animal models, including Akt, MAPK, NF-κB, PKC, Ca^{2+} and JAK/STAT. However, the close relationship and crosstalk among these pathways and the significance of anti-apoptotic mechanisms in cardioprotection have not been illustrated. It is unknown whether inhibiting apoptosis for cardioprotection against various heart diseases may subsequently lead to non-apoptotic cell death [49]. Given the multiple targets of luteolin in various cells, the mechanisms associated with cardiomyocyte apoptosis are complex. Therefore, it is interesting and important to determine the mechanism of luteolin-induced selective protection and anti-apoptosis in rat cardiomyocytes during I/R.

It is clear that distinct mechanisms are adopted to modulate signaling pathways in different cells. For example, luteolin suppresses Akt in vascular smooth muscle cells [50], whereas it activates Akt in cardiac cells [19]. Similarly, luteolin inhibits NF-κB through suppressing IKK activation in epithelial cells and macrophages during inflammation, whereas it inhibits NF-κB in the nucleus of cancer cells. It remains to be determined whether these discrepancies are due to differences in cellular contexts. Additionally, many studies have been conducted to explore the cardioprotection mechanisms of luteolin treatment during myocardial IRI in rats, and some consensus has been achieved [19-21]. For instance, luteolin can exert the anti-apoptotic effect through the PI3K/Akt and caspase signaling pathways, therefore protecting rat myocardium against I/R. However, it is not yet clear whether the effects of luteolin treatment on myocardial IRI protection and anti-apoptosis involve the death receptor, mitochondria or MAPK signaling pathways [16]. Mechanisms for cardiomyocyte protection during myocardial IRI by the JAK/STAT and LOX-1 signaling pathways in rats following luteolin treatment are not known either [30, 32]. Many further studies are required to address these questions.

Understanding the mechanisms will undoubtedly facilitate the therapeutic application of luteolin in treating IRI. Thus, further investigation is required to determine whether the mechanisms of cardioprotection and anti-apoptosis of luteolin in I/R rat cardiomyocytes involve MAPK, PKC, PKG, small G protein, JAK/STAT and LOX-1 signaling pathways. Moreover, the exact cardioprotective mechanisms of luteolin require detailed illustration, such as the cooperation or crosstalk among Akt, MAPK, PKC, PKG, small G protein and JAK/STAT signaling pathways. In summary, luteolin can protect the myocardium against IRI. However, the exact mechanism warrants further investigation.

Some questions need to be addressed in future studies. First, most studies so far were performed in cells, not in vivo. Moreover, drug treatment in rats needs to be advanced to a more clinically relevant stage. However, there has been little attention to this issue in animal models that are more relevant to physiological and pathological processes in vivo. Second, there is a lack of direct evidence supporting the connection between luteolin and some signaling pathways, such as PKC, PKG and JAK/STAT, and its role in anti-apoptosis during I/R. Since the role of these signaling pathways in luteolin-induced anti-apoptosis has not been elucidated, it may still be premature to draw any conclusion regarding its implication. Third, there is the question of possible side effects in cardiac treatment by luteolin pretreatment, as some results have shown that a 20μg/mL concentration of luteolin has a toxic effect on rat cardiomyocytes in I/R and other adverse effects have not been clearly reported. Therefore, the significance of this potential connection is unclear. By the way, we should clarify that the cardiomyocytes are the major cell type damaged during I/R, and the main target in this manuscript. Moreover, whether IPC works against apoptotic pathways or luteolin acts through IPC pathways need be explained. The main topic in this chapter is the role of luteolin in the apoptotic pathways during IRI, the many part of the role of luteolin is from speculation based on the observation from other cell types etc. In this regard, the main part of this chapter scientific evidence and how the present novel research showed the cardio-protective effect of luteolin in IRI should be further studied. In all, more efforts are required to clarify the exact effects and mechanisms of luteolin on cardioprotection and anti-apoptosis in rat cardiomyocytes during I/R.

References

[1] Fukuyama N., Tanaka E., Tabata Y., Fujikura H., Hagihara M., Sakamoto H., Ando K., Nakazawa H., Mori H. Intravenous injection of phagocytes transfected ex vivo with FGF4 DNA/biodegradable gelatin complex promotes angiogenesis in a rat myocardial ischemia/reperfusion injury model. *Basic Res. Cardiol.*, 2007; 102(3):209-216.

[2] Kim D. S., Kwon D. Y., Kim M. S., Kim H. K., Lee Y. C., Park S. J., Yoo W. H., Chae S. W., Chung M. J., Kim H. R., Chae H. J. The involvement of endoplasmic reticulum stress in flavonoid-induced protection on cardiac cell death caused by ischaemia/reperfusion. *J. Pharm. Pharmacol.*, 2010; 62(2): 197-204.

[3] Yong Lin, Ranxin Shi, Xia Wang,and Han-Ming Shen. Luteolin, a flavonoid with potentials for cancer prevention and therapy. *Curr. Cancer Drug Targets*, 2008; 8(7): 634-646.

[4] López-Lázaro M. Distribution and biological activities of the flavonoid Luteolin. *Mini. Rev. Med. Chem.*, 2009, 9(1): 31-59.

[5] Gottlieb R. A., Burleson K. O., Kloner R. A., Babior B. M., Engler R. L. Reperfusion injury induces apoptosis in rabbit cardiomyocytes. *J. Clin. Invest.*, 1994; 94(4): 1621-1628.

[6] Fliss H., Gattinger D. Apoptosis in ischemic and reperfused rat myocardium. *Cire Res.*, 1996; 79(5): 949-956.

[7] Chakrabarti S., Hoque A. N., Karmazyn M. A rapid ischemia-induced apoptosis in isolated rat hearts and its attenuation by the sodium-hydrogen exchange inhibitor HOE 642(cariporide). *J. Mol. Cell Cardiol.*, 1997; 29(11): 3169-3174.

[8] Youngil Lee, Asa B. Gustafsson. Role of apoptosis in cardiovascular disease. *Apoptosis,* 2009; 14: 536-548.

[9] Yue T. L., Ma X. L., Wang X., Romanic A. M., Liu G. L., Louden C., Gu J. L., Kumar S., Poste G., Ruffolo R. R. Jr., Feuerstein G. Z. Possible involvement of stress-activated protein kinase signaling pathway and Fas receptor expression in prevention of ischemia/reperfusion-induced cardiomyocyte apoptosis by carvedilol. *Circ. Res.*, 1998; 82(2): 166-174.

[10] Chipuk J. E., Kuwana T., Bouchier-Hayes L. et al. Direct activation of Bax by p53 mediates mitochondrial membrane permeabilization and apoptosis. *Science,* 2004; 303: 1010-1014.

[11] Nathan Susnow, Liyun Zeng, Daciana Margineantu et al. Bcl-2 family proteins as regulators of oxidative stress. *Seminars in Cancer Biology*, 2009;19: 42-49.

[12] Lin K. M., Lin B., Lian I. Y., Mestril R., Scheffler I. E., Dillmann W. H. Combined and individual mitochondrial HSP60 and HSP10 expression in cardiac myocytes protects mitochondrial function and prevents apoptotic cell deaths induced by simulated ischemia-reoxygenation. *Circulation,* 2001; 103(13): 1787-1792.

[13] Lancel S., Joulin O., Favory R., Goossens J. F., Kluza J., Chopin C., Formstecher P., Marchetti P., Neviere R. Ventricular myocyte caspases are directly responsible for endotoxin-induced cardiac dysfunction. *Circulation*, 2005; 111(20): 2596-2604.

[14] Joseph W. Gordon, James A. Shaw, Lorrie A. Kirshenbaum. Multiple facets of NF-kappaB in the heart: to be or not to NF-kappaB. *Circ. Res.*, 2011; 108: 1122-1132.

[15] Jamerson M. H.; Johnson M. D.; Dickson R. B. Dual regulation of proliferation and apoptosis: c-myc in bitransgenic murine mammary tumor models. *Oncogene,* 2000; 19(8):1065-1071.

[16] Nam Y. J., Mani K., Ashton A. W., Peng C. F., Krishnamurthy B., Hayakawa Y., Lee P., Korsmeyer S. J., Kitsis R. N. Inhibition of both the extrinsic and intrinsic death pathways through nonhomotypic death-fold interactions. *Mol. Cell.,* 2004; 15(6): 901-912.

[17] Michae l A. Frohman. Mitochondria as integrators of signal transduction and energy production in cardiac physiology and disease. *J. Mol. Med.*, 2010; 88: 967-970.

[18] Song J., Liu K., Yi J., Zhu D., Liu G., Liu B. Luteolin inhibits lysophosphatidylcholine-induced apoptosis in endothelial cells by a calcium/mitocondrion/caspases-dependent pathway. *Planta Med.*, 2010; 76(5): 433-438.

[19] Fang F., Li D., Pan H., Chen D., Qi L., Zhang R., Sun H. Luteolin inhibits apoptosis and improves cardiomyocyte contractile function through the PI3K/Akt pathway in simulated ischemia / reperfusion. *Pharmacology,* 2011; 88(3-4): 149-158.

[20] Qi L., Pan H., Li D., Fang F., Chen D., Sun H. Luteolin improves contractile function and attenuates apoptosis following ischemia-reperfusion in adult rat cardiomyocytes. *Eur. J. Pharmacol.*, 2011; 668(1-2): 201-207.33.

[21] Yang X. M., Proctor J. B., Cui L., Krieg T., Downey J. M., Cohen M. V. Multiple, brief coronary occlusions during early reperfusion protect rabbit hearts by targeting cell signaling pathways. *J. Am. Coll. Cardiol.*, 2004; 44(5): 1103-1110.

[22] Mullonkal C. J., Toledo-Pereyra L. H. Akt in ischemia and reperfusion. *J. Invest. Surg.*, 2007; 20(3): 195-203.

[23] Li C., Tian J., Li G., Jiang W., Xing Y., Hou J., Zhu H., Xu H., Zhang G., Liu Z., Ye Z. Asperosaponin VI protects cardiac myocytes from hypoxia-induced apoptosis via activation of the PI3K/Akt and CREB pathways. *Eur. J. Pharmacol.*, 2010; 649(1-3): 100-107.

[24] Matsui T., Tao J., del Monte F., Lee K. H., Li L., Picard M., Force T. L., Franke T. F., Hajjar R. J., Rosenzweig A. Akt activation preserves cardiac function and prevents injury after transient cardiac ischemia in vivo. *Circulation*, 2001; 104(3): 330-335.

[25] Rose B. A., Force T., Wang Y. Mitogen-activated protein kinase signaling in the heart angels versus demons in a heart-breaking tale. *Physiol. Rev.*, 2010; 90(4): 1507-1546.

[26] Young Choi, Ji Hyun Choi, Hana Yoon et al. Luteolin induces apoptosis through endoplasmic reticulum stress and mitochondrial dysfunction in Neuro-2a mouse neuroblastoma cells. *European Journal of Pharmacology*, 2011;668: 115-126.

[27] Gutie ´rrez-Venegas G., Bando-Campos C. G. The flavonoids luteolin and quercetagetin inhibit lipoteichoic acid actions on H9c2 cardiomyocytes. *International Immunopharmacology,* 2010;10: 1003–1009.

[28] Xin Wu, Tongda Xu, Dongye Li, Shasha Zhu, Qiuping Chen, Wenjing Hu, Defeng Pan, Hong Zhu, Hong Sun. ERK/PP1a/PLB/SERCA2a and JNK Pathways Are Involved in Luteolin-Mediated Protection of Rat Hearts and Cardiomyocytes following Ischemia/Reperfusion. *PLoS One*, 2013;8(12);e82957.

[29] Boengler K., Hilfiker-Kleiner D., Drexler H., Heusch G., Schulz R. The myocardial JAK/STAT pathway: from protection to failure. *Pharmacol. Ther.*, 2008; 120(2): 172-185.

[30] Lecour S., Suleman N., Deuchar G. A., et al. Pharmacological preconditioning with tumor necrosis factor-alpha activates signal transducer and activator of transcription-3 at reperfusion without involving classic prosurvival kinases (Akt and extracellular signal-regulated kinase). *Circulation,* 2005; 112(25): 3911-3918.

[31] Wagner M.; Siddiqui M. A. Signaling networks regulating cardiac myocyte survival and death. *Curr. Opin. Investig. Drugs*, 2009; 10(9): 928-937.

[32] Hu C., Chen J., Dandapat A., Fujita Y., Inoue N., Kawase Y., Jishage K., Suzuki H., Li D., Hermonat P. L., Sawamura T., Mehta J. L. LOX-1 abrogation reduces myocardial ischemia-reperfusion injury in mice. *J. Mol. Cell. Cardiol.*, 2008; 44 (1):76-83.

[33] Lv L., Lv L., Zhang Y., Kong Q. Luteolin Prevents LPS-Induced TNFα Expression in Cardiac myocytes through inhibiting NF-κB signaling pathway. *Inflammation,* 2011; 34(6): 620-629.

[34] Juan-Zhang, Hong-Jun Bian, Xiao-Xing Li et al. ERK-MAPK signaling opposes rho-kinase to reduce cardiomyocyte apoptosis in heart ischemic preconditioning. *MOL MED.*, 2010; 16 (7-8): 307-315.

[35] Zhang J., et al. Inhibition of the activity of Rho-kinase reduces cardiomyocyte apoptosis in heart ischemia/reperfusion via suppressing JNK-mediated AIF translocation. *Clin. Chim. Acta.,* 2009; 401: 76–80.

[36] E. Shen, Yanwen Li, Ying Li et al. Rac1 is required for cardiomyocyte apoptosis during hyperglycemia. *Diabetes*, 2009; 58: 2386-2395.

[37] SunnyYang Xiang, Davy Vanhoutte, Dominic P. Del et al. RhoA protects the mouse heart against ischemia/reperfusion injury. *J. Clin. Invest.*, 2011; 121(8): 3269-3276.

[38] Zeenat S. Hakim, Laura A. DiMichele, Mauricio Rojas et al. FAK regulates cardiomyocyte survival following ischemia/reperfusion. *Journal of Molecular and Cellular Cardiology,* 2009; 46: 241-248.

[39] Youngil Lee Asa B. Gustafsson. Role of apoptosis in cardiovascular disease. *Apoptosis,* 2009; 14: 536-548.

[40] Soochan Bae, Bhargavi Yalamarti, Peter M. Kang. Role of caspase-independent apoptosis in cardiovascular diseases.*Frontiers in Bioscience*, 2008; 13: 2495-2503.

[41] Liao P. H., Hung L. M., Chen Y. H., Kuan Y. H., Zhang F. B., Lin R. H., Shih H. C., Tsai S. K., Huang S. S. Cardioprotective effects of luteolin during ischemia reperfusion injury in rats. *Circ. J.,* 2011;75: 443-450.

[42] Qian L. B., Lu J. F., Ye Z. G., Wang H. P., Xia Q. Luteolin reduces cardiac dysfunctions in streptozotocin-induced diabetic rats. *Zhongguo Ying Yong Sheng Li Xue Za Zhi[Article in Chinese]*, 2011; 27(4): 409-414.

[43] futao Zhou, Lina Qu, Ke Lv et al. Luteolin protects against reactive oxygen species-mediated cell death induced by zinc toxicity via the PI3K-Akt-NF-kappaB-ERK-dependent pathway. *Journal of Neuroscience Research*, 2011; 89: 1859-1868.

[44] Prema S. Rao, Arun Satelli, Majid Moridani et al. Luteolin induces apoptosis in multidrug resistant cancer cells without affecting the drug transporter function: involvement of cell line-specific apoptotic mechanisms. *Int. J. Cancer*, 2011; 1-12.

[45] Gutiérrez-Venegas G., Bando-Campos C. G. The flavonoids luteolin and quercetagetin inhibit lipoteichoic acid actions on H9c2 cardiomyocytes. *Int. Immunopharmacol.,* 2010; 10(9):1003-1009.

[46] Guo Guang Wang, Xiao Hua Lu, Wei Li et al. Protective effects of luteolin on diabetic nephropathy in STZ-induced diabetic rats. *Evidence-Based Complementary and Alternative Medicine,* 2011; 1-7.

[47] Kim H. S., Cho J. E., Hwang K. C., Shim Y. H., Lee J. H., Kwak Y. L. Diabetes mellitus mitigates cardioprotective effects of remifentanil preconditioning in ischemia-reperfused rat heart in association with anti-apoptotic pathways of survival. *Eur. J. Pharmacol.*, 2010; 628(1-3): 132-139.

[48] Sun D., Huang J., Zhang Z., Gao H., Li J., et al. Luteolin limits infarct size and improves cardiac function after myocardium ischemia/reperfusion injury in diabetic rats. *PLoS One*, 2012; 7(3): e33491.

[49] Liam Portt, Grant Norman, Caitlin Clapp,et al. Anti-apoptosis and cell survival: a review. *Biochimica et Biophysica Acta.*, 2011; 1813: 238 –259.

[50] Lang Y,, Chen D,, Li D,, et al. Luteolin inhibited hydrogen peroxide-induced vascular smooth muscle cells proliferation and migration by suppressing the Src and Akt signaling pathways. *J. Pharm. Pharmacol.*, 2012; 64(4): 597-603.

In: Myocardial Infarctions
Editor: Pattie Wilkonson

ISBN: 978-1-63321-726-3

Chapter 7

Essential Roles of Monocytes/Macrophages in Acute Myocardial Infarction

Makoto Orii, MD, Toshio Imanishi*[*]*, MD, PhD
and Takashi Akasaka, MD, PhD
Department of Cardiovascular Medicine, Wakayama Medical University, Wakayama, Japan

Abstract

Despite improvements in interventional and pharmacological therapy of acute coronary syndrome (ACS), it is still the leading cause of death.

Hence, there is a need for further development of effective therapeutic approaches. This requires better understanding of the molecular mechanisms and pathophysiology of the disease.

During the long-term process of initiation and progression of an atherosclerotic plaque, monocytes/macrophages plays a major role in this process. Macrophages, which are differentiated from circulating monocytes, give rise to foam cells by excessive accumulation of modified lipoproteins. Atherogenesis subsequently progress through necrotic core expansion associated with the death of macrophage, followed by the transition to vulnerable plaques.

The transition from stable atherosclerotic plaques to rupture of the atherosclerotic plaque, finally resulting in acute thrombus formation in ACS is the consequence of an inflammatory process. It is well recognized that plaque growth is not continuous and plaque rupture may suddenly occur during the acute inflammatory phase.

Here, we discuss the impact of monocytes/macrophages on both advanced plaque progression and onset of ACS, focusing on the potential targeting of inflammatory process in atherosclerosis.

[*] Name and complete address for correspondance: Toshio Imanishi, MD, PhD. Department of Cardiovascular Medicine, Wakayama Medical University; 811-1, Kimiidera, Wakayama, 641-8510, Japan. Phone: +81-73-441-0621, Fax: +81-73-446-0631; E-mail: t-imani@wakayama-med.ac.jp.

1. Introduction

Acute coronary syndrome (ACS) refers to a clinical spectrum ranging from those for ST-segment elevation myocardial infarction (STEMI) to non-STEMI or unstable angina. ACS is almost always associated with rupture of an atherosclerotic plaque and partial or complete thrombosis of the infarct-related artery. Most cases of ACS occur from disruption of a previously non-occlusive but vulnerable plaque. The characteristic features of a vulnerable plaque include a thin fibrous cap, a higher predominance of macrophages in the cap, smaller collagen content, and a large, lipid-rich necrotic core with overlying thrombus and platelet aggregates. An understanding of the pathogenesis of ACS may provide novel strategies to target against inflammatory processes in ACS.

1. Experimental Lessons

Inflammatory Professionals

Neutrophils, mast cells, and platelets are detectable in lesions and may impact on atherosclerosis and its complications. Neutrophils, the inflammatory granulocytes, circulate in large numbers and accumulate early on at sites of injury or infection. In experimental atherosclerosis, increased recruitment of neutrophils from bone marrow help monocyte adhesion and other preformed granular proteins [1]. Neutrophils also contain large quantities of myeloperoxidase, nicotinamide adenine dinucleotide phosphate (NADPH) oxidase, and lipoxygenases, which contribute to oxidative stress, a major determinant of endothelial cell dysfunction, lesion growth, and vulnerability. Mast cells, best known for their role in allergy and anaphylaxis, also promote atherosclerosis by releasing the contents of their protease-cytokine-autacoid–rich granules [2]. Platelets play an essential, dual role. During atherosclerosis, they adhere to the endothelium and help monocytes enter lesions [3]. During plaque rupture, they form the thrombus through interaction with red blood cells that causes ischemia of downstream tissue [4]. Thus, neutrophils, mast cells, and platelets all promote atherosclerosis by intensifying inflammation.

Leukocytes

Small atherosclerotic lesions that do not affect blood flow are found in many people. If coronary arterial stenosis reaches more than 80%, cardiac ischemia occurs, especially when a high cardiac work load increases oxygen demand. On the other hands, plaque rupture, which is precipitated by leukocyte action, suddenly occludes the artery and causes ACS. In contrast to atherosclerosis, where chronic low-grade stimulation by native and oxidized lipoproteins mobilizes leukocytes to the vessel wall, in ACS, acutely dying myocytes elicit different triggers that nevertheless recruit similar classes of leukocytes. In response to the ACS, the leukocyte profile in the myocardium changes drastically. The population of macrophages [5] and dendritic cells (DC) [6] that reside in the healthy heart is quickly overwhelmed by inflammatory leukocytes. Shortly after onset of ischemia, endothelial cells up-regulate adhesion molecules that, along with released chemokines, trigger neutrophil extravasation.

Rapid accumulation leads to an early neutrophil peak after injury [7]. In the ischemic heart, neutrophils phagocytose dead tissue and release inflammatory mediators: an immunological misfire aimed at myocytes that survived the ischemic injury. It is believed that neutrophils are deleterious in ACS, but they eventually undergo apoptosis and are removed by macrophages.

Circulating Monocyte Recruitment

Monocytes account for 3% to 8% of peripheral blood leukocytes. They are mononuclear cells often characterized by typical kidney-like shaped nuclei, but they are more accurately described by their expression of various surface receptors [8].

High trafficking ability is another characteristic feature of monocytes. A hallmark of monocyte trafficking is the capacity of monocytes to traverse from the circulation into areas of injury/inflammation, aiming for resolution of inflammation and contribution to the restoration of the tissue integrity via differentiation of different types of tissue macrophages and DC. However, "reparative" properties of the monocytes might fail and lead to a disease state, with atherosclerosis being an example. Indeed, monocytes are precursors of lipid-laden "foam" cell macrophages, which are a critical component of atherosclerotic plaques. Even mature monocyte-derived macrophages do not lose their mobility entirely, under certain circumstances monocyte/macrophages, including "foam cells" can migrate from the vascular wall back into the circulation [9].

Atherogenesis and Plaque Neovascularization

Atherosclerosis is characterized by monocyte adherence to endothelial cell, migration into the arterial wall, and lipid accumulation [10]. The earliest detectable atherosclerotic change is pathological intimal thickening [11]. Enlargement of the plaque results in intraplaque hypoxia that triggers the inflammatory cell infiltration, thus promoting local neovascularization [12]. Evidence of the role of ischemia in the initiation of angiogenesis stems from the demonstration of increased levels of hypoxia inducible factor (HIF-1), which ultimately promotes vascular endothelial growth factor (VEGF) production [13,14]. As a potent stimulator of angiogenesis, VEGF is consequently able to create a local pro-angiogenic environment by mobilizing endothelial progenitor cells (EPCs) [15]. Furthermore, aggressive plaque development and accelerated neovascularization of the vascular wall have been seen following the administration of VEGF in laboratory experiments [16]. Hypoxia-independent pathways triggered by an inflammatory stimulation within the vascular wall have also been recognized as modulators of angiogenesis [17]. The density of intraplaque vessels corresponds to the focal accumulation of monocytes/macrophages forming a pathological circle [18]. Switching between this inflammatory/angiogenic cascade may be responsible for enhanced plaque progression related to local plaque inflammation and plaque destabilization. This hypothesis is supported by increased expression of leukocyte adhesion molecules, such as vascular adhesion molecule-1 (VCAM-1) and intracellular adhesion molecule-1 (ICAM-1), on the intimal side of vascular endothelium as opposed to the adventitial side [19]. Therefore, these observations suggest that the presence of these adhesion molecules on the newly formed vessels is associated with the enhanced accumulation of leukocytes [19]. The primary pathological focus of this evidence has been on understanding the atherosclerosis-related angiogenesis in plaque formation, and the inhibition of neovascularization thereby attempting to slow the disease progression [20]. VEGF expressed by macrophages and T-lymphocytes stimulate endothelial cells to produce monocyte chemoattractant protein (MCP)-1, hence attracting monocytes and enhancing cell migration by increasing the permeability of the endothelial layer [21,22]. Angiogenesis is defined by the sprouting of new vessels from pre-existing vasculatureis. Angiogenic signals from surrounding cells lead to vasodilatation and an increase in vascular permeability [23, 24]. Ultimately, the newly formed capillaries become part of the existing circulation in a process in which shear stress is a critical factor [25]. The behavior of endothelial cells is significantly influenced by inflammatory leukocytes, which release the number of proangiogenic factors, such as VEGF, hepatocyte growth factor, and tumor necrosis factor- (TNF)-α, and interleukin (IL)-8 [26,27]. In atherogenic lesions, chronic infection, cigarette smoking, free radicals, hypertension, and diabetes have all been implicated as causes in the activation of endothelial cells (Figure 1) [25,28]. The increased shear stress acting through both membrane structures and cell junction molecules, stimulate quiescent endothelial cells lining the vascular wall [29]. This intracellular signaling triggers the expression of genes such as MCP-1 mRNA, involved in induction of transcription factors responsible for shear stress-mediated effects [24,30]. This sequence of events in the presence of hypercholesterolemia triggers expression of adhesion molecules, particularly P-selectin, E-selectin, VCAM-1, ICAM-1, and MCP-1 release and activation of genes responsible for the expression of CCR2 (MCP-1 receptor) (Figure 1) [24,31].

Monocytes in Angiogenesis

VEGF, expressed by macrophages activates the production of MCP-1 by the endothelial cells and an increase in the permeability of the endothelial layer [25]. The chronic low-grade inflammation inside the vascular wall has been shown to be associated with monocyte infiltration. The monocyte maturation to macrophages is accompanied by the production of cytokines and growth factors [27,32]. The monocytes produce platelet-derived growth factor, which induces mitotic activity of the endothelial cells and vascular smooth muscle cells (VSMCs) [33]. Activated plaque monocytes/macrophages ingest the oxidized lipids and become lipid-laden " foam" cells (Figure 1). It is believed that "foam" cells promote vascular remodeling by stimulation of VSMCs migration and a subsequent shift in endothelial dysfunction [34]. Once monocytes have infiltrated the tissue layers, a proportion of them will differentiate into DC triggering the activation of antigen specific T lymphocytes associated with creation of the local inflammatory environment [35]. A large proportion of circulating EPCs was found to be of monocytic origin [36]. Human monocytes include a population of cells able to obtain endothelial cell phenotype in culture [37]. Cultures of so-called "early" EPCs are mainly comprised of monocytes and T-cells and their formation is strictly dependent upon monocyte presence [38]. Cells bearing CD14 are capable of improving re-endothelialization after carotid balloon injury in animals and this process depends on the levels of a major factor stimulating monocyte mobilization, MCP-1 [39].

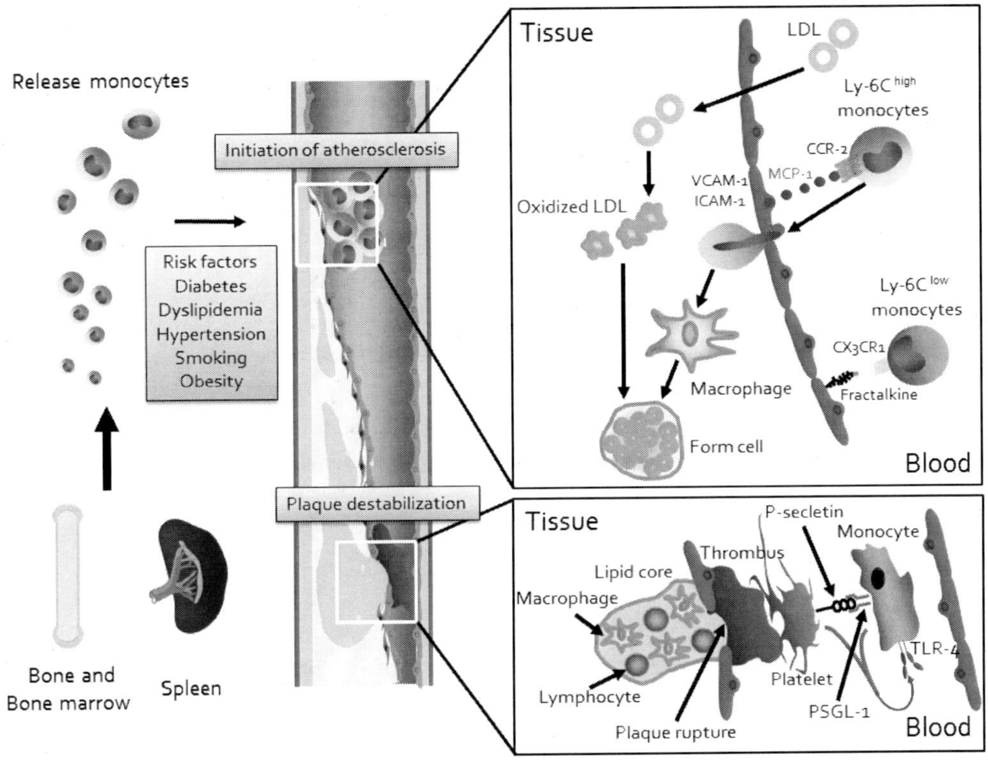

Figure 1. Monocytes at different stages of the atherosclerotic process.
Monocytes are made in bone marrow (medullary hematopoiesis) and spleen (extra-medullary hematopoiesis). Monocytes patrolling in the circulation are activated by a number of chemokines and cytokines. They traffic to the damaged and/or activated endothelium. The dysfunctional endothelium over-express monocyte chemotactic protein-1 ligand and adhesion molecules (vascular cell adhesion molecule [VCAM]-1, intercellular adhesion molecule [ICAM]-1) on its surface. Ly-6C^{high} monocytes are recruited via monocyte chemoattractant protein (MCP)-1. After attachment to the endothelium, the monocytes cross the endothelial surface. Ly-6C^{high} monocytes accumulate preferentially in the lesion and differentiate to macrophages via macrophage colony stimulating factor. The macrophages ingest oxidized low-density lipoprotein (LDL) via scavenger receptors forming "foam" cells. These undergo a process of apoptosis/necrosis that perpetuates the formation of further lipid-laden macrophages. Ly-6C^{low} monocytes patrol the vasculature and enter lesions less frequently. During an acute coronary syndrome (ACS) with plaque rupture, thinning of the fibrous cap on plaque surface, and monocyte platelet aggregates are shown. Monocytes have a role in thrombus propagation contributing to the coagulation cascade during an ACS. Moreover, monocytes accumulated within thrombus specifically overexpress Toll-like receptor (TLR)-4. CCR: CC chemokine receptor, MCP: monocyte chemoattractant protein, TLR: Toll-like receptor, PSGL-1: P-selectin glycoprotein ligand-1.

Monocyte Subset in Early Atherosclerosis

Monocytes contribute to atherogenesis through promoting leukocyte recruitment to plaques, and their roles are also mediated by activation of downstream signaling pathways, such as nuclear factor kappa-B pathway [40]. In mice, monocytes are divided into a Ly-6C^{high} CX3CR1^{low} CCR2+ subset that is actively recruited into inflamed tissue and a Ly-6C^{low} CX3CR1^{high} CCR2- subset that home into non-inflamed tissues (Figure 1) [41]. The Ly-6C^{high}

monocytes are increased in blood during hypercholesterolaemia and are preferentially recruited to atherosclerotic plaques by the use of CCR2 and CX3CR1 receptors [42,43]. In contrast, Ly-6C^{low} monocytes have been shown to enter plaques less frequently than Ly-6C^{high} monocytes, but they are, on the other hand, more prone to develop into plaque resident cells [43]. Despite a high expression of CX3CR1, the Ly-6C^{low} monocytes depend mainly on CCR5 to enter plaques [43]. The mobilization of classical Ly-6C^{high} monocytes from bone marrow is severely impaired in the absence of CCR2, resulting in reduced numbers of this monocyte subset in blood, which could contribute to reduced atherosclerosis [44]. Absence of CX3CR1 affects survival of Ly-6C^{low} monocytes, as CX3CR1 seems to mediate growth factor like signals, resulting in reduced Ly-6C^{low} monocyte levels [45]. Notably, when the three chemokine pathways CCR2, CX3CR1 and CCR5 are simultaneously targeted, atherosclerosis in mice is almost completely abrogated [46]. During atherosclerosis development in mice, the spleen supplements the haematopoietic function of the bone marrow by producing Ly-6C^{high} monocytes that readily accumulate in the aorta [47].

Monocytes in Atherosclerosis Progression

Uncontrolled lipid accumulation followed by rapid monocyte infiltration and phagocytosis of low-density lipoprotein mediated by scavenger receptors subsequently results in macrophage apoptosis. This process increases the atherosclerotic plaque core with ensuing necrotic tissue, collagen deposition and VSMCs migration [24]. Monocyte activation by the interaction with toll-like receptors (TLR) promotes both angiogenesis and plaque growth and destabilization.

Toll-like Receptor

Monocytes accumulated within thrombus following by percutaneous coronary interventions, specifically overexpress TLR-4, chemokines and inflammatory cytokines compared with circulating monocytes (Figure 1) [48,49]. TLRs are key pattern-recognition receptors expressed by innate immunity cells, and they can recognize a large number of molecules named pathogen-associated molecular patterns; they are usually expressed by pathogens but are absent in normal mammal tissues. Niessner et al. [50] demonstrated that interferon (IFN)-α produced by plasmacytoid DC in atherosclerotic plaques could enhance TLR-4 signaling by sensitizing these cells to lipopolysaccharide and other microbial molecules but also to endogenous molecules, all abundantly present in the atherosclerotic lesion microenvironment. These sensitized antigen-presenting cells strongly up-regulate the production of cytokines such as tumor necrosis factor (TNF)-α, interleukin (IL)-12, IL-23, and matrix metalloproteinases (MMPs)-9, thus enhancing plaque instability.

Plaque Instability and Rupture

An atheromatous plaque is responsible for approximately 75% of ACS. Neovascularization has been implicated as a possible contributor to the process by the progression of fibroatheromatous plaque into plaque rupture, although the precise mechanism remains unclear. As the plaque progresses, the adventitial vasa vasorum plays a pivotal role in the formation of vessels [51]. Indeed, the presence of neo-vessels within the plaque has been associated to its rupture [51]. In a comparison of stable plaques to those in both vulnerable and ruptured plaques, there is a 2- to 4-fold increase in the number of vasa vasorum, respectively [52]. Although plaque deposits themselves may be localized and unique, the changes found in the arterial wall vascularization are known to be systemically widespread, lending to the notion of atherosclerosis being a panarterial disease [53]. However the factors that trigger the change, from a nonthreatening to unstable plaque remains poorly understood.

The synthesis of pro-inflammatory molecules such as IL-6 and TNF-α, mediated by stimulation of TLR4 are augmented by activated monocytes [38]. The interaction among CD14, a monocyte endotoxin receptor, acting together with a coreceptor, TLR, results in monocytic activation [54]. This monocyte activation subsequently enhances the affinity of monocyte ligands to adhesion molecules, thus promoting monocyte–endothelium adhesion [54]. This has been demonstrated by the presence of microvessels within lipid-rich plaques strongly expressing adhesion molecules (ICAM-1, VCAM-1) thereby facilitating transendothelial migration of monocytes into the plaque microenvironment (Figure 1) [19]. This implicates the potential involvement of monocytes and their role in plaque neovascularization and plaque rupture.

Monocyte Subset in ACS

Monocytes promote destabilization of the fibrous cap leading to the plaque rupture. This is mainly orchestrated by MMPs [55,56]. Activated macrophages produce a wide range of lytic enzymes, including MMPs (e.g., MMP-1, -2, -3, -8, -9, and -14) [57]. Increased expression and activity of MMPs has been noted in vulnerable plaque regions, whereas elevated serum MMPs have been demonstrated in patients with ACS [58]. Plaque rupture could lead to downstream occlusion of coronary flow to the myocardium, the principle mechanism of ACS. Monocytes have a role in thrombus propagation contributing to the coagulation cascade during the acute event. Patients with ACS show features of procoagulant monocyte activation with exposure of tissue factor [59]. Monocyte-platelet aggregates, and markers of monocyte and platelet activation involved in regulation of their function are also increased in ACS patients, persisting even after one month of the acute event [60]. Also, microparticles derived from monocytes are abundant in ACS and support faster fibrin formation [61]. Monocyte adherence to extracellular matrix and extravasation to the injured tissue induces the expression of a multitude of cytokines, including TNF-α, IL-1 and IL-6; platelet-derived endothelial cell growth factor; transforming growth factor (TGF)-α and -β; macrophage colony-stimulating factor, and insulin-like growth factor [62,63].

ACS is a severe traumatic event that mobilizes multiple organ systems. A substantial number of the initially recruited monocytes derives from a reservoir in the splenic red pulp, where increased renin-angiotenssin system triggers their mobilization within hours after injury [64]. For the first few days after infarction, leukocyte recruitment remains at astonishing levels [65]. To meet the demand, cell production increases in the bone marrow and the spleen. Pain and anxiety during ACS alert the sympathetic nervous system and activate neuroimmune synapses [66].

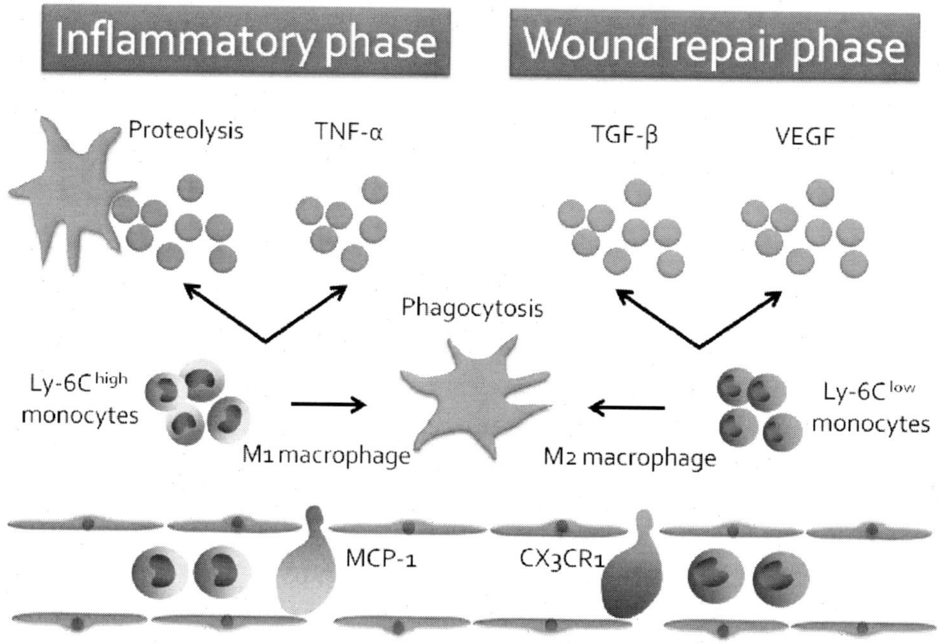

Figure 2. Biphasic monocyte and macrophage response.
In a first phase, inflammatory Ly-6C^{high} monocytes are recruited via monocyte chemoattractant protein (MCP)-1. Ly-6C^{high} monocytes differentiate into M1 type, classically activated macrophages that affect proteolysis and inflammation. In a second phase, Ly-6C^{low} monocytes accumulate via CX3CL1. Ly-6C^{low} monocytes differentiate into M2 type, alternatively activated macrophages that involved in wound repair and tissue remodeling. MCP: monocyte chemoattractant protein, TNF: tumor necrosis factor, TGF: transforming growth factor, VEGF: vascular endothelial growth factor.

A mouse model of ACS has demonstrated substantial functional differences between monocyte subsets in the course of the infarction (Figure 2). For instance, inflammatory Ly-6C^{high} monocytes (considered to be equivalent to CD14++ CD16- CCR2+ human cells) are among the earliest responders. Distressed tissue expresses CCL2 [67], which attracts Ly-6C^{high} monocytes during the first several days, after which the wounded heart switches to CX3CL1-mediated recruitment of Ly-6C^{low} monocytes (considered to be the equivalent of human CD14^{+}CD16^{++}CCR2^{-} cells) (Table 1) [7]. The cause of the switch is unknown, but sequentially accumulating monocyte subsets do pursue differential functions in the infarct. Although both are phagocytic, the early inflammatory subset is particularly rich in proinflammatory mediators. These include proteases, which are tightly regulated to balance wound debridement with tissue destabilization, because unchecked proteolysis may cause infarct expansion or even rupture. During resolution of inflammation, reparative Ly-6C^{low} monocytes support angiogenesis and extracellular matrix synthesis by providing VEGF and TGF-β (Figure 2) (Table 1) [7]. Whether Ly-6C^{high} and Ly-6C^{low} monocytes give rise to distinct macrophage subsets in the infarcted myocardium is unknown, but more intriguing is the possibility that monocytes, as monocytes, impose a lasting effect on the tissue environment before differentiating (or dying or exiting). Decades of research have argued that macrophages are highly susceptible to micro-environmental cues. Perhaps recruited monocytes influence a tissue in a manner that long-seeded, sessile macrophages no longer can. Lymphocytes are present in low numbers in the infarct and proliferate in draining lymph nodes shortly after ischemic injury [68]. $CD4^+$ T cell deficiency delays the transition from Ly-$6C^{high}$ to Ly-$6C^{low}$ monocyte presence and impairs healing of the heart. Likewise, depletion of DC disturbs resolution of inflammation [69]. At the other end of the monocyte differentiation spectrum, levels of circulating DC (both plasmacytoid as well as myeloid DCs) have been found to be significantly reduced in patients after an ACS, compared with healthy control subjects [70]. It is thought that this is due to increased recruitment of DC to the infarcted tissue. This hypothesis was supported with immunohistochemistry findings indicating an increase in the DC and T-cell infiltration of peri-infarct zone [71]. These observations suggest a link to adaptive immunity, but it is unclear, given that ACS is a form of sterile injury, whether any processed peptide antigens are recognized and presented. ACS may be mobilizing elements of adaptive immunity without necessarily relying on its essential mechanisms. The emerging picture positions leukocytes as both protective and harmful in ACS. Ly-$6C^{high}$ monocytes, for example, are required during the initial response to ischemia but can also be destructive if they persist in the infarct too long. Ly-$6C^{low}$ monocytes, on the other hand, are probably essential to wound repair (Figure 2) [7,65]. Optimal healing requires balance: Sequential and coordinated cell recruitment that removes dead tissue and strengthens the wound so that the heart performs its vital function is a manifestation of that balance [7].

Table 1. Comparison of different monocyte subsets and functions

Characteristic		Inflammatory/Classical	Newly Described Intermediate Population	Resident/Non classical
Human		CD14++CD16-CCR2+	CD14++CD16+CCR2+	CD14+CD16++CCR2-
Mice		Ly6-C^{high} CX3CR1^{low} CCR2+	No distinct model is available; however, has characteristics of Ly6-C^{high} models	Ly6C^{low} CX3CR1^{high} CCR2-
Recruitment		Early in acute inflammation	Early in acute inflammation	Late in acute inflammation
Reservoirs		Spleen	Unknown	Unknown
Function	Acute	Accumulate in injured myocardium and perform inflammatory and proteolytic function	Inflammation?	Assumed role in granulation tissue formation and angiogenesis, later mobilization
	Chronic	Accumulate in atherosclerotic plaque in response to activated endothelium		Accumulate in atherosclerotic plaque via CCR5 and CX3CR1

Monocyte Heterogeneity in Human

Over the last 30 years, human monocyte subsets were distinguished based on their surface CD14 and CD16 expressions as " classical" $CD14^{++}CD16^-$ cells and less frequent "nonclassical" $CD14^+CD16^{++}$ blood monocytes [72]. More accurate delineation of $CD14^{++}CD16^+$ and $CD14^+CD16^{++}$ monocytes can be achieved by additional marker CCR2

[73], with "intermediate" monocytes being "$CD14^{++}CD16^{+}$ $CCR2^{+}$" and "non-classical" monocytes being "$CD14^{+}CD16^{++}CCR2^{-}$" (Table 1). These $CD14^{++}CD16^{+}CCR2^{+}$ monocytes phenotypically resemble the previously reported pro-angiogenic monocytes [73]. The identification of each subset thus allows further research into their respective physiological functions. Ziegler-Heitbrock et al. [74] showed that $CD14^{+}CD16^{+}$ monocytes have some features common with mature tissue macrophages. However, animal-based studies on monocyte subsets are controversial due to substantial differences between human and murine monocyte subsets [75]. Nahrendorf et al. [7] compared monocytes in a model of mouse myocardial infarction and suggested that specific signaling may depend on site and type of hypoxia/ischemia insult and time of recovery from this injury.

Although 3 monocyte subsets are now recognized, the majority of published studies only refer to 2 monocyte subpopulations (i.e., $CD14^{+}CD16^{-}$ and $CD14^{+}CD16^{+}$ monocytes) without further subdivision of the $CD16^{+}$ cells, and thus careful interpretation of such data is required. The $CD16^{+}$ monocytes are infrequent (less than 15% in healthy humans), but their proportions are increased in patients with stable angina pectoris, and ACS, being related to the up-regulation of inflammatory cytokines [60,76]. These data may indicate a possible role of $CD16^{+}$ monocytes for the advanced inflammation-mediated intraplaque angiogenesis. However, the relation of monocyte populations to systemic atherosclerosis (intima-media thickness, adventitial vasa vasorum) and high-risk indices for plaque destabilization remains unclear. Subset specificity may also be dependent on expression of multiple receptors and MCP-1 mediated signaling [77]. Indeed, angiogenesis and monocyte subset involvement is a multiple stepwise process, which consists of 2 areas of recruitment, local and bone marrow, which are specific to the stimulating environment [77]. Further studies would be needed to delineate the specific functions of each of the monocyte subsets, their specific roles in plaque progression, stability, and rupture.

Macrophage

The relative contribution of macrophage exit and/or death may indeed be critical to how disease progresses. On the one hand, efficient macrophage exit [78], or reduced monocyte influx [79], is central to regression; when lesions regress, macrophage numbers diminish. On the other hand, limited macrophage death, effective efferocytosis (phagocytosis of dead cells), and active autophagy are fundamental to lesional stability [80]; lesions with large necrotic cores are most vulnerable. A macrophage is not simply "a big eater," however, and it does not exist in isolation. Regional macrophages are poly-functional and interact with other leukocytes and non-leukocyte client cells. Macrophage poly-functionality represents either dedicated behavior of individually specialized cells (distinct macrophage subsets) or adaptive behavior elicited by the tissue environment (macrophage plasticity).

Macrophages are currently considered to comprise 2 types: the classically activated (pro-inflammatory M1 type), which are differentiated from Ly-$6C^{high}$ monocyte and promote inflammation, are typically activated by lipopolysaccharide in the presence of IFN-γ, leading to the production of high level of IL-2, IL-23, IL-6, IL-1, and TNF-α; and the alternatively activated M2, which are differentiated from Ly-$6C^{low}$ monocyte acting as anti inflammatory cells (Figure 2) [62]. The M1 macrophages promote inflammation and extracellular matrix destruction. The IL-1b secretion from M1 induces MMP-9 and TGF-β secretion and stimulates fibroblast proliferation [62]. Macrophage phagocytosis of dying cells also triggers TGF-β production [81]. An imbalance in macrophage subsets (relative increase M1 macrophages) may result in coronary plaque vulnerability.

Aside from, or perhaps in addition to, controlling LDL levels, a therapeutic goal for atherosclerosis may be to coax macrophage responses away from inflammation and proteolysis and toward robust cholesterol transport, intelligent cellular flux, and sustained efferocytosis. Therapeutic strategies should therefore aim to recalibrate the leukocyte response toward optimal healing. *In vivo* RNA interference is one strategy that can selectively silence CCR2 at defined time points, thus limiting the accumulation of Ly-6C^{high} monocytes in atherosclerotic plaques and the infarcted myocardium [65].

2. Clinical Studies and Therapy

In several studies monocyte migration from atherosclerotic plaques led to plaque regression under experimental conditions [82, 83]. In a mouse model, statin therapy augmented the regression of the plaque macrophages via removing the inhibitory effect on CCR7 and independently of lipid levels [84], possibly representing an additional pleiotropic effect of statins. In human, administration of statins to subjects with hypercholesterolemia inhibited the expression of monocyte proinflammatory cytokines (TNF and IL1β) and the treatment has been effective to reduce risk of unfavorable events in patients with stable coronary heart disease [85]. Moreover, although the relative magnitude of lipid independent pleiotropic effects of the statins remains unclear, long-term treatment with statins can prevent progression or even lead to regression of the atheroma.

CX3CR1 knockout mice fed on a high-fat diet showed a significant reduction in monocyte recruitment to the vascular wall and reduced atherosclerotic plaque formation. In fact, genetic deletions of CCL2, CX3CL1, or their cognate receptors, CCR2 and CX3CR1, markedly reduced atherosclerotic lesion size in murine models of atherosclerosis [86]. When the 3 chemokine receptors CCR5, CCR2, and CX3CR1 were blocked, the maximal reduction in the atherosclerotic plaque formation was evident, suggesting that all monocyte subpopulations are involved in atherogenesis [87].

Despite strong evidence in mice, Berg et al. found no association between CX3CR1 and CCR2 expression on monocytes and cardiovascular risk [88]. CCR5 expression on non-classical CD14^{+}CD16^{++} monocytes was, however, negatively associated to carotid IMT. Increased levels of classical CD14^{++}CD16^{-} monocytes at baseline were also associated with an increased risk for suffering cardiovascular events during a 15-year follow-up of 700 subjects from the Malmö Diet and Cancer Study population cohort [88]. The hazard ratio for suffering a cardiovascular event in the highest tertile of classical monocytes was 1.66 compared to the lowest tertile even after adjustment for common risk factors. The classical monocytes did not, however, associate with the extent of atherosclerosis, measured as intima-media thickness (IMT), at baseline. In contrast, the percentage of monocytes expressing CD16 was negatively associated to the extent of carotid atherosclerosis at baseline. This association was independent of other common risk factors. These data might indicate that different monocyte subsets have different biological functions in cardiovascular disease in humans. CD14^{++} CD16^{-} classical monocytes might cause inflammation that weakens the fibrous cap covering plaques and thus be associated with increased risk of clinical events, whereas $CD16^-$ expressing monocytes might play a role in determining the size of the plaque, perhaps even having a protective, or reparative, rather than plaque promoting function. Although the association of chemokine receptor expression on monocytes to cardiovascular risk is poorly understood, the potential to treat human disease by targeting chemokine receptors is emphasized by the fact that polymorphisms in the CX3CR1 gene have been found to protect against atherosclerosis [89-91]. Evidence also indicates that a naturally occurring frame-shift mutation in the human CCR5 gene is associated with lower carotid intima-media thickness in the common carotid artery and reduced cardiovascular disease risk [92]. Also, in mice, pharmacological intervention of several chemokine receptors has been proven to reduce atherosclerosis [93]. In addition, it has been speculated that several approved chemokine receptor antagonists, such as CCR5 antagonists approved for HIV therapy, could also limit plaque development [94]. At present, clinical studies targeting atherosclerosis with these compounds have, although not been initiated.

Limitations

The varying nomenclature used to describe monocytes poses a problem in unified interpretation of animal and human data. Because most of the current knowledge in the field originates from murine models, effort is directed toward establishment of parallels between monocyte subsets across species. Scarce information on their functions adds to the complexity of drawing reliable conclusions on the physiological and pathological roles of monocyte subsets in humans. For example, features of "intermediate" being "$CD14^{++}CD16^{+}CCR2^{+}$" and "non-classical" monocytes being "$CD14^{+}CD16^{++}CCR2^{-}$" are increasingly demonstrated and recognized in a wide range of pathological conditions. An "intermediate" pattern of the subset might be partly due to some overlap with "non-classical" monocytes, when their definition is solely based on their CD14 and CD16 expression. Of note, $CD14^{++}CD16^{+}$ monocytes show the highest of all monocyte expression of many surface receptors, particularly those involved in reparative processes. This, together with the evidence of specific enrichment of this subset in bone marrow, indicates that it is unlikely to just represent an "intermediate" state between the other 2 subsets but rather a unique and distinct monocyte subpopulation. Although it is not yet entirely clear whether specific monocyte subsets are pre-determined to differentiate into particular types of tissue macrophages and DC, published data suggest existence of common features and links between $CD14^{++}CD16^{-}$ and $CD14^{++}CD16^{+}$ monocytes and M1 and M2 polarized macrophages, respectively. Also in vivo, Ly-$6C^{low}$ and Ly-$6C^{high}$ monocytes from mice differentiate more readily into M2-like cells and M1-like macrophages, respectively, but macrophage development also depends on surrounding microenvironment and interaction with other cell types, such as lymphocytes [95, 96]. Accordingly, the assignment of numerical dominators for human monocyte subsets might not be appropriate until more data are available on the relationships between the subsets.

Conclusion

The development from stable atherosclerotic plaques to vulnerable plaque finally resulting in the onset ACS is the consequence of an inflammatory process. Detailed understanding of the mechanism of this process may provide us the novel therapeutic strategies in ACS patients.

References

[1] Drechsler M, Megens RT, et al. Hyperlipidemia-triggered neutrophilia promotes early atherosclerosis. *Circulation.* 2010;122:1837-45.

[2] Sun J, Sukhova GK, et al. Mast cells promote atherosclerosis by releasing proinflammatory cytokines. *Nat Med.* 2007;13:719-24.

[3] Huo Y, Schober A, et al. Circulating activated platelets exacerbate atherosclerosis in mice deficient in apolipoprotein E. *Nat Med.* 2003;9:61-7.

[4] Hansson GK, Libby P. The immune response in atherosclerosis: a double-edged sword. *Nat Rev Immunol.* 2006;6:508-19.

[5] Pinto AR, Paolicelli R, et al. An abundant tissue macrophage population in the adult murine heart with a distinct alternatively-activated macrophage profile. *PLoS One.* 2012;7:e36814.

[6] Choi JH, Do Y, et al. Identification of antigen-presenting dendritic cells in mouse aorta and cardiac valves. *J Exp Med.* 2009;206:497-505.

[7] Nahrendorf M, Swirski FK, et al. The healing myocardium sequentially mobilizes two monocyte subsets with divergent and complementary functions. *J Exp Med.* 2007;204:3037-47.

[8] Shalhoub J, Falck-Hansen MA, et al. Innate immunity and monocyte-macrophage activation in atherosclerosis. *J Inflamm* (Lond) 2011;8:9.

[9] Gratchev A, Sobenin I, et al. Monocytes as a diagnostic marker of cardiovascular diseases. *Immunobiology* 2012;217:476–82.

[10] Pietsch A, Erl W, et al. Lovastatin reduces expression of thecombined adhesion and scavenger receptor CD36 in human monocytic cells. *Biochem Pharmacol* 1996;52:433–9.

[11] de Groot E, van Leuven SI, et al. Measurement of carotid intima-media thickness to assess progression and regression of atherosclerosis. *Nat Clin Pract Cardiovasc Med* 2008;5:280–8.

[12] Kwon HM, Sangiorgi G, et al. Enhanced coronary vasa vasorum neovascularization in experimental hypercholesterolemia. *J Clin Invest* 1998;101:1551–6.

[13] Bjornheden T, Levin M, et al. Evidence of hypoxic areas within the arterial wall in vivo. *Arterioscler Thromb Vasc Biol* 1999;19:870–6.

[14] Kuwahara F, Kai H, et al. Hypoxia-inducible factor-1alpha/vascular endothelial growth factor pathway for adventitial vasa vasorum formation in hypertensive rat aorta. *Hypertension* 2002;39:46–50.

[15] Inoue M, Itoh H, et al. Vascular endothelial growth factor (VEGF) expression in human coronary atherosclerotic lesions: possible pathophysiological significance of VEGF in progression of atherosclerosis. *Circulation* 1998;98:2108–16.
[16] Celletti FL, Hilfiker PR, et al. Effect of human recombinant vascular endothelial growth factor 165 on progression of atherosclerotic plaque. *J Am Coll Cardiol* 2001;37:2126–30.
[17] Carmeliet P. Angiogenesis in health and disease. *Nat Med* 2003;9:653–60.
[18] Moulton KS, Vakili K, et al. Inhibition of plaque neovascularization reduces macrophage accumulation and progression of advanced atherosclerosis. *Proc Natl Acad Sci U S A* 2003;100:4736–41.
[19] O'Brien KD, McDonald TO, et al. Neovascular expression of E-selectin, intercellular adhesion molecule-1, and vascular cell adhesion molecule-1 in human atherosclerosis and their relation to intimal leukocyte content. Circulation 1996;93:672–82.
[20] Johnstone CC, Farley A. The physiological basics of wound healing. *Nurs Stand* 2005;19:59–65.
[21] Melter M, Reinders ME, et al. Ligation of CD40 induces the expression of vascular endothelial growth factor by endothelial cells and monocytes and promotes angiogenesis in vivo. *Blood* 2000;96:3801–8.
[22] Hong KH, Ryu J, et al. Monocyte chemoattractant protein-1-induced angiogenesis is mediated by vascular endothelial growth factor-A. *Blood* 2005;105:1405–7.
[23] Kimura H, Esumi H. Reciprocal regulation between nitric oxide and vascular endothelial growth factor in angiogenesis. *Acta Biochim Pol* 2003;50:49–59.
[24] Pamukcu B, Lip GY, et al. The role of monocytes in atherosclerotic coronary artery disease. *Ann Med* 2010;42:394–403.
[25] Marumo T, Schini-Kerth VB, et al. Vascular endothelial growth factor activates nuclear factor-kappaB and induces monocyte chemoattractant protein-1 in bovine retinal endothelial cells. *Diabetes* 1999;48:1131–7.
[26] Hoeben A, Landuyt B, et al. Vascular endothelial growth factor and angiogenesis. *Pharmacol Rev* 2004;56:549–80.
[27] Hoefer IE, van Royen N, et al. Direct evidence for tumor necrosis factor-alpha signaling in arteriogenesis. *Circulation* 2002;105:1639–41.
[28] Ross R. Atherosclerosisdan inflammatory disease. *N Engl J Med* 1999;340:115–26.
[29] Resnick N, Yahav H, et al. Fluid shear stress and the vascular endothelium: for better and for worse. *Prog Biophys Mol Biol* 2003;81:177–99.
[30] Ojeifo JO, Forough R, et al. Angiogenesisdirected implantation of genetically modified endothelial cells in mice. *Cancer Res* 1995;55:2240–4.
[31] Sadhu C, Ting HJ, et al. CD11c/CD18: novel ligands and a role in delayed-type hypersensitivity. *J Leukoc Biol* 2007;81:1395–403.
[32] Hoefer IE, van Royen N, et al. Arteriogenesis proceeds via ICAM-1/Mac-1- mediated mechanisms. *Circ Res* 2004; 94:1179–85.
[33] Polverini PJ, Cotran PS, et al. Activated macrophages induce vascular proliferation. *Nature* 1977;269:804–6.
[34] Kruth HS. Macrophage foam cells and atherosclerosis. *Front Biosci* 2001;6:D429-55.
[35] Randolph GJ, Beaulieu S, et al. Differentiation of monocytes into dendritic cells in a model of transendothelial trafficking. *Science* 1998;282:480–3.

[36] Shantsila E, Watson T, et al. Endothelial progenitor cells in cardiovascular disorders. *J Am Coll Cardiol* 2007;49:741–52.
[37] Fernandez Pujol B, Lucibello FC, et al. Endotheliallike cells derived from human CD14 positive monocytes. *Differentiation* 2000;65:287–300.
[38] Shantsila E, Lip GY. Monocytes in acute coronary syndromes. *Arterioscler Thromb Vasc Biol* 2009;29:1433–8.
[39] Fujiyama S, Amano K, et al. Bone marrow monocyte lineage cells adhere on injured endothelium in a monocyte chemoattractant protein-1-dependent manner and accelerate reendothelialization as endothelial progenitor cells. *Circ Res* 2003;93:980–9.
[40] de Winther MP, Kanters E, et al. Nuclear factor kappaB signaling in atherogenesis. *Arterioscler Thromb Vasc Biol* 2005;25:904–14.
[41] Geissmann F, Jung S, et al. Blood monocytes consist of two principal subsets with distinct migratory properties. *Immunity* 2003;19:71-82.
[42] Swirski FK, Libby P, et al. Ly-6Chi monocytes dominate hypercholesterolemia-associated monocytosis and give rise to macrophages in atheromata. *J Clin Invest* 2007;117:195-205.
[43] Tacke F, Alvarez D, et al. Monocyte subsets differentially employ CCR2, CCR5, and CX3CR1 to accumulate within atherosclerotic plaques. *J Clin Invest* 2007;117:185-94.
[44] Tsou CL, Peters W, et al. Critical roles for CCR2 and MCP-3 in monocyte mobilization from bone marrow and recruitment to inflammatory sites. *J Clin Invest* 2007;117:902-9.
[45] Landsman L, Bar-On L, et al. CX3CR1 is required for monocyte homeostasis and atherogenesis by promoting cell survival. *Blood* 2009;113:963-72.
[46] Combadiere C, Potteaux S, et al. Combined inhibition of CCL2, CX3CR1, and CCR5 abrogates Ly6C(hi) and Ly6C(lo) monocytosis and almost abolishes atherosclerosis in hypercholesterolemic mice. *Circulation* 2008;117:1649-57.
[47] Robbins CS, Chudnovskiy A, et al. Extramedullary hematopoiesis generates Ly-6C(high) monocytes that infiltrate atherosclerotic lesions. *Circulation* 2012;125:364-74.
[48] Wyss CA, Neidhart M, et al. Cellular actors, Toll-like receptors, and local cytokine profile in acute coronary syndromes. *Eur Heart J* 2010;31:1457–69.
[49] Yonekawa K, Neidhart M, et al. Myeloid related proteins activate Toll-like receptor 4 in human acute coronary syndromes. *Atherosclerosis* 2011;218:486–92.
[50] Niessner A, Shin MS, et al. Synergistic proinflammatory effects of the antiviral cytokine interferon-alpha and Toll-like receptor 4 ligands in the atherosclerotic plaque. *Circulation* 2007;116:2043–52.
[51] Kumamoto M, Nakashima Y, et al. Intimal neovascularization in human coronary atherosclerosis: its origin and pathophysiological significance. *Hum Pathol* 1995;26:450–6.
[52] Virmani R, Kolodgie FD, et al. Atherosclerotic plaque progression and vulnerability to rupture: angiogenesis as a source of intraplaque hemorrhage. *Arterioscler Thromb Vasc Biol* 2005;25:2054–61.
[53] Fleiner M, Kummer M, et al. Arterial neovascularization and inflammation in vulnerable patients: early and late signs of symptomatic atherosclerosis. *Circulation* 2004;110:2843–50.
[54] Lauener RP, Geha RS, et al. Engagement of the monocyte surface antigen CD14 induces lymphocyte function-associated antigen-1/intercellular adhesion molecule-1-dependent homotypic adhesion. *J Immunol* 1990;145:1390–4.

[55] Newby AC, George SJ, et al. Vulnerable atherosclerotic plaque metalloproteinases and foam cell phenotypes. *Thromb Haemost* 2009;101:1006–11.
[56] Medbury HJ, Tarran SL, et al. Monocytes contribute to the atherosclerotic cap by transformation into fibrocytes. *Int Angiol* 2008;27:114–23.
[57] Newby AC. Metalloproteinases and vulnerable atherosclerotic plaques. *Trends Cardiovasc Med 2007*;17:253–8.
[58] Momiyama Y, Ohmori R, et al. High plasma levels of matrix metalloproteinase-8 in patients with unstable angina. *Atherosclerosis* 2010;209:206–10.
[59] Altieri DC, Morrissey JH, et al. Adhesive receptor Mac-1coordinates the activation of factor X on stimulated cells of monocytic and myeloid differentiation: an alternative initiation of the coagulation protease cascade. *Proc Natl Acad Sci U S A* 1988;85:7462–6.
[60] Tapp LD, Shantsila E, et al. The CD14++CD16+ monocyte subset and monocyte-platelet interactions in patients with ST-elevation myocardial infarction. *J Thromb Haemost* 2012;10:1231–41.
[61] Aleman MM, Gardiner C, et al. Differential contributions of monocyte- and platelet-derived microparticles towards thrombin generation and fibrin formation and stability. *J Thromb Haemost* 2011;9:2251–61.
[62] Lambert JM, Lopez EF, et al. Macrophage roles following myocardial infarction. *Int J Cardiol* 2008;130:147–58.
[63] Frangogiannis NG, Mendoza LH, et al. MCSF expression is induced in healing myocardial infarcts and may regulate monocyte and endothelial cell phenotype. *Am J Physiol Heart Circ Physiol* 2003;285:H483–92.
[64] Swirski FK, Nahrendorf M, et al. Identification of splenic reservoir monocytes and their deployment to inflammatory sites. *Science.* 2009;325:612-6
[65] Leuschner F, Rauch PJ, et al. Rapid monocyte kinetics in acute myocardial infarction are sustained by extramedullary monocytopoiesis. *J Exp Med.* 2012;209:123-37.
[66] Dutta P, Courties G, et al. Myocardial infarction accelerates atherosclerosis. *Nature.* 2012;487:325-9.
[67] Dewald O, Zymek P, et al. CCL2/Monocyte Chemoattractant Protein-1 regulates inflammatory responses critical to healing myocardial infarcts. *Circ Res.* 2005;96:881-9.
[68] Hofmann U, Beyersdorf N, et al. Activation of CD4+ T lymphocytes improves wound healing and survival after experimental myocardial infarction in mice. *Circulation.* 2012;125:1652-63.
[69] Anzai A, Anzai T, et al. Regulatory role of dendritic cells in postinfarction healing and left ventricular remodeling. *Circulation.* 2012;125:1234-45.
[70] Fukui D, Yasukawa H, et al. Transient reduction and activation of circulating dendritic cells in patients with acute myocardial infarction. *Int J Cardiol* 2012;160:216–9.
[71] Kretzschmar D, Betge S, et al. Recruitment of circulating dendritic cell precursors into the infarcted myocardium and proinflammatory response in acute myocardial infarction. *Clin Sci (Lond)* 2012;123:387–98.
[72] Grage-Griebenow E, Flad HD, et al. Heterogeneity of human peripheral blood monocyte subsets. *J Leukoc Biol* 2001;69:11–20.

[73] Shantsila E, Wrigley B, et al. Immunophenotypic characterization of human monocyte subsets: possible implications for cardiovascular disease pathophysiology. *J Thromb Haemost* 2011;9:1056–66.

[74] Ziegler-Heitbrock HW, Fingerle G, et al. The novel subset of CD14+/CD16+ blood monocytes exhibits features of tissue macrophages. *Eur J Immunol* 1993;23:2053–8.

[75] Auffray C, Sieweke MH, et al. Blood monocytes: development, heterogeneity, and relationship with dendritic cells. *Annu Rev Immunol* 2009;27:669–92.

[76] Schlitt A, Heine GH, et al. CD14.CD16. monocytes in coronary artery disease and their relationship to serum TNF alpha levels. *Thromb Haemost* 2004;92:419–24.

[77] Capoccia BJ, Gregory AD, et al. Recruitment of the inflammatory subset of monocytes to sites of ischemia induces angiogenesis in a monocyte chemoattractant protein-1-dependent fashion. *J Leukoc Biol* 2008;84:760–8.

[78] Feig JE, Pineda-Torra I, et al. LXR promotes the maximal egress of monocyte-derived cells from mouse aortic plaques during atherosclerosis regression. *J Clin Invest.* 2010;120:4415-24.

[79] Potteaux S, Gautier EL, et al. Suppressed monocyte recruitment drives macrophage removal from atherosclerotic plaques of Apoe-/- mice during disease regression. *J Clin Invest.* 2011;121:2025-36.

[80] Liao X, Sluimer JC, et al. Macrophage autophagy plays a protective role in advanced atherosclerosis. *Cell Metab.* 2012;15:545-53.

[81] Singer AJ, Clark RA. Cutaneous wound healing. *N Engl J Med* 1999;341:738–46.

[82] Feig JE, Quick JS, et al. The role of a murine transplantation model of atherosclerosis regression in drug discovery. *Curr Opin Investig Drugs* 2009;10:232–8.

[83] Llodra J, Angeli V, et al. Emigration of monocyte-derived cells from atherosclerotic lesions characterizes regressive, but not progressive, plaques. *Proc Natl Acad Sci U S* A 2004;101:11779–84.

[84] Feig JE, Shang Y, et al. Statins promote the regression of atherosclerosis via activation of the CCR7-dependent emigration pathway in macrophages. *PLoS One* 2011;6:e28534.

[85] Ferro D, Parrotto S, et al. Simvastatin inhibits the monocyte expression of proinflammatory cytokines in patients with hypercholesterolemia. *J Am Coll Cardiol* 2000;36:427–31.

[86] Saederup N, Chan L, et al. Fractalkine deficiency markedly reduces macrophage accumulation and atherosclerotic lesion formation in CCR2-/- mice: evidence for independent chemokine functions in atherogenesis. *Circulation* 2008;117:1642–8.

[87] Combadiere C, Potteaux S, et al. Combined inhibition of CCL2, CX3CR1, and CCR5 abrogates Ly6C(hi) and Ly6C(lo) monocytosis and almost abolishes atherosclerosis in hypercholesterolemic mice. *Circulation* 2008;117:1649–57.

[88] Berg KE, Ljungcrantz I, et al. Elevated CD14++CD16- monocytes predict cardiovascular events. *Circ Cardiovasc Genet* 2012;5:122-31.

[89] McDermott DH, Fong AM, et al. Chemokine receptor mutant CX3CR1-M280 has impaired adhesive function and correlates with protection from cardiovascular disease in humans. *J Clin Invest* 2003;111:1241-50.

[90] Apostolakis S, Baritaki S, et al. Effects of polymorphisms in chemokine ligands and receptors on susceptibility to coronary artery disease. *Thromb Res* 2007;119:63-71.

[91] Norata GD, Garlaschelli K, et al. Effects of fractalkine receptor variants on common carotid artery intima-media thickness. *Stroke* 2006;37:1558-61.
[92] Afzal AR, Kiechl S, et al. Common CCR5-del32 frameshift mutation associated with serum levels of inflammatory markers and cardiovascular disease risk in the Bruneck population. *Stroke* 2008;39:1972-8.
[93] Koenen RR, Weber C. Chemokines: established and novel targets in atherosclerosis. *EMBO Mol Med* 2011;3:713-25.
[94] Weber C. Obstacles and options in the quest for drug candidates against vascular disease. *Thromb Haemost* 2010;104:1-3.
[95] Geissmann F, Manz MG, et al. Development of monocytes, macrophages, and dendritic cells. *Science* 2010;327:656–61.
[96] Gratchev A, Sobenin I, et al. Monocytes as a diagnostic marker of cardiovascular diseases. *Immunobiology* 2012;217:476–82.

In: Myocardial Infarctions
Editor: Pattie Wilkonson

ISBN: 978-1-63321-726-3

Chapter 8

Comprehensive Management in the Acute Phase for Improving the Long-Term Clinical Outcomes of Acute Myocardial Infarction

Kiyoshi Kume[1,•], Yoshinori Yasuoka[1] and Tatsuya Sasaki[1]
[1]Cardiovascular Division, Osaka Minami Medical Center, Osaka, Japan

Abstract

Acute myocardial infarction (AMI) remains the leading cause of mortality in Western countries as well as in Asia. The remarkable progress achieved in the treatment of cardiovascular disease over the past few decades has resulted in decreased mortality worldwide. In particular, advances in intensive management in patients with AMI, such as the use of primary percutaneous coronary intervention (PCI) and development of coronary care units, have contributed to increases in in-hospital survival rates. However, increases in the rates of postinfarction morbidity and mortality are a growing problem, especially with respect to the frequency of admission for congestive heart failure.

AMI pathologically progresses in the coronary arteries in sequence from plaque formation to destabilization to rupture. A predisposition toward atherosclerosis and the effects of a hyperinflammatory state play important roles in the onset of AMI. In-hosital mortality due to AMI, particularly in cases of ST-segment elevation myocardial infarction, is primarily caused by arrhythmias, acute heart failure and/or cardiac rupture, whereas the severity of postinfarction complications depends on the magnitude of left ventricular remodeling, consequently resulting in a reduced left ventricular function.

In this chapter, we review the potentially predictive risk factors for long-term outcomes and suggest preventive measures at each stage: before a PCI-capable hospital, before primary PCI, during primary PCI, after primary PCI and before hospital discharge. Finally, we propose acute-phase strategies for improving long-term outcomes in patients with AMI.

• Tel.: 81-721-53-5761, Fax: 81-721-53-5843, E-mail: k_kume@ommc-hp.jp.

Introduction

Recent advances, including the application of primary percutaneous coronary intervention (PCI) in the management of acute myocardial infarction (AMI) [1], have decreased short-term mortality to approximately 15% in Western countries [2] and 6% in Japan [3]. However, as the number of survivors with AMI has increased, so too have the rates of postinfarction morbidity and mortality [4]. In particular, the global pandemic burden of heart failure due to ischemic heart disease is a growing the problem. Left ventricular (LV) remodeling after AMI is associated with worse postinfarction outcomes, including mortality, arrhythmic events and admissions for congestive heart failure. Therefore, the preventive management of LV remodeling in the acute phase of AMI has potentially beneficial effects on long-term outcomes.

AMI pathologically progresses in the coronary arteries in a sequence from plaque formation to destabilization to rupture, ultimately resulting in coronary artery obstruction due to thrombus formation. In addition, the severity of postinfarction complications is dependent on the magnitude of LV remodeling, leading to a reduced left ventricular function, while a hyperinflammatory state plays an important role in the outcomes of morbidity and mortality after AMI.

In this chapter, we review potentially predictive risk factors for long-term outcomes and suggest preventive measures at each stage: before a PCI-capable hospital, before primary PCI, during primary PCI, after primary PCI and before hospital discharge. Finally, we propose acute-phase strategies for improving long-term outcomes in patients with AMI.

The acute-phase risk factors for a worse long-term outcome and preventive measures for AMI management are summarized in Table 1.

LV Remodeling after AMI (Figure 1)

LV remodeling after AMI involves changes in both the cardiac structure and function that contribute to worse postinfarction outcomes, including mortality, myocardial reinfarction and admission for congestive heart failure. Therefore, the use of an intensive strategy to prevent LV remodeling in the acute phase of AMI is associated with improved long-term outcomes.

The LV exhibits an adaptive response to an increased load in order to maintain the pump capacity in the early stages of AMI. Initially, sites of infarction develop myocardial wall thinning and dilation. Then, immediately after the onset of AMI, ventricular myocardial necrosis develops in the infarct regions, with necrotic myocytes replacing collagen fibers over a period of a few weeks. Infarct sites without sufficient collagen fibers are very fragile and extend outward due to stress on the LV wall. Consequently, gaps develop between myocytes with and without necrosis due to the actions of activated matrix metalloproteases (MMPs). The infarct areas then display focal expansion, with associated ventricular myocyte dislodgement and myocardial thinning. This process is influenced by three factors: the infarct size, rate of infarct healing and degree of ventricular wall stress. The grade of ventricular enlargement is strongly determined by the infarct size, with greater enlargement being more frequent in patients with anteroseptal myocardial infarction and sometimes leading to the development of ventricular aneurysms.

Table 1. Preventive measures and acute-phase risk factors for long-term outcomes

Risk factors	Before PCI hospital	Before primery PCI	During primary PCI	After primary PCI	Before hospital discharge
Non-modifiable	Advanced age Women Cardiac arrest/Shock state Long distance to PCI center	Advanced age Women Renal insufficiency Anemia Previous MI STEMI Statin-naïve HF with Killip class ≥ II Cardiogenic shock	LAD culprit lesion LMT lesion Multivessel lesions		
Potentially modifiable	Nondiagnostic MI			Acute kidney injury Bleeding Transfusion	
Modifiable			Final TIMI 3		Reduced LVEF Residual lesions Insufficient drugs
Preventive measurements	Education for patients Training for medical crews Facillitated PCI	Facillitated PCI High dose statin Intravenous nicorandil Intravenous bicarbonate	Aspiration intracoronary nicorandil (intracoronary nitroprusside) IABP insertion	Low-dose carperitide/ nesiritide Intravenous nicorandil ACE inhibitors Beta blockers	Staged PCI Additional drugs

PCI: percutaneous coronary intervention, MI: myocardial infarction, STEMI: ST-segment elevation myocardial infarction, HF: heart failure, LAD: left anterior descending coronary artery, LMT: left main trunk, TIMI: Thrombolysis in Myocardial Infarction, IABP: intraaortic balloon pumping, ACE: angiotensin converting enzyme, LVEF: left ventricular ejection fraction.

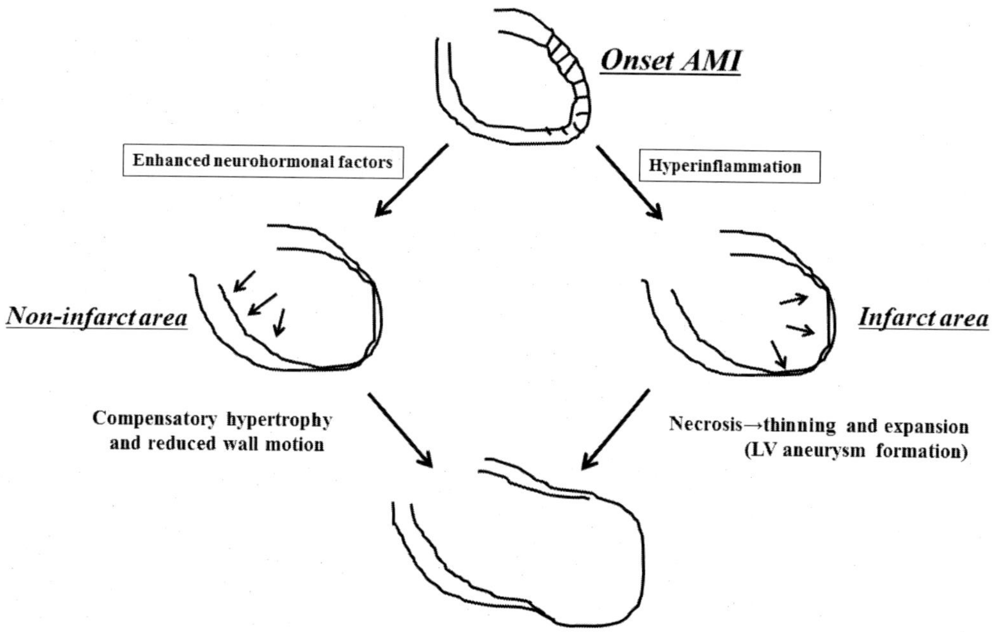

AMI: Acute myocardial infarction, LV: Left ventricle.

Figure 1. LV remodeling after AMI.

Second, compensatory ventricular hypertrophy and fibrosis occur in non-infarct areas in the chronic stage of LV remodeling. Abnormal enlargement of the non-infarcted LV induces longitudinal hypertrophy of the remaining myocytes in order to reduce wall stress. In addition, compensatory stimulation of neurohumoral factors (i.e. catecholamines, angiotensin and aldosterone) plays an important role in the progression of LV remodeling in both infarct and non-infarct areas. Finally, the LV becomes enlarged, which reduces the cardiac systolic function, resulting in worse long-term outcomes, including the potential for admission due to congestive heart failure.

The main points for preventing LV remodeling after AMI include reducing the infarct size with the early administration of reperfusion therapy and inhibiting the activation of neurohumoral factors. Therefore, providing comprehensive intensive treatment in the acute phase of AMI can achieve improved postinfarction outcomes.

Before a PCI-Capable Hospital

A shortened door-to-balloon time has been reported to be significantly associated with in-hospital mortality [5]. However, recent reports have demonstrated no significant correlations between a shortened door-to-balloon time and better outcomes [6]. Patients with AMI have a rate of sudden death that is four to six times higher than that of the general population, and half of AMI patients die before arriving at the hospital. In particular, males are more likely to die outside of the hospital than females [7]. Therefore, shortening the time to recanalization after AMI onset (onset-to-balloon time) naturally contributes to improving the survival rate, as myocardial necrosis begins to develop immediately after onset.

Shiomi et al. demonstrated the importance of a shortened onset-to-balloon time based on the results of the CREDO-Kyoto registry in Japan. Among the 3,391 retrospectively analyzed patients with ST-segment elevation myocardial infarction (STEMI) who underwent primary PCI within 24 hours of symptom onset, a shorter door-to-balloon time was found to be independently associated with better outcomes in the subjects with early presentation (an onset-to-balloon time of ≤ 3 hours), but not those with delayed presentation (an onset-to-balloon time of > 3 hours) [8]. Predictors of delayed presentation to the hospital after symptom onset generally include an older age and female gender. In that study, delays occurred most frequently at non PCI-capable hospitals (64.0%), and the most common reason for delay at a non PCI-capable hospital was the need to wait for transportation (26.4%). Interestingly, delays due to cardiac arrest and/or cardiogenic shock was associated with the highest in-hospital mortality (30.6%), whereas nondiagnostic initial ECG findings did not affect mortality (0%) [9].

Both fibrinolytic therapy and primary PCI have been reported to be associated with decreased in-hospital mortality rates in patients with STEMI. Primary PCI has become the predominant reperfusion strategy, as a fibrinolytic strategy is less likely to achieve Thrombolysis in Myocardial Infarction (TIMI) grade 3 reperfusion, with a higher rate of hemorrhagic complications [10]. However, the administration of a half-dose of thrombolytic agents and/or the use of PCI have been shown to improve outcomes in patients with early presentation [11], compared with the application of full-dose fibrinolytic drugs [12].

There are few PCI-capable hospitals in the US, compared to that observed in Japan. Fibrinolytic treatment is therefore an effective strategy for shortening the onset-to-balloon time (total ischemic time), thus resulting in improved long-term outcomes.

Before Primary PCI

Early invasive reperfusion treatment for STEMI helps to reduce the rate of in-hospital mortality. As the door-to-balloon time decreases, so too does the in-hospital mortality rate, in a linear fashion [9]. For example, the rate of in-hospital mortality among patients with STEMI who receive invasive treatment within 90 minutes after arriving at a PCI-capable hospital is 3.0%. However, this rate increases to 4.2%, 5.7% and 7.4% when treatment is delayed for 91 to 120 minutes, 121 to 150 minutes and more than 150 minutes, respectively [13]. Therefore, recent guidelines recommend a treatment goal of a door-to-balloon time of 90 minutes or less. Bradley et al. proposed a strategy for reducing the door-to-balloon time in the US [14]. Consequently, the proportion of STEMI patients who undergo primary PCI within 90 minutes significantly increased from 44% in 2005 to 91% in 2010, while the door-to-balloon time decreased from 96 to 64 minutes (median), respectively [15]. Furthermore, many reports have demonstrated a positive correlation between a shortened door-to-balloon time and clinical outcomes.

Successful early invasive treatment is defined as the attainment of a final TIMI 3 grade flow in the culprit vessel, resulting in a reduction in the expansion of the infarct area. Therefore, it is necessary to quickly and accurately define primary PCI strategies for achieving a final TIMI 3 grade flow in the culprit vessel and preventing complications after primary PCI.

There are several prerequisites for a PCI-capable hospital: for example, an annual primary PCI volume up to 25 patients is particularly essential [16]. On the other hand, there are no differences in rates of treatment success or complications of primary PCI between PCI-capable hospitals with and without cardiovascular surgeons [17]. Major risk scores and post-PCI complications (e.g. contrast-induced nephropathy; CIN, bleeding and transfusion) are shown in Table 2. Some variables overlap, as described in the table.

Table 2. Risk scores for outcomes in patients with ACS and simple scores for post-PCI complications

Variables	*TIMI risk*	*Zwolle risk*	*CADILLAC risk*	CIN	Bleeding
Advanced age	○	○	○	○	○
Low systolic blood pressure	○			○	
Heart rate	○				
Killip class II-IV	○	○	○	○	
Anterior MI	○	○			
Body weight	○				
Time delay to reperfusion	○	○			
Final TIMI grade < 3		○	○		
Triple vessel disease		○	○		
LVEF < 40%			○		
Renal insufficiency			○		○
Anemia			○	○	○
STEMI					○
Female					○
WBC count					○
Diabetes				○	
IABP				○	
Contrast dose				○	

CIN: contrast-induced nephropathy. TIMI risk score [70], Zwolle score [71], CADILLAC score [72], CIN risk score [73], Bleeding risk score [74].

Importantly, a hyperinflammatory state contributes to LV remodeling and post-PCI complications; therefore, the administration of anti-inflammatory agents prior to primary PCI is essential for improving outcomes.

1) Risk Factors

Advanced Age

The number of elderly patients is increasing, particularly in developed countries. Such patients are more likely to have additional comorbidities, such as renal insufficiency, anemia and dementia, as well as an increased rate of heart failure due to concomitant LV diastolic dysfunction, resulting in more frequent delays in arrival to a PCI-capable hospital and the development of post-PCI complications, such as CIN, bleeding and the need for transfusions. Moreover, coronary interventionists tend to hesitate in performing invasive treatments in this population. However, aggressive treatment improves short-term outcomes, even in nonagenarians.

Female Gender

The in-hospital mortality of female patients with STEMI remains relatively high. Female subjects display unique characteristics, including an older age, atypical anginal symptoms, mode frequent delays to arrival at a PCI-capable hospital and an increased frequency of post-PCI complications. Moreover, female patients are less likely to receive evidence-based management, including invasive pharmacological and interventional reperfusion therapy and medical treatments. Invasive therapy has a beneficial effect on one-year outcomes in males and patients with acute coronary syndrome, whereas conflicting results are observed in females. The non-superiority of invasive treatment in females is influenced by worse outcomes in the acute phase, that is, it is important to improve acute-phase outcomes with a combination of pharmacological and interventional treatments, thereby improving the long-term outcomes.

Renal Insufficiency

Renal insufficiency is significantly associated with cardiovascular disease and mortality [18]. Patients with renal insufficiency exhibit enhanced inflammation, oxidative stress and sympathetic nervous system activation [19]. In addition, they are more likely to receive invasive treatment and less likely to receive cardiovascular protective drugs.

Anemia

The addition of anemia to cardiorenal interactions (cardio-renal-anemia interactions) in the setting of cardiovascular disease has recently been highlighted. Patients with anemia also display enhanced activation of neurohormonal factors. The preprocedural hemoglobin level is an independent predictor of cardiovascular events in patients with acute coronary syndrome [20]. In addition, a low baseline hemoglobin value and decrease in the hemoglobin level during follow-up are independently associated with a higher risk of mortality and hospitalization for heart failure, even in patients without baseline anemia.

STEMI

Compared with patients with non-ST-segment elevation myocardial infarction (NSTEMI), those with STEMI exhibit high short-term mortality. The appropriate timing for invasive reperfusion therapy in patients with NSTEMI has been discussed, although no consensus has been reached. However, some data have demonstrated worse long-term outcomes in patients with NSTEMI than in those with STEMI, likely due to the increased prevalence of comorbidities and multivessel coronary artery disease in the former group.

A Statin-Naïve Status

Statins act by inhibiting of 3-hydroxy-3-methylglutaryl coenzyme A (HMG-CoA) reductase, thereby lowering the low-density lipoprotein (LDL) cholesterol level. In addition, statins exert cholesterol-independent effects (pleiotropic effects) by reducting the level of isoprenoids (farnesyl pyrophosphate and geranylgeranyl pyrophosphate), which subsequently improves the vascular function (e.g. anti-inflammatory effects) [21] (Figure 3).

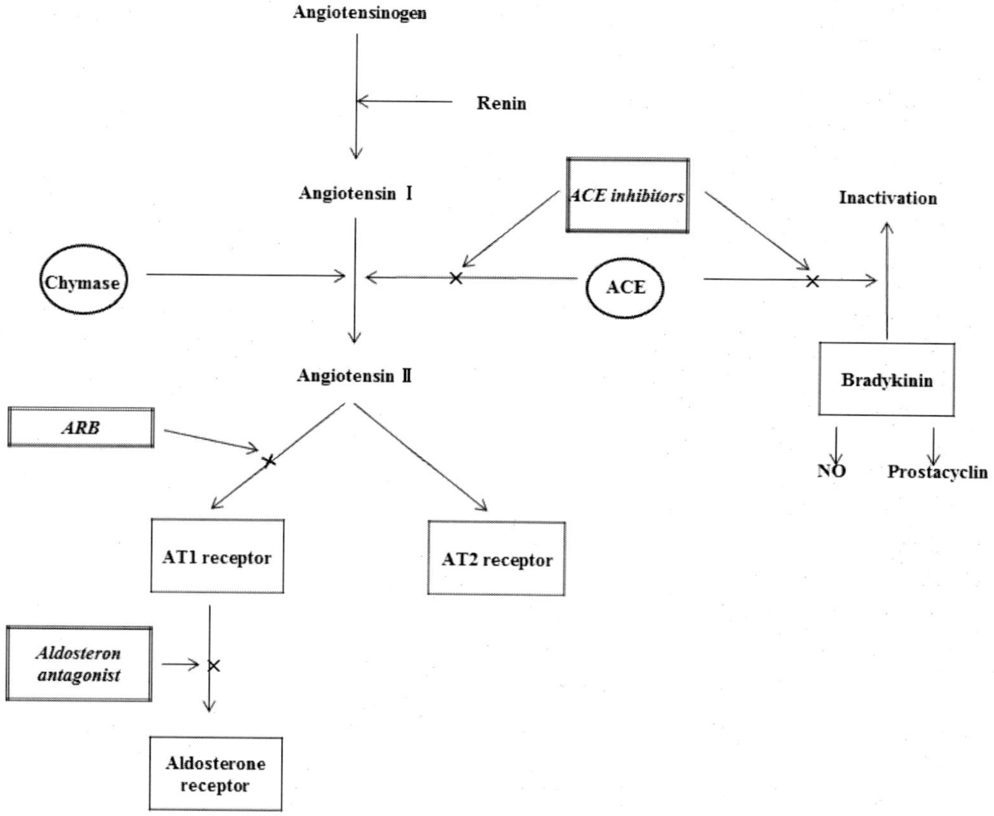

ACE: angiotensin-converting enzyme, ARB: angiotensin receptor blocker, AT: angiotensin.

Figure 2. Renin-angiotensin-aldosterone system (RAAS).

Statin therapy is established in the primary and secondary treatment of coronary artery disease, and a hyperinflammatory state plays an important role in the pathogenesis of acute coronary syndrome and postinfarction remodeling. Patients without a history of statin treatment (statin-naïve) more frequently experience adverse periprocedural events than those who have previously received statin therapy. Moreover, the preprocedural administration of high-dose statins is effective for reducing the rate of periprocedural myocardial injury in statin-naïve patients with stable angina and acute coronary syndrome [22,23]. Notably, these strategies are especially effective in patients with high C-reactive protein levels [23]. The acute effects of statins may depend on their isoprenoid-dependent effects, which rapidly prevent oxidative stress. Therefore, the single administration of high-dose statin therapy prior to primary PCI is acceptable in acute situations, although it remains unclear whether this strategy results in better outcomes in STEMI patients.

2) Post-PCI Complications and Potentially Preventive Measures

No-Reflow Phenomenon

The no-reflow phenomenon involves a flow limitation in the epicardial coronary arteries and has been reported to be an independent predictor of in-hospital mortality [24]. Complications of the no-reflow phenomenon have been reported to independently predict both short- and long-term mortality in patients with STEMI, regardless of the infarct size. Therefore, preventing such complications is essential for improving survival in STEMI patients. The no-reflow phenomenon is caused by the following mechanisms of pathological microvascular dysfunction: 1) coronary occlusion, resulting in damage to the vascular endothelium, tissue edema and platelet aggregation, 2) coronary artery reperfusion, resulting in the activation of oxygen free radicals, and 3) atheroembolism, resulting in microvascular (arteriole or capillary) occlusion and spasms [25]. Hence, understanding the pathophysiology of the no-reflow phenomenon is important for preventing of this condition. Nicorandil, which has both nitrate-like properties and the ability to function as a potassium-channel (KATP) opener, exerts numerous cardioprotective effects, including pharmacological preconditioning (reducing infarct expansion), effectively restoring the coronary blood flow to ischemic area (cardiac protection), preventing Ca^{2+} overload (reducing the risk of the no-reflow phenomenon), suppressing cardiac sympathetic nerve injury and improving tolerance to treatment. In contrast, patients treated with KATP-channel closers (e.g. sulfonylureas) exhibit an increased risk of developing congestive heart failure. The single intravenous administration of 12 mg of nicorandil 30 minutes prior to primary PCI has beneficial effects, including a higher rate of achievement of a final TIMI 3 flow and reduced incidence of both cardiovascular death and admission for congestive heart failure [26]. Therefore, the infusion of nicorandil is an effective strategy for improving outcomes by preventing periprocedural cardiovascular injury.

Contrast-Induced Nephropathy (CIN)

CIN occurs in 2% to 25% of patients with coronary artery disease undergoing PCI. The pathophysiology of CIN involves an increase in systemic oxidative stress resulting from a decreased renal blood flow and direct renal injury induced by the contrast agent. The development of CIN after AMI exhibits a graded association with long-term mortality [27], and both transient and persistent renal dysfunction contribute to worse long-term outcomes [28]. Therefore, preventing CIN may help to improve outcomes. There is no reliable prophylaxis for CIN, with the exception of normal saline fluid hydration. However, there is not enough time to perform this procedure in the emergent setting. Recently, various prospective studies have demonstrated the potentially beneficial effects of intravenous and oral N-acetylcysteine as well as the single intravenous administration of sodium bicarbonate.

Bleeding and Transfusion

Post-PCI bleeding occurs in 2% to 14% of cases. Bleeding (major bleeding defined as any intracranial bleed and/or a reduction in hemoglobin of ≥ 5 g/dL or > 15% decrease in hematocrit) is significantly associated with both morbidity and mortality [29]. Acute bleeding has direct hemodynamic effects, including a reduced oxygen supply associated with an increased oxygen demand, elevated neurohormonal levels and the need to discontinue antithrombotic and anticoagulant therapy. On the other hand, the use of blood transfusions is independently associated with worse outcomes. The administration of stored red blood cells induces adverse effects, such as microvascular occlusion and erythrocyte dysfunction due to the depletion of 2,3-diphosphoglycerate [30]. The best method for preventing post-PCI bleeding is to properly select the access route and sheath size for primary PCI. Transradial coronary intervention is associated with decreased mortality, major bleeding, vascular complications and blood transfusions in STEMI patients. Moreover, the use of a smaller sheath size (5 > 6 > 7 >8 French) may help to reduce bleeding complications after primary PCI. However, it is difficult to treat serious conditions using these strategies in unexpected situations, such as those involving cardiogenic shock and/or cardiac arrest in the emergent setting.

During Primary PCI

The goal of treatment with primary PCI is to achieve a final TIMI 3 flow as quickly as possible, thereby reducing the degree of infarct expansion. In addition to successful reperfusion, the prevention of post-PCI adverse events may improve survival in patients with AMI.

1) No-Reflow Phenomenon

What can we do during primary PCI to prevent the no-reflow phenomenon?

1.1) Aspiration Catheter and Distal Protection Devices

Acute coronary syndrome frequently occurs in patients with lipid-rich plaques covered with a thin fibrous cap (unstable plaque); coronary artery occlusion subsequently results from plaque rupture and thrombus formation.

In addition, atherosclerotic embolization frequently occurs due to dilatation of the balloon catheter and/or deployment of the coronary stent, thus inducing the no-reflow phenomenon. In contrast, the aspiration of plaque components (including thrombi) reduces the incidence of the no-reflow phenomenon.

Aspiration catheters are easy to use, and a higher one-year rate of survival has been documented in STEMI patients treated with aspiration catheters. Moreover, a meta-analysis demonstrated the beneficial effects of aspiration catheter use on outcomes in patients with STEMI [31].

However, distal protective devices (PercuSurge and filter-type devices) have not been found to be effective in improving post-PCI outcomes due to the time delay required to use the devices and the Dotter effect.

1.2) Intracoronary Administration of Nicorandil Prior to Dilatation of Culprit Lesions Using a Balloon Catheter

If the microvessel coronary artery is adequately dilated so as not to be occluded by atherosclerotic components, the no-reflow phenomenon does not occur. The intracoronary administration of 2 mg of nicorandil before balloon dilatation or stent deployment or after the occurrence of the no-reflow phenomenon has beneficial effects in preventing and reversing the no-reflow phenomenon [32].

1.3) Intra-Aortic Balloon Pumping (IABP) Insertion

If successful reperfusion (a final TIMI 3 flow) is not achieved, the coronary flow can be increased by inserting an IABP and flushing out the atherosclerotic components occluding the microvessels. However, this strategy has not been demonstrated to result in superior outcomes and may actually increase the risk of bleeding and CIN.

2)-CIN

The preventive strategy is to reduce the amount of contrast media as much as possible. The maximum allowable contrast volume (ml, ≤ 400 ml) has been demonstrated to be 5 x body weight (kg) / serum creatinine value (mg/dl) [33].

3)-Culprit Vessel Only Versus One-Time Multivessel PCI?

Culprit vessel only primary PCI is associated with better outcomes in patients with STEMI [34]. However, some reports demonstrated that one-time multivessel primary PCI is superior to staged PCI for non-culprit vessels with respect to long-term outcomes [35]. On the other hand, in patients with NSTEMI, multivessel coronary intervention potentially results in better outcomes [36], likely due to the relatively high rate of complications of heart failure. One-time multivessel PCI has no effect on the survival rate in patients with STEMI complicated with cardiogenic shock. However, this strategy improves hemodynamics [37], especially in patients with severe residual stenosis in the LAD.

After Primary PCI

The main point for improving long-term outcomes in this period is the early administration of anti-remodeling agents. ANP and BNP, which belong to the natriuretic peptide family and exhibit various bioactivities, including natriuresis, dieresis, vasodilation and inhibition of the renin-angiotensin-aldosterone (RAAS) and sympathetic nervous systems, thus playing an important role in preventing cardiac toxicity. The plasma levels of both ANP and BNP generally increase according to the severity of chronic heart failure. Two patterns for the plasma BNP level are observed after admission in patients with AMI: a monophasic pattern with one peak at approximately 16 hours and a biphasic pattern with two peaks at approximately 16 hours and five days [38]. Patients with anterior infarction, congestive heart failure, higher levels of maximal creatine kinase-MB isoenzymes and a lower left ventricular ejection fraction (LVEF) are likely to display a biphasic BNP pattern. Therefore, the second BNP peak has been suggested to reflect the infarct size and subsequent degree of LV remodeling after AMI [39]. Therefore, inhibiting the second peak in the plasma BNP level helps to prevent LV remodeling.

1.1) RAAS Inhibitors: Angiotensin-Converting Enzyme (ACE) Inhibitors, Angiotensin Receptor Blockers (ARBs) and Aldosterone Antagonists

The RAAS is demonstrated in Figure 2. The activation of the RAAS contributes to the aggravation of heart failure and onset of AMI. Several clinical trials have demonstrated that the early administration of ACE inhibitors (within 24 hours after AMI onset) is significantly associated with reductions in LV remodeling and mortality in patients with AMI, without excessive blood pressure lowering [40]. The beneficial effects of ACE inhibitors for the outcomes of AMI include enhancement of nitric oxide production due to an increased bradykinin level and inhibition of the activated sympathetic nervous system as well as both myocardial MMPs and circulating angiotensin II (AT II). However, ARBs inhibit tissue-specific AT II, whereas ACE inhibitors do not. Nevertheless, both ACE inhibitors and ARBs are effective for improving post-MI outcomes, although ACE inhibitors are superior to ARBs with respect to blood pressure-independent effects in patients with coronary artery disease according to the BPLTTC meta-analysis [41]. Meanwhile, although this strategy is theoretically more effective, the administration of ARBs in combination with ACE inhibitors demonstrates no efficacy as to postinfarction outcomes, likely due to excessive blood pressure-lowering effects.

1.2) Beta-Blockers

In 1975, Waagstein et al. reported the effects of metoprolol in reducing the size of the heart in seven patients with dilated cardiomyopathy [42]. Since then, large randomized controlled trials have documented the beneficial effects of beta-blockers in improving the cardiac function and survival in patients with chronic heart failure of NYHA class I to IV. Potential mechanisms underlying the beneficial effects of beta-blockers in patients with cardiovascular dysfunction include: 1) a reduction in myocardial oxygen consumption following a reduction in heart rate, 2) protection against direct catecholamine-induced myocyte toxicity, 3) improvements in intramyocardial calcium handling in cardiac myocytes, 4) inhibition of the activated sympathetic nervous and RAA systems, 5) antioxidative effects [43]. These effects potentially contribute to improving both the LV function and size, that is, so-called "reverse remodeling." According to the results of a meta-analysis, similar effects of beta-blockers on survival are noted in patients with both ischemic and non-ischemic heart failure [44], although patients with non-ischemic heart failure achieve greater improvements in the LVEF than those with ischemic heart failure [45]. Reverse remodeling of the LV by beta-blockers is observed significantly more frequently in patients with larger non-infarct areas, as reverse remodeling does not occur in areas of infraction. Moreover, carvedilol has beneficial effects on the hibernating and/or ischemic myocardium [46]. For example, the CAPRICORN trial [47] demonstrated the beneficial effects of the early administration of carvedilol on mortality after AMI in patients with LV systolic dysfunction (average LVEF: 32%, previous myocardial infarction: 30%). According to the results of the echocardiographic studies performed at six months, the LV systolic volume reductions and LVEF improvements were greater in the patients treated with carvedilol. Moreover, carvedilol has an antiarrhythmic effect on the postinfarction heart [both atrial (risk reduction: 52%) and ventricular arrhythmia (risk reduction: 63%)] in addition to a preventive effect against adverse coronary events, thus resulting in better outcomes. The STEMI treatment guidelines proposed by the ACCF/AHA in 2013 recommend the use of oral beta-blockers in the first 24 hours [48]. Recently, conflicting retrospective data from the j-Cypher registry in Japan showed beneficial effects of beta-blockers in patients with a reduced LV systolic function (EF $< 40\%$), but not in those with a preserved LV systolic function (EF $\geq 40\%$) [49]. Nevertheless, beta-blockers should generally be administered in patients with cardiovascular disease.

1.3) Low-Dose Intravenous Nesiritide (BNP) and Carperitide (hANP)

B-type natriuretic peptide (BNP, nesiritide) is approved in the US, whereas human atrial natriuretic peptide (hANP, carperitide) is approved only in Japan. Both ANP and BNP increase the intracellular cyclic guanosine monophosphate levels by linking to guanylyl cyclase A receptors and exhibit various bioactivities, including natriuresis, vasodilation, antioxidative effects and inhibitive effects on the RAAS [50, 51], activated sympathetic nervous system, cardiac hypertrophy and interstitial fibrosis, thus resulting in protective effects against LV remodeling. According to the results of the J-WIND trial, the administration of intravenous low-dose carperitide (less than 0.025γ) for 72 hours results in a reduction in the infarct size with consequent better outcomes [52]. Notably, the infusion of carperitide does not induce blood pressure-lowering effects.

1.4) Intravenous Nicorandil

Microangiopathy sometimes occurs following successful reperfusion (a final TIMI 3 grade flow), especially in diabetic patients. The administration of low-dose nicorandil (4 mg per day) was found to have negative outcomes in the J-WIND trial; however, the continuous infusion of intravenous nicorandil (2 mg per hour), if not associated with excessive blood pressure lowering, has been suggested to improve the microvascular circulation, thereby reducing the infarct size.

1.5) Aldosterone Antagonist: Eplerenone

The serum aldosterone levels may remain high if the RAAS is inhibited by both ACE inhibitors and ARBs (aldosterone breakthrough phenomenon). The addition of eplerenone to an ACE inhibitor and/or beta-blocker contributes to reductions in both morbidity and mortality in patients with MI and LV systolic dysfunction.

Before Hospital Discharge

The duration of hospital stay in the US differs from that observed in Japan; an average five days in the US, in comparison to less than 14 days in 40% cases in Japan [3]. Are there additional strategies for improving long-term outcomes prior to hospital discharge?

1) Staged PCI for Residual Lesions in Patients with Multivessel Disease

A reduced incidence of residual stenotic lesions is associated with better outcomes in patients with multivessel coronary artery disease. A regional dysfunctional hibernating myocardium induces left ventricular remodeling [53], while revascularization via either PCI or CABG improves the cardiac function and survival.

How does the prognosis of PCI differ according to the target vessel? Claessen et al. examined the prognostic effect of successful revascularization using PCI in chronic total occlusion (CTO) in patients with one CTO lesion in the left anterior descending (LAD), left circumflex (LCx) or right coronary (RCA) artery. One comparison of patients treated with successful vs. unsuccessful PCI showed long-term mortality rates in LAD, LCx, and RCA patients of 6.7% vs. 11.0%, 5.5% vs. 13.9% and 6.6% vs. 4.1%, respectively [54]. These results support the use of aggressive revascularization of the left coronary artery in order to improve the long-term survival.

2) Optimal Medical Therapy for Secondary Prevention of Coronary Artery Disease

PCI has beneficial effects on target, but not non-target, coronary stenotic lesions. Among patients treated with PCI, clinical plaque progression is noted in approximately 6% of non-target lesions, requiring repeated PCI within one year. The PROSPECT trial, a prospective observational study of patients with acute coronary syndrome who underwent three-vessel coronary angiography and gray-scale intravascular ultrasonographic imaging of both culprit and non-culprit lesions demonstrated rates of adverse coronary events in the culprit and non-culprit lesions of 12.9% and 11.6% over 3.4 years, respectively [55]. These results are in concordance with those of the REACH registry (approximately 4% per year) [56]. In addition, Asakura et al. reported that vulnerable plaques, presenting as yellow areas on angioscopy, are detected in both culprit and non-culprit vessels in patients with acute coronary syndrome [57]. Furthermore, the rate of plaque progression significantly increases as the number of diseased vessels increases. The most important treatment for adverse coronary events is the secondary prevention of classical cardiovascular risk factors, which remain undertreated and undercontrolled based on the findings of the REACH registry [58]. Meanwhile, the COURAGE trial emphasized the use of optimal medical therapy (intensive pharmacologic therapy and lifestyle intervention) as an important strategy in patients with coronary artery disease [59]. Guideline-based treatment goals for the secondary prevention of coronary artery disease generally include: 1) a systolic blood pressure of < 130 mmHg, 2) a hemoglobin A1c level of < 7.0%, 3) an LDL cholesterol level of < 100 mg/dl and 4) smoking cessation [60]. However, in several large clinical trials of patients with diabetes, the rates of achievement of the treatment goals for all four specific risk factors at one year of follow-up were only 18%, 23% and only 8% (COURAGE [59] diabetes subgroup, BARI 2D [61] patients and FREEDOM [62] patients, respectively [60]). Aggressive LDL cholesterol-lowering therapy with statins is correlated with the regression and stabilization of coronary atherosclerotic plaque. The target level for LDL cholesterol is 60 to 80 mg/dL. However, both excessive blood pressure lowering and intensive blood glucose control result in higher mortality rates among postinfarction patients (J-shaped phenomenon).

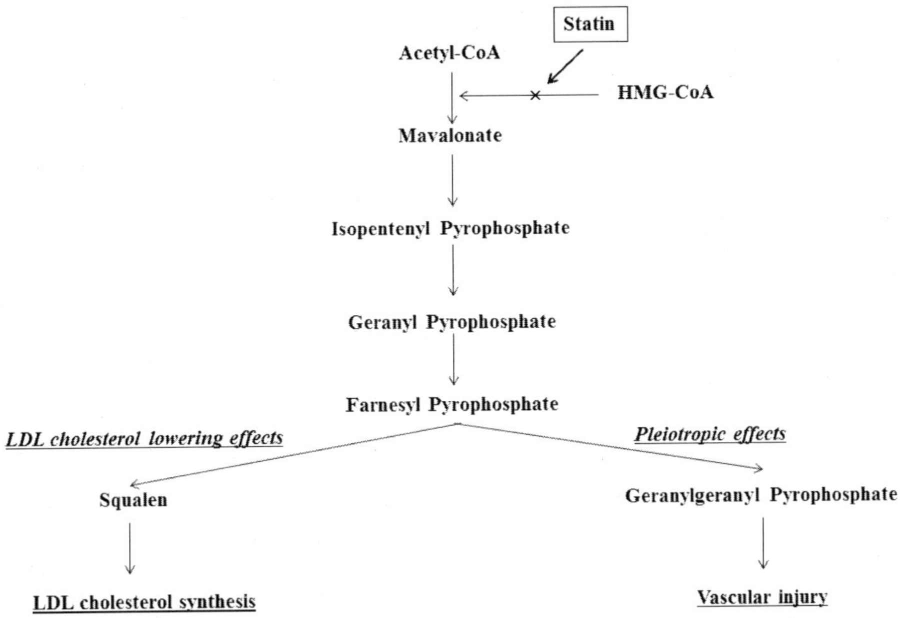

CoA: coenzyme A, HMG-CoA: 3-hydroxy-3-methylglutaryl coenzyme A.

Figure 3. Pathways affected by statins.

Hypotension and hypoglycemia are thought to activate the sympathetic nervous system, thus increasing the rate of cardiovascular events.

3) Additional Drugs

3.1) Thiazolidinediones (TZDs): Rosiglitazone and Pioglitazone

Peroxisome-proliferator-activated receptor gamma (PPARγ) is a member of the nuclear-receptor superfamily, which is expressed predominantly in adipose tissue, pancreatic beta cells, vascular endothelium and macrophages. Thiazolidinediones, PPARγ agonists, improve insulin resistance as well as exert antiatherosclerotic effects. According to the results of the PROactive trial, treatment with pioglitazone results in an approximately 28% reduction in the risk of recurrence of acute coronary syndrome in patients with a previous history of MI [63]. Furthermore, in the PERISCOPE trial, a randomized trial comparing the effects of pioglitazone and glimepiride on the progression of coronary atherosclerotic plaque, as assessed on coronary intravascular ultrasonography, pioglitazone achieved regression of coronary atherosclerotic plaque [64] under an LDL cholesterol level of 93.5 mg/dL. Moreover, according to the results of a meta-analysis of randomized trials, pioglitazone is significantly associated with a reduction in the rate of adverse cardiovascular events, whereas rosiglitazone is associated with a significantly increased risk of cardiovascular events [65]. Although previous reports have demonstrated the superiority of pioglitazone to rosiglitazone with respect to the incidence of cardiovascular events, various adverse effects of thiazolidinediones present a growing problem, including the development of heart failure and cancers. Thiazolidinedione increase sodium reabsorption in the proximal nephron via the PPARγ-dependent nongenomic stimulation of renal proximal transport, which subsequently results in volume expansion. Elderly females treated with this drug are likely to develop edema and heart failure, in a dose-dependent fashion. However, a consensus statement from the American Heart Association and American Diabetes Association regarding the use of thiazolidinediones published in 2003 recommends against the administration of thiazolidinediones in patients with heart failure with a NYHA class of 3 to 4 or a LVEF of < 40% [66].

Compared with patients treated with rosiglitazone, subjects treated with pioglitazone demonstrate a lower risk of heart failure and improvement in the cardiac function. The relationship between the administration of thiazolidinediones and various cancers, in particular, bladder cancer, has been highlighted. For example, pioglitazone has been withdrawn in some countries due to reports of an increased incidence of bladder cancer; however, the controversy regarding this issue is ongoing [67].

3.2) Dipeptidyl Peptidase-4 Inhibitors (DPP-4 Inhibitors)

DPP-4 inhibitors increase the incretin levels, inhibit glucagon release and enhance insulin secretion, thereby decreasing the blood glucose level. Hypoglycemia is a growing serious problem increasing the incidence of cardiovascular adverse events [68]. DPP-4 inhibitors potentially exert both antiatherosclerotic and cardioprotective effects [69] and carry a relatively low risk of hypoglycemia.

Therefore, DPP-4 inhibitors are easy for non-diabetic specialists to use without inducing hypoglycemia in patients with diabetes and MI.

Conclusion

Proposed acute-phase strategies for improving long-term outcomes in patients with AMI are summarized in Table 1. Intensive acute-phase management during hospitalization, particularly the inhibition of LV remodeling, may be associated with improved long-term outcomes in patients with AMI.

References

[1] Nabel E. G. and Braunwald E. (2012) A tale of coronary artery disease and myocardial infarction. *N. Engl. J. Med.*, 366(1):54-63.

[2] Beller G. A. (2001) Coronary heart disease in the first 30 years of the 21st century: challenges and opportunities: The 33rd Annual James B. Herrick Lecture of the Council on Clinical Cardiology of the American Heart Association. *Circulation*, 103(20): 2428-35.

[3] Takii T. and Yasuda S. (2010) MIYAGI-AMI. Trends in acute myocardial infarction incidence and mortality over 30 years in Japan: report from the MIYAGI-AMI Registry Study. *Circ. J.*, 74(1):93-100.

[4] Ezekowitz J. A. and Kaul P. (2009) Declining in-hospital mortality and increasing heart failure incidence in elderly patients with first myocardial infarction. *J. Am. Coll. Cardiol.*, 53(1):13-20.

[5] McNamara R. L. and Wang Y. (2006) NRMI Investigators. Effect of door-to-balloon time on mortality in patients with ST-segment elevation myocardial infarction. *J. Am. Coll. Cardiol.*, 47(11):2180-6.

[6] Flynn A. and Moscucci M. (2010) Trends in door-to-balloon time and mortality in patients with ST-elevation myocardial infarction undergoing primary percutaneous coronary intervention. *Arch. Intern. Med.*, 170(20):1842-9.

[7] Rosamond W. and Flegal K. (2010) American Heart Association. Heart disease and stroke statistics--2008 update: a report from the American Heart Association Statistics Committee and Stroke Statistics Subcommittee. *Circulation,* 117(4):e25-146.

[8] Shiomi H. and Nakagawa Y. (2012) CREDO-Kyoto AMI. Association of onset to balloon and door to balloon time with long term clinical outcome in patients with ST elevation acute myocardial infarction having primary percutaneous coronary intervention: observational study. *BMJ,* 344:e3257.

[9] Miedema M. D. and Newell M. C. (2011) Causes of delay and associated mortality in patients transferred with ST-segment-elevation myocardial infarction. *Circulation,* 124(15):1636-44.

[10] Keeley E. C. and Boura J. A. (2003) Primary angioplasty versus intravenous thrombolytic for acute myocardial infarction: a quantitative review of 23 randomised trials. *Lancet,* 361(9351):13–20.

[11] Keeley E. C. and Boura J. A. (2006) Comparison of primary and facilitated percutaneous coronary interventions for ST-elevation myocardial infarction: quantitative review of randomised trials. *Lancet,* 367(9510):579-88.

[12] Assessment of the Safety and Efficacy of a New Treatment Strategy with Percutaneous Coronary Intervention (ASSENT-4 PCI) investigators. (2006) Primary versus tenecteplase-facilitated percutaneous coronary intervention in patients with ST-segment elevation acute myocardial infarction (ASSENT-4 PCI): randomised trial. *Lancet,* 367(9510):569-78.

[13] Nallamothu B. K. and Bradley E. H. (2007) Time to treatment in primary percutaneous coronary intervention. *N. Engl. J. Med.*, 357(16):1631-8.

[14] Bradley E. H. and Herrin J. (2006) Strategies for reducing the door-to-balloon time in acute myocardial infarction. *N. Engl. J. Med.*, 355(22):2308-20.

[15] Krumholz H. M. and Herrin J. (2011) Improvements in door-to-balloon time in the United States, 2005 to 2010. *Circulation,* 124(9):1038-45.

[16] Weaver W. D. (2003) All hospitals are not equal for treatment of patients with acute myocardial infarction. *Circulation,* 108(15):1768-71.

[17] Ting H. H. and Raveendran G. (2006) A total of 1,007 percutaneous coronary interventions without onsite cardiac surgery: acute and long-term outcomes. *J. Am. Coll. Cardiol.*, 47(8):1713-21.

[18] Keith D. S. and Nichols G. A. (2004) Longitudinal follow-up and outcomes among a population with chronic kidney disease in a large managed care organization. *Arch. Intern. Med.*, 164(6):659-63.

[19] McCullough P. A. (2003) Why is chronic kidney disease the "spoiler" for cardiovascular outcomes? *J. Am. Coll. Cardiol.*, 41(5): 725-728.

[20] Sabatine M. S. and Morrow D. A. (2005) Association of hemoglobin levels with clinical outcomes in acute coronary syndromes. *Circulation,* 111(16):2042-9.

[21] Mason R. P. and Walter M. F. (2005) Intermolecular differences of 3-hydroxy-3-methylglutaryl coenzyme a reductase inhibitors contribute to distinct pharmacologic and pleiotropic actions. *Am. J. Cardiol.,* 96(5A):11F-23F.

[22] Pasceri V. and Patti G. (2004) ARMYDA Investigators. Randomized trial of atorvastatin for reduction of myocardial damage during coronary intervention: results from the ARMYDA (Atorvastatin for Reduction of MYocardial Damage during Angioplasty) study. *Circulation,* 110(6):674-8.

[23] Di Sciascio G. and Patti G. (2009) Efficacy of atorvastatin reload in patients on chronic statin therapy undergoing percutaneous coronary intervention: results of the ARMYDA-RECAPTURE (Atorvastatin for Reduction of Myocardial Damage During Angioplasty) Randomized Trial. *J. Am. Coll. Cardiol.,* 54(6):558-65.

[24] Resnic F. S. and Wainstein M. (2003) No-reflow is an independent predictor of death and myocardial infarction after percutaneous coronary intervention. *Am. Heart J.,* 145(1):42-6.

[25] Rezkalla S. H. and Kloner R. A. (2002) No-reflow phenomenon. *Circulation,* 105(5): 656-62.

[26] Ishii H. and Ichimiya S. (2005) Impact of a single intravenous administration of nicorandil before reperfusion in patients with ST-segment-elevation myocardial infarction. *Circulation,* 112:1284-8.

[27] Parikh C. R. and Coca S. G. (2008) Long-term prognosis of acute kidney injury after acute myocardial infarction. *Arch. Intern. Med.,* 168(9):987-95.

[28] Wi J. and Ko Y. G. (2011) Impact of contrast-induced acute kidney injury with transient or persistent renal dysfunction on long-term outcomes of patients with acute myocardial infarction undergoing percutaneous coronary intervention. *Heart,* 97(21): 1753-7.

[29] Steg P. G. and Huber K. (2011) Bleeding in acute coronary syndromes and percutaneous coronary interventions: position paper by the Working Group on Thrombosis of the European Society of Cardiology. *Eur. Heart J.,* 32(15):1854-64.

[30] Jolicoeur E. M. and O'Neill W. W. (2009) APEX-AMI. Transfusion and mortality in patients with ST-segment elevation myocardial infarction treated with primary percutaneous coronary intervention. *Eur. Heart J.,* 30(21):2575-83.

[31] Burzotta F. and De Vita M. (2009) Clinical impact of thrombectomy in acute ST-elevation myocardial infarction: an individual patient-data pooled analysis of 11 trials. *Eur. Heart J.,* 30(18):2193-203.

[32] Inoue F. and Hashimoto T. (1998) Estimation of coronary flow reserve by intracoronary administration of nicorandil: comparison with intracoronary administration of papaverine. *Heart Vessels,* 13(5):229-36.

[33] Marenzi G. and Assanelli E. (2009) Contrast volume during primary percutaneous coronary intervention and subsequent contrast-induced nephropathy and mortality. *Ann. Intern. Med.,* 150(3):170-7.

[34] Prasad A. and Gersh B. J. (2009) Prognostic significance of periprocedural versus spontaneously occurring myocardial infarction after percutaneous coronary intervention in patients with acute coronary syndromes: an analysis from the ACUITY (Acute

Catheterization and Urgent Intervention Triage Strategy) trial. *J. Am. Coll. Cardiol.*, 54(5):477-86.

[35] Vlaar P. J. and Mahmoud K. D. (2011) Culprit vessel only versus multivessel and staged percutaneous coronary intervention for multivessel disease in patients presenting with ST-segment elevation myocardial infarction: a pairwise and network meta-analysis. *J. Am. Coll. Cardiol.*, 58:692-703.

[36] Shishehbor M. H. and Lauer M. S. (2007) In unstable angina or non-ST-segment acute coronary syndrome, should patients with multivessel coronary artery disease undergo multivessel or culprit-only stenting? *J. Am. Coll. Cardiol.*, 49(8):849-54.

[37] Wald D. S. and Morris J. K. (2013) PRAMI Investigators. Randomized trial of preventive angioplasty in myocardial infarction. *N. Engl. J. Med.*, 369(12):1115-23.

[38] Morita E. and Yasue H. (1993) Increased Plasma Levels of Brain Natriuretic Peptide in Patients With Acute Myocardial Infarction. *Circulation*, 88:82-91.

[39] Garcia-Alvarez A. and Sitges M. (2009) Relation of plasma brain natriuretic peptide levels on admission for ST-elevation myocardial infarction to left ventricular end-diastolic volume six months later measured by both echocardiography and cardiac magnetic resonance. *Am. J. Cardiol.*, 104(7):878-82.

[40] Pfeffer M. A. and Braunwald E. (1992) Effect of captopril on mortality and morbidity in patients with left ventricular dysfunction after myocardial infarction. Results of the survival and ventricular enlargement trial. The SAVE Investigators. *N. Engl. J. Med.*, 327(10):669-77.

[41] Blood Pressure Lowering Treatment Trialists' Collaboration, Turnbull F. and Neal B. (2007) Blood pressure-dependent and independent effects of agents that inhibit the renin-angiotensin system. *J. Hypertens.*, 25(5):951-8.

[42] F. Waagstein and A. Hjalmarson. (1975) Effect of chronic beta-adrenergic receptor blockade in congestive cardiomyopathy. *Br. Heart J.*, 37(10):1022-1036.

[43] J. Alderman and W. Grossman. (1985) Are beta-adrenergic-blocking drugs useful in the treatment of dilated cardiomyopathy? *Circulation,* 71(5):854-857.

[44] Fauchier L. and Pierre B. (2007) Comparison of the beneficial effect of beta-blockers on mortality in patients with ischaemic or non-ischaemic systolic heart failure: a meta-analysis of randomised controlled trials. *Eur. J. Heart Fail.*, 9(11):1136-9.

[45] O'Keefe J. H. Jr. and Magalski A. (2000) *Predictors of improvement in left ventricular ejection fraction with carvedilol for congestive heart failure* 7(1):3-7.

[46] Cleland J. G. and Pennell D. J. (2003) Carvedilol hibernating reversible ischaemia trial. Myocardial viability as a determinant of the ejection fraction response to carvedilol in patients with heart failure (CHRISTMAS trial): randomised controlled trial. *Lancet,* 362(9377):14-21.

[47] Dargie H. J. (2001) Effect of carvedilol on outcome after myocardial infarction in patients with left-ventricular dysfunction: the CAPRICORN randomised trial. *Lancet,* 357(9266):1385-90.

[48] American College of Emergency Physicians; Society for Cardiovascular Angiography and Interventions, O'Gara P. T. and Kushner F. G. (2013) 2013 ACCF/AHA guideline for the management of ST-elevation myocardial infarction: a report of the American College of Cardiology Foundation/American Heart Association Task Force on Practice Guidelines. *J. Am. Coll. Cardiol.*, 61:e78-140.

[49] Ozasa N. and Kimura T. (2010) j-Cypher Registry. Lack of effect of oral beta-blocker therapy at discharge on long-term clinical outcomes of ST-segment elevation acute myocardial infarction after primary percutaneous coronary intervention. *Am. J. Cardiol.,* 106(9):1225-33.

[50] Hayashi M. and Tsutamoto T. (2001) Intravenous atrial natriuretic peptide prevents left ventricular remodeling in patients with first anterior acute myocardial infarction. *J. Am. Coll. Cardiol.,* 37(7):1820-6.

[51] Chen H. H. and Martin F. L. (2009) Low-dose nesiritide in human anterior myocardial infarction suppresses aldosterone and preserves ventricular function and structure: a proof of concept study. *Heart,* 95(16):1315-9.

[52] Kitakaze M. and Asakura M. (2007) J-WIND investigators. Human atrial natriuretic peptide and nicorandil as adjuncts to reperfusion treatment for acute myocardial infarction (J-WIND): two randomised trials. *Lancet,* 370(9597):1483-93.

[53] Chen C. and Ma L. (1997) Left ventricular remodeling in myocardial hibernation. *Circulation,* 96(9 Suppl.):II-46-50.

[54] Claessen B. E. and Dangas G. D. (2013) Multinational CTO Registry. Impact of target vessel on long-term survival after percutaneous coronary intervention for chronic total occlusions. *Catheter Cardiovasc. Interv.,* 82(1):76-82.

[55] Stone G. W. and Maehara A. (2011) PROSPECT Investigators. A prospective natural-history study of coronary atherosclerosis. *N. Engl. J. Med.,* 364(3):226-35.

[56] Bhatt D. L. and Eagle K. A. (2010) REACH Registry. Comparative determinants of 4-year cardiovascular event rates in stable outpatients at risk of or with atherothrombosis. *JAMA,* 304(12):1350-7.

[57] Asakura M. and Ueda Y. (2001) Extensive development of vulnerable plaques as a pan-coronary process in patients with myocardial infarction: An angioscopic study. *J. Am. Coll. Cardiol.*, 37: 1284 - 1288.

[58] Bhatt D. L. and Steg P. G. (2006) REACH Registry. International prevalence, recognition, and treatment of cardiovascular risk factors in outpatients with atherothrombosis. *JAMA,* 295(2):180-9.

[59] Boden W. E. and O'Rourke R. A. (2007) COURAGE Trial Research Group. Optimal medical therapy with or without PCI for stable coronary disease. *N. Engl. J. Med.,* 356(15):1503-16.

[60] Farkouh M. E. and Boden W. E. (2013) Risk factor control for coronary artery disease secondary prevention in large randomized trials. *J. Am. Coll. Cardiol.,* 61(15):1607-15.

[61] BARI 2D Study Group, Frye R. L. and August P. (2009) A randomized trial of therapies for type 2 diabetes and coronary artery disease. *N. Engl. J. Med.,* 360(24): 2503-15.

[62] Farkouh M. E. and Domanski M. (2012) FREEDOM Trial Investigators. Strategies for multivessel revascularization in patients with diabetes. *N. Engl. J. Med.,* 367(25): 2375-84.

[63] Erdmann E. and Dormandy J. A. (2007) PROactive Investigators. The effect of pioglitazone on recurrent myocardial infarction in 2,445 patients with type 2 diabetes and previous myocardial infarction: results from the PROactive (PROactive 05) Study. *J. Am. Coll. Cardiol.,* 49(17):1772-80.

[64] Nissen S. E. and Nicholls S. J. (2008) PERISCOPE Investigators. Comparison of pioglitazone vs glimepiride on progression of coronary atherosclerosis in patients with type 2 diabetes: the PERISCOPE randomized controlled trial. *JAMA,* 299(13):1561-73.

[65] Nissen S. E. and Wolski K. (2007) Effect of rosiglitazone on the risk of myocardial infarction and death from cardiovascular causes. *N. Engl. J. Med.,* 356(24):2457-71.

[66] Nesto R. W. and Bell D. (2003) American Heart Association; American Diabetes Association. Thiazolidinedione use, fluid retention, and congestive heart failure: a consensus statement from the American Heart Association and American Diabetes Association. *Circulation,* 108(23):2941-8.

[67] Ferrara A. and Lewis J. D. (2011) Cohort study of pioglitazone and cancer incidence in patients with diabetes. *Diabetes Care,* 34(4):923-9.

[68] Desouza V. C. and Bolli G. B. (2010) Hypoglicemia, Diabetes, and Cardiovascular Events. *Diabetes Care,* 33(6):1389-1394.

[69] Scheen A. J. (2013) Cardiovascular effects of gliptins. *Nat. Rev. Cardiol.,* 10(2):73-84.

[70] Morrow D. A. and Antman E. M. (2000) TIMI risk score for ST-elevation myocardial infarction: A convenient, bedside, clinical score for risk assessment at presentation: An intravenous nPA for treatment of infarcting myocardium early II trial substudy. *Circulation,* 102(17):2031-7.

[71] De Luca G. and Suryapranata H. (2004) Prognostic assessment of patients with acute myocardial infarction treated with primary angioplasty: implications for early discharge. *Circulation,* 109(22):2737-43.

[72] Halkin A. and Singh M. (2005) Prediction of mortality after primary percutaneous coronary intervention for acute myocardial infarction: the CADILLAC risk score. *J. Am. Coll. Cardiol.,* 45(9):1397-405.

[73] Mehran R. and Aymong E. D. (2004) A simple risk score for prediction of contrast-induced nephropathy after percutaneous coronary intervention: development and initial validation. *J. Am. Coll. Cardiol.,* 44(7):1393-9.

[74] Mehran R. and Pocock S. J. (2010) A risk score to predict bleeding in patients with acute coronary syndromes. *J. Am. Coll. Cardiol.,* 55(23):2556-66.

In: Myocardial Infarctions
Editor: Pattie Wilkonson

ISBN: 978-1-63321-726-3

Chapter 9

Address to Critical Issues in a Cardiogenic Shock Complicating Acute Myocardial Infarction

Makoto Suzuki[*]
Department of Cardiovascular Medicine, Sakakibara Heart Institute. Tokyo, Japan

Abstract

Cardiogenic shock is a well-recognized leading cause of death in patients with an acute myocardial infarction even in the era of early prompt percutaneous coronary intervention (PCI). So far the intensive strategy such as an early use of mechanical circulatory support with PCI also failed to provide significant clinical benefits in those with a cardiogenic shock complicating acute myocardial infarction. As one of the main considerations, systemic mal-perfusion and also high incidence of failed myocardial tissue-level reperfusion may have a critical role in the fatal pathogenesis of a cardiogenic shock complicating acute myocardial infarction. Recently we found an association of exaggerated inflammation with systemic and myocardial tissue-level mal-perfusion in patients treated with PCI for a cardiogenic shock complicating acute myocardial infarction. Here we present an overview of critical issues and then think of the best challenges to provide better clinical outcomes in patients with a cardiogenic shock complicating acute myocardial infarction.

Keywords: Cardiogenic shock, multi-organ dysfunction syndromes, systemic inflammatory response syndrome, ischemia-reperfusion injury, therapeutic hypothermia

[*] Corresponding author: Makoto Suzuki, MD, Department of Cardiovascular Medicine, Sakakibara Heart Institute, 3-16-1 Asahi, Fuchu Tokyo 183-0003 Japan, +81-42-314-3111, fax +81-42-314-3133, E-mail: msuzuki@shi.heart.or.jp.

Introduction

A presence of cardiogenic shock plays the critical role in limiting the rewarding clinical benefits in patients with an acute myocardial infarction despite promptly undergoing percutaneous coronary intervention (PCI). Complication of cardiogenic shock has been diagnosed by three parts of viewpoints, namely hemodynamic, clinical and biochemical manifestations: persistent hypo-perfusion (the systolic arterial pressure less than 90 mm Hg or the mean arterial pressure less than 70 mm Hg or 30 mm Hg lower than baseline, cardiac index less than 1.8 L/min/m^2 without support or less than 2.0 to 2.2 L/min/m2 with support), cold and clammy skin with altered mental state and oliguria, and hyper-lactatemia over 1.5 mmol/L [1,2]. Recently we demonstrated an association of exaggerated inflammation with systemic and myocardial tissue-level mal-perfusion in patients treated with PCI for a cardiogenic shock complicating acute myocardial infarction [3]. Hence, the main feature of a cardiogenic shock complicating acute myocardial infarction is a critical systemic illness that reveals systemic mal-perfusion resulting in inadequate whole-body cellular oxygen utilization with exaggerated systemic inflammation. In this chapter, we address an overview of critical issues [4] and then think of the best challenges to provide better clinical outcomes in patients with a cardiogenic shock complicating acute myocardial infarction.

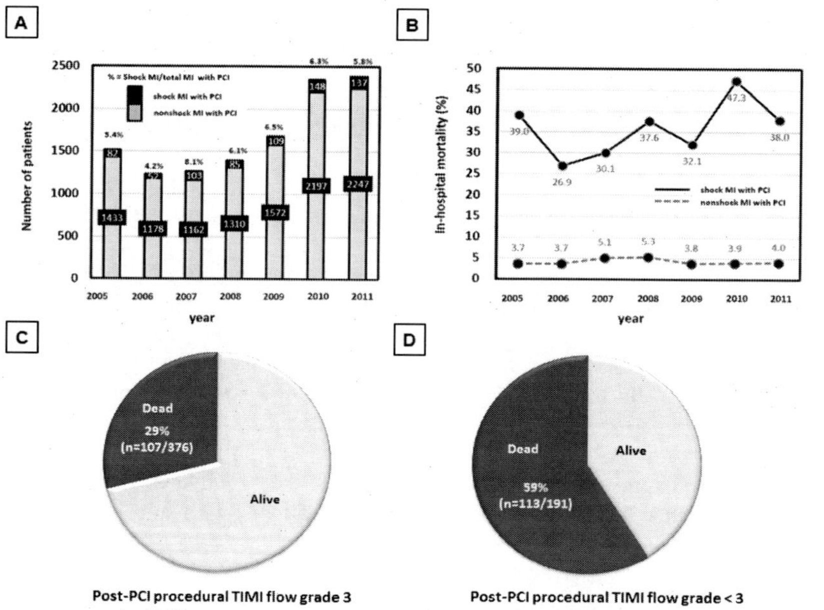

CCU, coronary care unit, PCI, percutaneous coronary intervention, TIMI, Thrombolysis in Myocardial Infarction.

Figure 1. A. Trends in the prevalence of a cardiogenic shock complicating acute myocardial infarction between 2005 and 2011 in the Tokyo CCU Network Councils. B. Trends in in-hospital mortality in patients treated with primary PCI between 2005 and 2011 in the Tokyo CCU Network Councils, in accordance with the presence or absence of cardiogenic shock. C and D. A difference in in-hospital mortality in patients with a cardiogenic shock complicating acute myocardial infarction between 2005 and 2011 in the Tokyo CCU Network Councils, in accordance with post-PCI-procedural TIMI flow grade 3 or less than 3.

Trends in the Prevalence of a Cardiogenic Shock Complicating Acute Myocardial Infarction

Even though a definite development of cardiovascular preventive medicine, any regional medical emergency system and timely reperfusion of patients with an acute myocardial infarction [5], an only modest declines from 7% to 6% in the incidence of a cardiogenic shock complicating acute myocardial infarction had been reported during the past three decades in the New England community [6]. As shown in our cohort analysis from the Tokyo CCU network councils which is operated in a growing number of hospitals from 54 in 2005 to 67 in 2011 supported with the Tokyo Fire Department [7], the percentage of PCI-treated cardiogenic shock complicating acute myocardial infarction also remains relatively unchanged over the periods (Figure 1A). Although an improvement in clinical outcomes under prompt coronary reperfusion has been recognized in those with a cardiogenic shock complicating acute myocardial infarction [8], in-hospital mortality with cardiogenic shock still remains unacceptably high as compared with those without cardiogenic shock (Figure 1B). In addition to the time periods from heart attack to PCI as a great determination of mortality in those with a cardiogenic shock complicating acute myocardial infarction [6], as shown in Figure 1C and 1D, Thrombolysis In Myocardial Infarction (TIMI) flow grades 0 to 2 following PCI which indicates lack of PCI-procedural success must be crucially associated with in-hospital mortality compared with those with post-PCI procedural TIMI flow grade 3 (i.e. optimal coronary reflow) [9]. Because of high prevalence of multi-vessel coronary artery diseases in those with cardiogenic shock [10], clinical significance of primary multi-vessel PCI remains an unresolved challenging issue to improve in-hospital clinical outcomes of those [11-13]. Furthermore, the available evidence does not support the routine use of mechanical circulatory support in those with a cardiogenic shock complicating AMI in whom PCI is attempted [14].

Critical Issues of Mechanical Circulatory Support

Possible advantages of the use of mechanical circulatory support such as intra-aortic balloon pump, percutaneous cardio-pulmonary bypass and also mechanical ventricular assist devices to improve hemodynamic parameters were well-known in contrast to a serious limitation of conservative managements with catecholamines, whereas survival benefit of those mechanical circulatory supports has not been proof in the treatment of a cardiogenic shock complicating acute myocardial infarction [15-20]. We addressed our hypothesis that mechanical circulatory support with optimal coronary reflow may ameliorate clinical outcomes in those with a cardiogenic shock complicating acute myocardial infarction. Nevertheless, we found in-hospital mortality of 36% in our cohort study of 376 patients with a cardiogenic shock complicating acute myocardial infarction with mechanical circulatory support irrespective of post-PCI procedural TIMI flow grade 3 in the Tokyo CCU Network Council between January 2005 and December 2010, suggesting a still high in-hospital mortality even under optimal coronary reflow. The main cause of in-hospital death of those was low output syndrome and/or multi-organ dysfunction syndromes (Figure 2A). Previous clinical studies validated that mortality is chiefly determined by the incidence of multi-organ dysfunction syndromes within a couple of days after the onset of cardiogenic shock in those with an acute myocardial infarction [4, 21]. Of note, the use of mechanical circulatory support does not ameliorate serum levels of lactate which indicate the severity of end-organ dysoxia and strongly impact on the risk of multi-organ dysfunction syndromes in those with a cardiogenic shock complicating acute myocardial infarction [4, 18, 21, 22]. Interestingly our multivariate analysis demonstrated that pre-PCI procedural TIMI flow grade 0 was mostly associated with in-hospital mortality in those with an anterior acute myocardial infarction with cardiogenic shock and optimal coronary reflow (Figure 2B). In view of these findings, we suppose a distinct possibility of total occlusion of initial coronary flow (i.e. pre-PCI procedural TIMI flow grade 0) as the key issues to produce lethal myocardial tissue-level reperfusion injury which may be one of the crucial basis of less clinical benefits of mechanical circulatory support irrespective of optimal culprit coronary reflow in those [23].

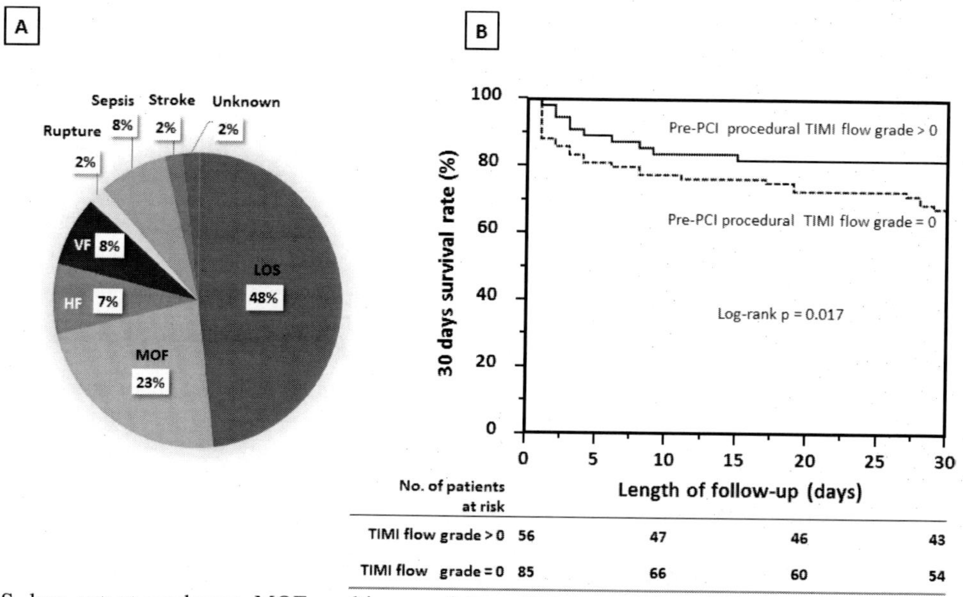

LOS, low output syndrome, MOF, multi-organ failure, HF, heart failure, VF, ventricular fibrillation, PCI, percutaneous coronary intervention, TIMI, Thrombolysis in Myocardial Infarction.

Figure 2. A. The cause of in-hospital death in a total of 53 of 141 patients with a cardiogenic shock complicating anterior acute myocardial infarction who achieved post-PCI procedural TIMI flow grade 3 in the Tokyo CCU Network Council between January 2005 and December 2010. B. A 30-days survival rate in 141 patients with a cardiogenic shock complicating anterior acute myocardial infarction who achieved post-PCI procedural TIMI flow grade 3 in the Tokyo CCU Network Council between January 2005 and December 2010, in accordance with pre-PCI procedural TIMI flow grade 0 or not.

Lethal Myocardial Ischemia-Reperfusion Injury and Multi-Organ Dysfunction Syndromes

Although several mechanisms for lethal myocardial ischemia-reperfusion injury have been proposed, those are activated within the first few minutes after coronary reperfusion [24]. At least four mechanisms are possibly considered to be composed of this injury [25].

Intracellular calcium overload during ischemia due to impaired calcium cycling and sarcolemmal damage can be exacerbated with reperfusion (*Calcium paradox*) [26]. The restoration of a normal extracellular pH after reperfusion produces a hydrogen gradient across the cell membrane. The sodium/hydrogen exchanger is activated and causes a net influx of sodium into the cytosol. Because the sodium/potassium ATPase may dysfunction due to a lack of energy and structural damages by ischemia, an influx of calcium with an outflux of sodium via the sodium/calcium exchanger produces further intracellular calcium overload (*pH paradox*). Reactive oxygen species are excessively produced within minutes of reperfusion and continue to be generated for hours after the restoration of blood flow to ischemic microvasculature [27]. Excess reactive oxygen species must directly damage both cardiomyocytes and vascular endothelial cells via altering membrane proteins and phospholipids and, in consequence, both of their membranes have malfunctioned as receptors, enzyme production, and ion channels (*Oxygen paradox*) [28]. The mitochondrial membrane is ordinarily impermeable to most ions and metabolites. With the restoration of blood flow with rapid oxygenation in the microvasculature, however, excess reactive oxygen species and calcium overload induce opening of the mitochondrial permeability transition pore and allows proteins to move freely across the mitochondrial membrane causing swell and then rupture of the outer membrane with subsequent release of mitochondrial proteins leading to induction of mitochondria distress. The subsequent fall in adenosine triphosphate levels further disrupts ionic and metabolic homeostasis and leads to the activation of degradative enzymes [29]. Influx of activated neutrophils throughout blood stream during reperfusion accelerates inflammation with subsequent adhesion to the endothelial surface and migration in the surrounding tissue of post-ischemic myocardium. Activated neutrophils furthermore overproduce reactive oxygen species, proteolytic enzymes, and pro-inflammatory mediators that can directly cause various cell injuries in myocardial tissue-levels (*Inflammatory attack*) [30]. Recently we demonstrated the presence of a great exaggeration of systemic and also coronary inflammation in the setting of a cardiogenic shock complicating acute myocardial infarction, and a possible role of those inflammations in the pathogenesis of excessive systemic as well as myocardial tissue-level mal-perfusion in those treated with PCI for a cardiogenic shock complicating acute myocardial infarction (Figure 3A-D) [3]. Importantly, fatal clinical outcomes in a cardiogenic shock complicating acute myocardial infarction were associated with the widespread systemic inflammatory response syndrome (SIRS) showing high serum levels of interleukin-6 [31, 32] with high scores of either Acute Physiology and Chronic Health Evaluation (APACHE) II [33] or Simplified Acute Physiology Score (SAPS) II [34] indicating severe multi-organ dysfunction syndromes, but less associated with cardiac function itself (Table) [20]. Thus, a course on the development of multi-organ dysfunction syndromes with SIRS in those with a cardiogenic shock complicating acute myocardial infarction must be the key issue which mimics the microcirculatory and cellular distress state underlying in septic shock [35] (Figure 4). In view of a bipolar action of inflammation as injury and repair in the pathogenesis of reperfused acute myocardial infarction with cardiogenic shock [36], we postulate to control the role of inflammation in accomplishing preserved systemic and myocardial tissue-level condition.

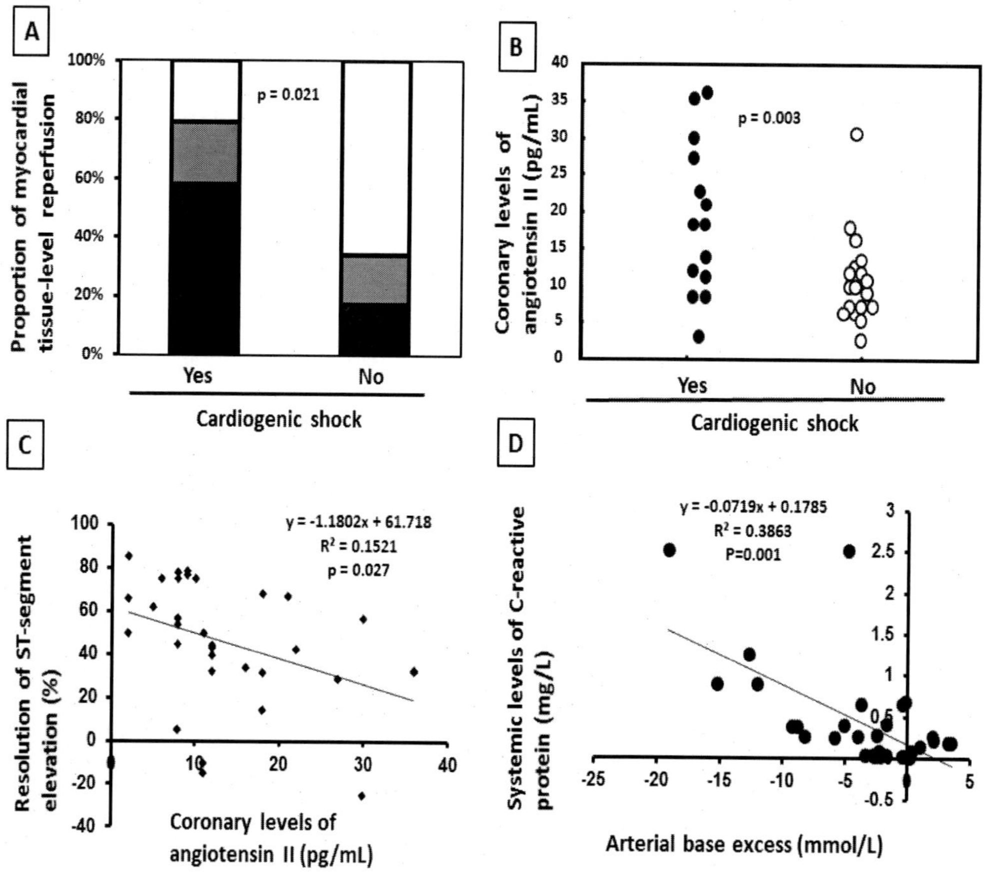

Figure 3. A. Proportion of myocardial tissue-level reperfusion in patients with a first anterior ST-segment elevation myocardial infarction, in accordance with the presence or absence of cardiogenic shock. White bar was a proportion of the presence of both ST-segment resolution ≥ 50% and myocardial blush grade 3, indicating well myocardial tissue-level reperfusion, gray bar presented a proportion of the presence of either ST-segment resolution < 50% or myocardial blush grade < 3, and black bar revealed a proportion of the presence of both ST-segment resolution < 50% and myocardial blush grade < 3, indicating failed myocardial tissue-level reperfusion. B. Coronary levels of angiotensin II in those with a first anterior ST-segment elevation myocardial infarction, in accordance with the presence or absence of cardiogenic shock C. Relationship between coronary levels of angiotensin II and resolution of ST-segment elevation in patients with a first anterior ST-segment elevation myocardial infarction with and without cardiogenic shock. D. Relationship between arterial base excess on admission and systemic levels of C-reactive protein in patients with a first anterior ST-segment elevation myocardial infarction with and without cardiogenic shock. Adapted from reference 3.

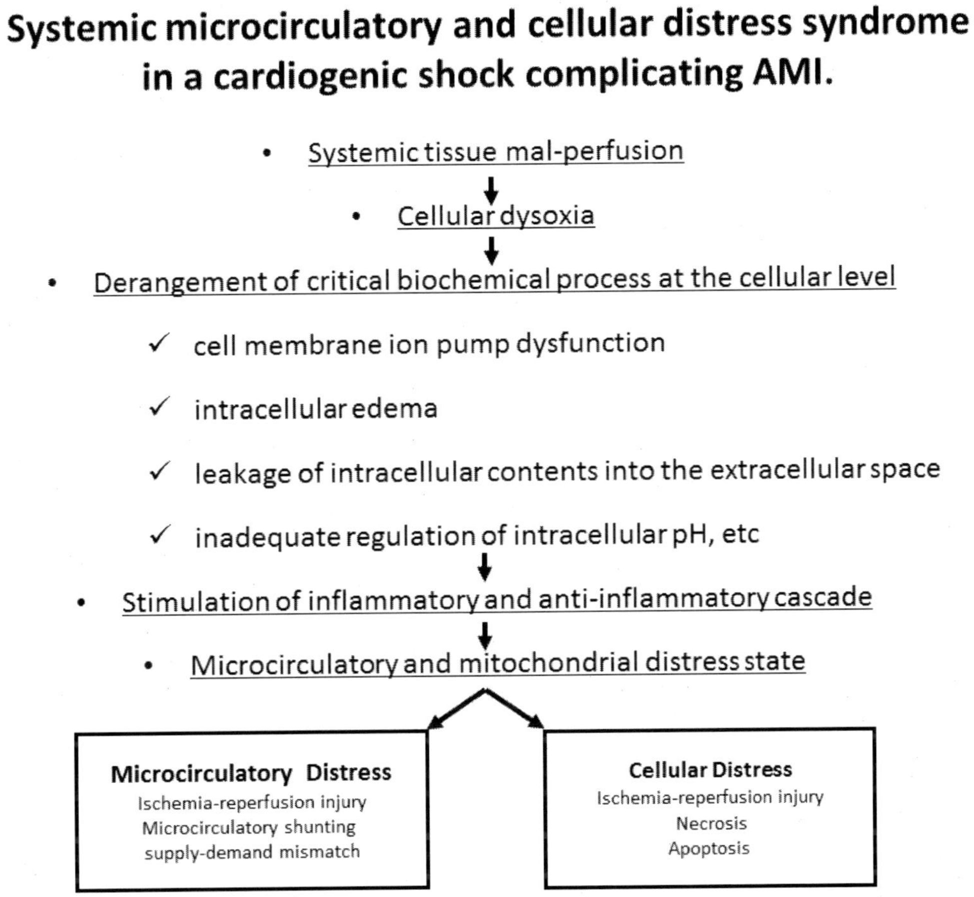

Figure 4. Potential pathogenesis of systemic microcirculatory and cellular distress syndrome in a cardiogenic shock complicating acute myocardial infarction.

Table. Predictive marker for in-hospital mortality in patients with a cardiogenic shock complicating acute myocardial infarction [17, 20]

Variable	Area under curve	p value
APACH score	0.850	< 0.001
SAPS score	0.873	< 0.001
Cardiac index	0.771	0.088
Cardiac power index	0.742	0.025
Plasma levels of interleukin-6	0.769	0.011
B-type natriuretic peptide	0.502	0.987
C-reactive protein	0.505	0.963

APACH=Acute Physiology and Chronic Health Evaluation, SAPS=Simplified Acute Physiology Score.

Address to these Critical Issues

Because of unacceptably high mortality despite rapid revascularization, optimal medications, and frequently use of mechanical circulatory support, novel therapeutic strategies must be developed in those with the critical systemic illness. Therapeutic hypothermia is widely available and has become an established standard of care for patients with post-cardiac arrest syndromes [37]. Non-randomized trials have also reported the feasibility of combination of therapeutic hypothermia with PCI in the setting of an acute myocardial infarction [38]. A clinical benefits of therapeutic hypothermia in the prevention of a systemic ischemia-reperfusion response as well as systemic inflammatory response in those with post-cardiac arrest syndromes have been proposed by several potential mechanisms such as an enhancing cellular membrane integrity through preserved adenosine triphosphate with a reduction in metabolic demand and glucose consumption [39], a prevention of mitochondrial damages via the inhibition of calcium-induced mitochondrial permeability transition pore [40], and an improvement in microcirculation [41]. Furthermore, the reduction in reactive oxygen species [42] and suppressions of pro-inflammatory mediators [43] during hypothermia may be of great benefit to ameliorate systemic and also myocardial tissue-level ischemia-reperfusion injury [44]. Although numerous pharmacologic interventions have been proposed and tested clinically to prevent myocardial ischemia-reperfusion injury in the setting of an acute myocardial infarction [45], a couple of clinical studies only showed clinical benefits over reperfusion alone [46,47]. A clinical advantages of therapeutic hypothermia has been assumed when treated with PCI in those with a cardiogenic shock complicating acute myocardial infarction, whereas there were only a few studies about treatment of hypothermia in patients complicated with cardiogenic shock [48-50]. We retrospectively recruited a total of 37 consecutive patients (28 men, 70 ± 13 years) who showed severe metabolic acidemia with the presence of arterial blood levels of lactate over 4 mmol/L on hospital admission or 30 minutes after resuscitation and underwent mechanical circulatory supported PCI for a cardiogenic shock complicating first anterior acute myocardial infarction and post-cardiac arrest syndromes to assess whether pre-reperfusion therapeutic hypothermia modify the myocardial tissue-level reperfusion and in-hospital clinical outcome. Of those, 13 patients were treated with pre-PCI procedural therapeutic hypothermia and 24 were not inducted with hypothermia treatments. All of 13 patients with therapeutic hypothermia had achieved target core temperature of 34°C when undergoing PCI. A total of 26 patients were dead in hospital, thereby overall in-hospital mortality was 70%. In detail, one patient with therapeutic hypothermia and 8 without hypothermia were dead within 24 hours after admission (8% vs. 33%, $p=0.063$), and 6 patients with therapeutic hypothermia and 20 without hypothermia were finally in-hospital dead (46% vs. 83%, $p=0.028$). A significant difference in In-hospital survival curve in accordance with the presence or absence of pre-PCI procedural therapeutic hypothermia was found in those with a severe refractory cardiogenic shock complicated anterior acute myocardial infarction (Figure 5A). Those with and without hypothermia showed a significant difference in the proportion of failed myocardial tissue-level reperfusion defined by a myocardial blush grade 0 or 1, which scored 0 to 3 with highest score indicating normal microvascular perfusion [51] (Figure 5B). Thus, we believe that systemic therapeutic hypothermia prior to coronary reperfusion may provide great possibilities to preserve myocardial tissue-level reperfusion as well as systemic mal-perfusion and so ameliorate in-hospital clinical outcomes in the setting of a severe refractory cardiogenic shock complicating acute myocardial infarction. Future investigations warrants cooling reperfusion using therapeutic hypothermia as a potential strategy in patients with PCI for a cardiogenic shock complicating acute myocardial infarction.

Conclusion and Future Perspectives

The main feature of a cariogenic shock complicating acute myocardial infarction is composed of the development of multi-organ dysfunction syndromes based on systemic microcirculatory and cellular distress state with exaggerated systemic inflammation. We hypothesize that an early initiation of therapeutic hypothermia, especially before coronary reperfusion, may be a promising strategy to address this critical systemic illness.

Acknowledgments

We deeply thank Dr. Morimasa Takayama and Ms. Nobuko Yoshida for their expert proposal in the preparation of data of the Tokyo CCU network councils.

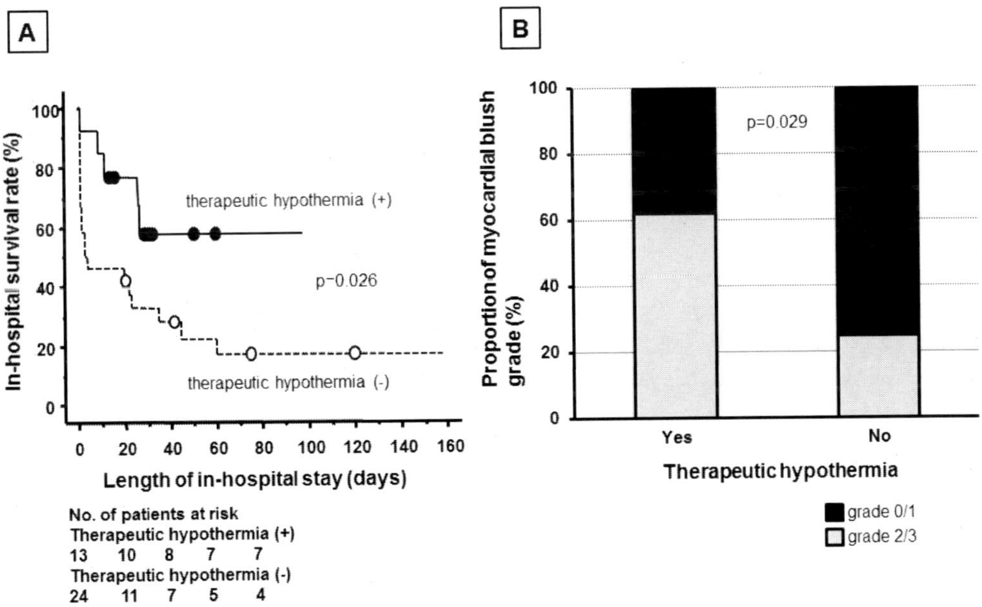

Figure 5. A. In-hospital survival rate in a total of 37 consecutive patients with a severe refractory cardiogenic shock complicating first anterior ST-segment elevation myocardial infarction, in accordance with the induction of pre-PCI procedural therapeutic hypothermia or not. Thirteen patients with pre-PCI procedural therapeutic hypothermia showed significantly low in-hospital mortality as compared with 24 patients without therapeutic hypothermia. B. Comparison of myocardial tissue-level reperfusion, in accordance with the induction of pre-PCI procedural therapeutic hypothermia or not.

References

[1] Reynolds, HR; Hochman, JS. Cardiogenic shock: Current concepts and improving outcomes. *Circulation.*, 2008, 117, 686-697.

[2] Vincent, J-L; De Backer, D. Circulatory shock. *N Engl J Med.*, 2013, 369, 1726-1734.

[3] Suzuki, M; Takamisawa, I; Seki, A; Tobaru, T; Seike, F; Shimizu, H; Takayama, M. Clinical evidence of exaggerated inflammation in patients with a cardiogenic shock complicating ST-segment elevation myocardial infarction. *Health.*, 2013, 5, 1648-1653.

[4] Thiele, H; Allam, B; Chatellier, G; Schuler, G; Lafont, A. Shock in acute myocardial infarction, the Cape Horn for trials? *Eur Heart J.*, 2010, 31, 1828-1835.

[5] O'Gara, PT; Kushner, FG; Ascheim, DD; Casey, DE; Jr. Chung, MK; de Lemos, JA; Ettinger, SM; Fang, JC; Fesmire, FM; Franklin, BA; Granger, CB; Krumholz, HM; Linderbaum, JA; Morrow, DA; Newby, LK; Ornato, JP; Ou, N; Radford, MJ; Tamis-Holland, JE; Tommaso, CL; Tracy, CM; Woo, YJ; Zhao, DX; Anderson, JL; Jacobs, AK; Halperin, JL; Albert, NM; Brindis, RG; Creager, MA; DeMets, D; Guyton, RA; Hochman, JS; Kovacs, RJ; Kushner, FG; Ohman, EM; Stevenson, WG; Yancy, CW. 2013 ACCF/AHA guideline for the management of ST-elevation myocardial infarction: a report of the American College of Cardiology Foundation/American Heart Association Task Force on Practice Guidelines. *J Am Coll Cardiol.*, 2013, 61, e78-e140.

[6] Goldberg, RJ; Spencer, FA; Gore, JM; Lessard, D; Yarzebski, J. Thirty-year trends (1975 to 2005) in the magnitude of, management of, and hospital death rates associated with cardiogenic shock in patients with acute myocardial infarction: a population-based perspective. *Circulation.*, 2009, 119, 1211-1219.

[7] Takano, T; Ida, T; Tanaka, K; Obayashi, K; Kimura, E. Prehospital care (CCU network) of acute myocardial infarction and treatment of cardiogenic shock by intra-aortic balloon pumping. *Jpn Circ J.*, 1981, 45, 623-635.

[8] Babaev, A; Frederick, PD; Pasta, DJ; Every, N; Sichrovsky, T; Hochman, JS. Trends in management and outcomes of patients with acute myocardial infarction complicated by cardiogenic shock. *JAMA.*, 2005, 294, 448-454.

[9] Mehta, RH; Ou, F-S; Peterson, ED; Shaw, RE; Hillegass, WB; Jr. Rumsfeld, JS; Roe, MT. Clinical significance of post-procedural TIMI flow in patients with cardiogenic shock undergoing primary percutaneous coronary intervention. *J Am Coll Cardiol intv.*, 2009, 2, 56-64.

[10] Sanborn, TA; Sleeper, LA; Webb, JG; French, JK; Bergman, G; Parikh, M; Wong, SC; Boland, J; Pfisterer, M; Stater, JN; Sharma, S; Hochman, JS. Correlates of one-year survival in patients with cardiogenic shock complicating acute myocardial infarction, angiographic findings from the SHOCK trial. *J Am Coll Cardiol.*, 2003, 42, 1373-1379.

[11] Cavender, MA; Milford-Beland, S; Roe, MT; Peterson, ED; Weintraub, WS; Rao, SV. Prevalence, predictors, and in-hospital outcomes of non-infarct artery intervention during primary percutaneous coronary intervention for ST-segment elevation myocardial infarction (from the National Cardiovascular Data Registry). *Am J Cardiol.*, 2009, 104, 507-513.

[12] Bauer, T; Zeymer, U; Hochadel, M; Möllman, H; Weidinger, F; Zahn, R; Nef, HM; Hamm, CW; Marco, J; Gitt, AK. Use and outcomes of multivessel percutaneous

coronary intervention in patients with acute myocardial infarction complicated by cardiogenic shock (from the EHS-PCI registry). *Am J Cardiol.*, 2012, 109, 941-946.

[13] Mylotte, D; Morice, MC; Eltchaninoff, H; Garot, J; Louvard, Y; Lefèvre, T; Garot, P. Primary percutaneous coronary intervention in patients with acute myocardial infarction, resuscitated cardiac arrest, and cardiogenic shock: the role of primary multivessel revascularization. *JACC Cardiovasc Interv.*, 2013, 6, 115-125.

[14] O'Connor, CM; Rogers, JG. Evidence for overturning the guidelines in cardiogenic shock. *N Engl J Med.*, 2012, 367, 1349-1350.

[15] Sjauw, KD; Engström, AE; Vis, MM; van der Schaaf, RJ; Baan, J: Jr. Koch, KT; de Winter, RJ; Piek, JJ; Tijssen, JG; Henriques, JP. A systematic review and meta-analysis of intra-aortic balloon pump therapy in ST-elevation myocardial infarction, should we change the guidelines? *Eur Heart J.*, 2009, 30, 459-468.

[16] Cheng, JM; den Uil, CA; Hoeks, SE; van der Ent, M; Jewbali, LS; van Domburg, RT; Serruys, PW. Percutaneous left ventricular assist devices vs. intra-aortic balloon pump counterpulsation for treatment of cardiogenic shock: a meta-analysis of controlled trials. *Eur Heart J.*, 2009, 30, 2102-2108.

[17] Prondzinsky, R; Lemm, H; Swyter, M; Wegener, N; Unverzagt, S; Carter, JM; Russ, M; Schlitt, A; Buerke, U; Christoph, A; Schmidt, H; Winkler, M; Thiery, J; Werdan, K; Buerke, M. Intra-aortic balloon counterpulsation in patients with acute myocardial infarction complicated by cardiogenic shock: the prospective, randomized IABP SHOCK Trial for attenuation of multiorgan dysfunction syndrome. *Crit Care Med.*, 2010, 38, 152-160.

[18] Thiele, H; Zeymer, U; Neumann, FJ; Ferenc, M; Olbrich, HG; Hausleiter, J; Richardt, G; Hennersdorf, M; Empen, K; Fuernau, G; Desch, S; Eitel, I; Hambrecht, R; Fuhrmann, J; Böhm, M; Ebelt, H; Schneider, S; Schuler, G, Werdan, K. Intraaortic balloon support for myocardial infarction with cardiogenic shock. *N Engl J Med.*, 2012, 367, 1287-1296.

[19] Thiele, H; Zeymer, U; Neumann, FJ; Ferenc, M; Olbrich, HG; Hausleiter, J; de Waha, A; Richardt, G; Hennersdorf, M; Empen, K; Fuernau, G; Desch, S; Eitel, I; Hambrecht, R; Lauer, B; Böhm, M; Ebelt, H; Schneider, S; Werdan, K; Schuler, G. Intra-aortic balloon counterpulsation in acute myocardial infarction complicated by cardiogenic shock (IABP-SHOCK II): final 12 month results of a randomized, open-label trial. *Lancet.*, 2013, 382, 1638-1645.

[20] Werdan, K; Gielen, S; Ebelt, H; Hochman, JS. Mechanical circulatory support in cardiogenic shock. *Eur Heart J.*, 2014, 35, 156-167.

[21] Kar, B; Basra, S; Shah, NR; Loyalka, P. Percutaneous circulatory support in cardiogenic shock. Interventional bridge to recovery. *Circulation.*, 2012, 125, 1809-1817.

[22] Den Uil, CA; Lagrand, WK; van der Ent, M; Jewbali, LSD; Cheng, JM; Spronk, PE; Simoons, ML. Impaired microcirculation predicts poor outcome of patients with acute myocardial infarction complicated by cardiogenic shock. *Eur Heart J.*, 2010, 31, 3032-3039.

[23] Hochman, JS. Cardiogenic shock complicating acute myocardial infarction. Expanding the paradigm. *Circulation.*, 2003, 107, 2998-3002.

[24] Prasad, A; Stone, GW; Holmes, DR; Gersh, B. Reperfusion injury, microvascular dysfunction, and cardioprotection: the "dark side" of reperfusion. *Circulation.*, 2009, 120, 2105-2112.

[25] Hausenloy, DJ; Yellon, DM. Myocardial ischemia-reperfusion injury: a neglected therapeutic target. *J Clin Invest.*, 2013, 123, 92-100.

[26] Meissner, A; Morgan, JP. Contractile dysfunction and abnormal Ca^{2+} modulation during postischemic reperfusion in rat heart. *Am J Physiol.*, 1995, 268, H100-H111.

[27] Boll, R; Jeroudi, MO; Patel, BS; DuBose, CM; Lai, EK; Roberts, R; McCay, PB. Direct evidence that oxygen-derived free radicals contribute to postischmic myocardial dysfunction in the intact dog. *Proc Natl Acad Sci USA.*, 1989, 86, 4695-4699.

[28] Toyokuni, S. Reactive oxygen species-induced molecular damage and its application in pathology. *Pathol Int.,* 1999, 49, 91-102.

[29] Halestrap, AP; Clarke, SJ; Javadov, SA. Mitochondrial permeability transition pore opening during myocardial reperfusion-a target for cardioprotection. Cardiovasc Res., 2004, 61, 372-385.

[30] Reffelmann, T; Kloner, RA. The no-reflow phenomenon: A basic mechanism of myocardial ischemia and reperfusion. *Basic Res Cardiol.*, 2006, 101, 359-372.

[31] Geppert, A; Dorninger, A; Delle-Karth, G; Zorn, G; Heinz, G; Huber, K. Plasma concntrations of interlukin-6, organ failure, vasopressor support, and successful coronary revascularization in predicting 30-day mortality of patients with cardiogenic shock complicating acute myocardial infarction. *Crit Care Med.,* 2006, 34, 2035-2042.

[32] Andrie, R; Becher, UM; Frommold, R; Tiyerili, V; Schrickel, JW; Nickenig, G; Schwab, JO. Interleukin-6 is the strongest predictor of 30-day mortality in patients with cardiogenic shock due to myocardial infarction. *Critical Care.*, 2012 Aug 13, 16, R152.[Epub ahead of print].

[33] Knaus, WA; Draper, EA; Wagner, DP; Zimmerman, JE. APACH II: A severity of disease classification system. *Crit Care Med.*, 1985, 13, 818-829.

[34] Le Gall, JR; Lemeshow, S; Saulnier, F. A new Simplified Acute Physiology Score (SAPS II) based on a European/North American multicenter study. *JAMA.*, 1993, 270, 2957-2963.

[35] Ince, C. The microcirculation is the motor of sepsis. *Critical care.*, 2005, 9(suppl 4), s13-s19.

[36] Suzuki, M. Acute coronary syndromes as auto-inflammatory disorders. *Curr Pharm Des.*, 2012, 18, 4370-4384.

[37] Hazinski, MF; Nolan, JP; Billi, JE; Böttiger, BW; Bossaert, L; de Caen, AR; Deakin, CD; Drajer, S; Eigel, B; Hickey, RW; Jacobs, I; Kleinman, ME; Kloeck, W; Koster, RW; Lim, SH; Mancini, ME; Montgomery, WH; Morley, PT; Morrison, LJ; Nadkarni, VM; O'Connor, RE; Okada, K; Perlman, JM; Sayre, MR; Shuster, M; Soar, J; Sunde, K; Travers, AH; Wyllie, J; Zideman, D. Part 1: executive summary: 2010 International consensus on cardiopulmonary resuscitation and emergency cardiovascular care science with treatment recommendations. *Circulation.*, 2010, 122, S250-S275.

[38] Stub, D; Bernard, S; Duffy, SJ; Kaye, DM. Post cardiac arrest syndrome: a review of therapeutic strategies. *Circulation.*, 2011, 123, 1429-1435.

[39] Simkhovich, BZ; Hale, SL; Kloner, RA. Metabolic mechanism by which mild regional hypothermia preserves ischemic tissue. *J Cardiovasc Pharmacol Ther.*, 2004, 9, 83-90.

[40] Tisser, R; Couvreur, N; Ghaleh, B; Bruunerval, P; Lidouren, F; Morin, D; Zini, R; Bize, A; Chenoune, M; Belair, MF; Mandet, C; Douheret, M; Dubois-Randel, JL; Parker, JC; Cohen, MV; Downey, JM; Berdeaux, A. Rapid cooling preserves the ischemic myocardium against mitochondrial damage and left ventricular dysfunction. *Cardiovasc Res.*, 2009, 83, 345-353.

[41] Ye, S; Weng, Y; Sun, S; Chen, W; Wu, X; Li, Z; Weil, MH; Tang, W. Comparison of the durations of mild therapeutic hypothermia on outcome after cardiopulmonary resuscitation in the rat. *Circulation.*, 2012, 125, 123-129.

[42] Khaliulin, I; Clarke, SJ; Lin, H; Parker, J; Suleiman, MS; Halestrap, AP. Temperature preconditioning of isolated rat hearts-a potent cardioprotective mechanism involving a reduction in oxidative stress and inhibition of the mitochondrial permeability transition pore. *J Physiol.*, 2007, 581, 1147-1161.

[43] Delhaye, C; Mahmoudi, M; Waksman, R. Hypothermia therapy. Neurological and cardiac benefits. *J Am Coll Caldiol.*, 2012, 59, 197-210.

[44] Kanemoto, S; Matsubara, M; Noma, M; Leshnower, BG; Parish, LM; Jackson, BM; Hinmon, R; Hamamoto, H; Gorman, JH; III. Gorman, RC. Mild hypothermia to limit myocardial ischemia-reperfusion injury: importance of timing. *Ann Thorac Surg.*, 2009, 87, 157-163.

[45] Yellon, DM; Hausenloy, DJ. Myocardial reperfusion injury. *N Engl J Med.*, 2007, 357, 1121-1135.

[46] Piot, C; Croisille, P; Staat, P; Thibault, H; Rioufol, G; Mewton, N; Elbelghiti, R; Cung, TT; Bonnefoy, E; Angoulvant, D; Macia, C; Raczka, F; Sportouch, C; Gahide, G; Finet, G; André-Fouët, X; Revel, D; Kirkorian, G; Monassier, J-P; Derumeaux, G; Ovize, M. Effect of cyclosporine on reperfusion injury in acute myocardial infarction. *N Engl J Med.*, 2008, 359, 473-481.

[47] Erlinge, D; Götberg, M; Lang, I; Holzer, M; Noc, M; Clemmensen, P; Jensen, U; Metzler, B; James, S; Bötker, HE; Omerovic, E; Engblom, H; Carlsson, M; Arheden, H; Ostlund, O; Wallentin, L; Harnek, J; Olivecrona, GK. Rapid endovascular catheter core cooling combined with cold saline as an adjunct to percutaneous coronary intervention for the treatment of acute myocardial infarction. The CHILL-MI trial: a randomized controlled study of the use of central venous catheter core cooling combined with cold saline as an adjunct to percutaneous coronary intervention for the treatment of acute myocardial infarction. *J Am Coll Cardiol.*, 2014, 63, 1857-1865.

[48] Hovdenes, J; Laake, JH; Aaberge, L; Haugaa, H; Bugge, JF. Therapeutic hypothermia after out-of-hospital cardiac arrest: experiences with patients treated with percutaneous coronary intervention and cardiogenic shock. *Acta Anaesthesiol Scand.*, 2007, 51, 137-142.

[49] Skulec, R; Kovarnik, T; Dostalova, G; Kolar, J; Linhart, A. Induction of mild hypothermia in cardiac arrest survivors presenting with cardiogenic shock syndrome. *Acta Anaesthesiol Scand.*, 2008, 52, 188-194.

[50] Zobel, C; Adler, C; Kranz, A; Seck, C; Pfister, R; Hellmich, M; Kochanek, M; Reuter, H. Mild therapeutic hypothermia in cardiogenic shock syndrome. *Crit Care Med.*, 2012, 40, 1715-1723.

[51] Suzuki, M; Sakaue, T; Tanaka, M; Hirose, E; Saeki, H; Matsunaka, T; Hiramatsu, S; Kazatani, Y. Association between right bundle branch block and impaired myocardial tissue-level reperfusion in patients with acute myocardial infarction. *J Am Coll Cardiol.*, 2006, 47, 2122-2124.

In: Myocardial Infarctions
Editor: Pattie Wilkonson

ISBN: 978-1-63321-726-3

Chapter 10

Management of Unstable Angina/ Non-ST Segment Myocardial Infarction

Sachin Mehta * ***and Tahir Mian***
Seton Family of Hospitals, Austin, TX, US

Abstract

Unstable angina is a classification of acute coronary syndrome (ACS). Indeed, ACS spans the spectrum of unstable angina, non-ST segment myocardial infarction, and ST segment elevation myocardial infarction. Millions of Americans present to medical care professionals with unstable angina. While the disease process and treatment varies with ACS presentation and degree of injury, there are certain characteristics that are common to each clinical scenario. A through history and physical examination, diagnostics including electrocardiogram, and biochemical markers help to establish the diagnosis and degree of ACS. By determining the extent of injury to a patient, physicians are able to guide appropriate treatment goals based on risk/benefit ratio. Medical treatment includes anti-ischemic, antiplatelet, antianginal, and statin therapies. Finally, invasive measures including revascularization plays a prominent role in treating unstable angina. Beyond revascularization, cardiac rehabilitation is increasingly recognized in treating patients who present with unstable angina.

Introduction

Every 34 seconds, an American will have a coronary event. [1] In an hour, approximately 60 Americans will die from coronary artery disease(CAD).(1) Due to the severe consequences and prevalence of ischemic heart disease, emergency room physicians rapidly attempt to diagnosis and treat patients who present with chest pain. In addition to a comprehensive history and physical, physicians use several diagnostic tools including chest x-

* Corresponding author: email is s.mehta.tx@gmail.com.

rays, electrocardiograms (EKGs), and laboratory tests to assist in diagnosing a patient who may present with symptomatic CAD.

The severity of coronary disease impacts treatment such that the burden of ischemia dictates medical and interventional approach. In managing patients with acute chest pain, a physician must consider if the patient has a previous history of CAD, EKG findings suggesting ischemia, or signs of congestive heart failure (CHF). Furthermore the patient's underlying heart rhythm and hemodynamic status must be evaluated and treated. Several scoring systems have been created to help risk-stratify patients. [2,3,4] These scoring systems were developed from the clinical presentation, diagnostic findings, and outcomes of patients who presented with coronary events. The systems are intended to assist in directing clinical management. Of course, this is assuming that the symptoms are due to angina, and not to another cause of chest pain.

Angina is typically divided into stable or unstable angina. There is considerable overlap in the medical treatment between these classifications. Intuitively, this makes sense since stable and unstable angina share the same underlying pathophysiology. However, the extent and degree of treatment varies according to the stability of angina. Essentially, the greater the degree of unstable symptoms, the more aggressive the treatment modality should be in treating CAD.

The term unstable angina encompasses a patient who presents with slightly worsening angina, to extreme chest pain with full coronary artery obstruction consistent with ST segment elevation on the standard 12 lead EKG. Recognizing this slope of disease burden, the term unstable angina is being replaced by the term "acute coronary syndrome" (ACS). ACS denotes a patient who is at a higher risk of having an ischemic coronary event, and therefore urges stronger consideration of aggressive management. The surface EKG is the first step in treatment direction when ACS is diagnosed. Typically, the EKG classifies patients into ST segment elevation myocardial infarction or non-ST segment myocardial infarction, with the former process requiring immediate and aggressive treatment.

This chapter will discuss the diagnosis and treatment of non-ST segment myocardial infarction. For a discussion regarding the management of ST segment myocardial infarction, please refer to chapter XXX. The utility of biochemical markers, role of distinct medical agents, and decision to pursue conservative or invasive strategies will be reviewed.

Laboratory Markers of Non-St Segment Myocardial Infarction Acute Coronary Syndrome

In the United States, there are about 5 million patient visits each year to the emergency department with the primary complaint of chest pain. [5] Identifying patients with chest pain caused by angina requires a careful assessment to exclude other causes of their symptoms. Furthermore, risk stratifying patients with acute coronary syndrome non-ST segment elevation myocardial infarction who are at a high risk for future coronary events is a difficult challenge. The development of sensitive biochemical markers were developed to assist in early risk stratification.

Troponin I and Troponin T are proteins that regulate the calcium mediated contractive process in cardiac muscle. These proteins are absent from circulation under normal conditions. Therefore, the detection of these proteins may signify signs of cardiac damage. Similarly, the proteins creatine kinase (CK) and the MB fraction of CK (CK-MB) are elevated in ACS; however these proteins can also be elevated in individuals who are not having coronary ischemia. Therefore the detection of serum troponins is a useful marker in detecting cardiac damage.

Positive levels of troponin blood levels can lag several hours after myocardial damage. Thus a patient who presents with chest pain from a non-ST segment elevation myocardial infarction may have cardiac ischemia despite negative troponins. The general approach is to check a troponin level from 6-12 hours after the initial blood draw. The difference/change in serial troponin values adds important prognostic information in diagnosing myocardial infarction. A recent study found that the delta change in troponin concentration within 3 hours from the baseline value increased the positive predictive value for ruling in myocardial infarction from 75.1% at admission to 95.8% after 3 hours. [6]

A negative troponin value does not exclude the diagnosis of CAD or ACS – the level may have been drawn too early for blood serum detection, or the disease process may not have caused enough myocardial damage to yield elevated cardiac enzymes. The Diagnostic Marker Cooperative study evaluated patients who presented to the emergency department and found that the most sensitive and specific markers were CK-MB at 10 hours and troponin at 18 hours from symptom onset. [7] This clearly demonstrates that in the absence of ischemic EKG changes, negative cardiac enzymes should not be used to exclude CAD or ACS. The goal of measuring cardiac enzymes in the emergency department is to assist in providing early identification of patients who present with chest pain without ST segment elevation myocardial infarction who may be at a high risk of adverse coronary events. [8] However, one should never underestimate the importance of clinical history and ECG findings. In a study evaluation of more than 10,000 patients admitted for acute chest pain, patients with a < 1% likelihood of cardiac complications could be identified utilizing the history and physical, admission ECG, and hemodynamic status of the patient. [9]

While troponin release signifies myocardial damage, detectible levels can confuse clinicians. Serum troponin levels represent myocardial stress, and therefore may be elevated in the setting of excessive myocardial demand rather than cardiac damage. For example, elevated cardiac enzymes can be seen in patients with renal insufficiency, cancer, rhabdomyolysis, pulmonary embolism, aortic dissection, endocarditis, and hypertensive crises. [10, 11, 12, 13]

Given the high sensitivity and specificity of troponin in relation to myocardial damage, perhaps the best yield of utilizing this enzyme may be in patients who have a moderate risk of ACS with negative EKG abnormalities. If serum troponin is elevated, the patient may need more aggressive treatment such as a cardiac catherization. Conversely, a negative troponin value suggests a more conservative approach. This noninvasive work up could include 24 hour observation, stress testing, or both.

While CK, CK-MB, and troponin are the conventional blood markers used to diagnose ACS, several other markers have shown remarkable sensitivity and specificity in detecting coronary ischemia. Heart fatty acid-binding protein (H-FABP) is released within 90 minutes of myocardial sarcolemma damage and has the same sensitivity and specificity of troponin in detecting ACS. [14, 15, 16, 17] Similarly, abnormal serum levels of myeloperoxidase, [18] soluble CD 40 ligand, [19] and copeptin [20] have been associated with ACS. While these biochemical markers show promise, they lack the evidence from large clinical trials.

Therefore, CK, CK-MB, and troponin remain the gold standard in the early identification of acute coronary syndrome.

Medical Therapy

Anti-Ischemic Therapy

Acute coronary syndrome can produce vasoconstriction and heart rate elevation due to catecholamine secretion. This can lead to a mismatch between the demand and supply of oxygen to the heart. The goal of anti-ischemic therapy is to alter the hemodynamics and improve the supply/demand balance of desired myocardial oxygen.

Beta-blockers are routinely used in treating acute coronary syndrome and have clinical data demonstrating a long term benefit. [21, 22] Contraindications include bradycardia, newly decompensated heart failure, hypotension, or high degree atrioventricular block. If beta-blockers cannot be used, non-dihydropyridine calcium channel blockers can be substituted provided there is no evidence of left ventricular dysfunction.

Antiplatelet Agents

Aspirin is standard therapy in treating coronary artery disease. The long-term benefits of aspirin have been demonstrated in many clinical trials. [23, 24] The dose of aspirin varies amongst providers, with standard formulations ranging from 81mg to 325mg. While controversy exists over which dose is optimal, literature does suggest that higher doses are associated with more bleeding complications. [25, 26] Since many patients are routinely treated with other agents that can cause bleeding, perhaps the most prudent dose is 81mg.

Ticlodipine, clopidogrel, and prasugrel are drugs that interfere with the ADP-mediated activation of platelet P2Y12. Ticlodipine has been replaced by the newer agents due to its side effect profile. The efficacy of clopidogrel in treating acute coronary syndrome was demonstrated in the CURE trial. When combined with aspirin, clopidogrel therapy led to a significant reduction in cardiovascular death, myocardial infarction, or stroke. [27] While the benefit of clopidogrel in ACS is evident, the timing and loading dose remain controversial. There is evidence that "upfront" loading (given before angiography) of clopidogrel is beneficial in unstable angina. [28, 29] Finally, there is considerable evidence that a higher loading dose of 600mg has more benefits than a 300mg loading dose. [30, 31]

Prasugrel has a faster onset of action and is able to achieve higher platelet inhibition than clopidogrel. In TRITON-TIMI-38, prasugrel demonstrated a significant reduction versus clopidogrel in the combined rate of death from cardiovascular causes, nonfatal myocardial infarction, or nonfatal stroke in patients who presented with ACS and who underwent percutaneous coronary intervention (PCI). [32] However, there was an increase in the rate of serious bleeding in the prasugrel group. It seems that the more effective anti-ischemic effect of prasugrel must be balanced against its higher rate of bleeding when compared to clopidogrel. The optimal use of prasugrel may be in certain patient subgroups such as those who present with a high thrombus burden or in diabetics. [33]

Ticagrelor is another oral antiplatelet agent that has efficacy in treating acute coronary syndrome. As compared to clopidogrel and prasugrel, ticagrelor has a shorter half-life. The PLATO study demonstrated a significant reduction of cardiovascular events for patients who received ticagrelor versus those treated with clopidogrel in the setting of ACS. [34]

In short, the antiplatelet agents clopidogrel, prasugrel, and ticagrelor are beneficial for patients who present with acute coronary syndrome. Each drug has a distinct pharmacokinetic profile, and the use of each one should be individualized to the particular patient and clinical scenario.

Glycoprotein IIb-IIIa antagonists are drugs that produce a blockade of the GPIIb-IIIα2β3 integrin platelet aggregation. The efficacy of these drugs in treating patients with ACS has been validated in several trials. [35, 36, 37] While the benefits of these drugs has been established, the decision when to start them is more controversial. Recently, there has been evidence to suggest that there is no benefit to upfront loading/upstream initiation of the Glycoprotein IIb-IIIa antagonists in ACS, and that a delayed strategy is associated with less bleeding. [38, 39]

In conclusion, antiplatelet therapy is clearly beneficial in treating patients with acute coronary syndrome. While the use of aspirin is almost always a certainty, the agents discussed above have their own distinct clinical benefits. This choice of a particular agent is dictated by the clinical scenario. The benefits of glycoprotein IIb-IIIa antagonists may be negated by the newer antiplatelet agents clopidogrel, prasugrel, and ticagrelor because of the rapid onset of action of these drugs at higher loading doses.

Antithrombotic Agents

Heparin has been used in the setting of acute coronary syndrome for decades. Several studies have shown the benefits of heparin in treating unstable angina. [40, 41] Generally, a bolus dose is given followed by an infusion drip. The most common complication of heparin is bleeding. Other side effects include heparin induced thrombocytopenia, skin necrosis, and urticaria.

The low molecular weight heparins (LMWHs) are processed from the fractionation of standard heparin. The uptake and bioavailability is rapid, achieving a more predictable anticoagulation effect. Several studies have compared the LWMH enoxaparin with standard heparin. [42, 43, 44] While some trials demonstrate a benefit of LMWH over standard heparin, other evidence suggests that there is no advantage. It is important to remember that the trials were not standardized to each other, and that there were different dosing regimens of agents along with the use of other ACS medications (anti-platelets) across a variety of doses. These factors may have had an effect on the outcomes of each particular trial. While controversy exists over the best agent, it is safe to say that the LMWHs are not inferior to heparin in treating patients with ACS. Similar to heparin and enoxaparin, fondaparinux, a synthetic heparin pentasaccharide, has shown efficacy in treating patients who present with unstable angina. [45]

The direct thrombin inhibitor bivalarudin is more capable than heparin in inhibiting clot-bound thrombin. The efficacy of this agent was demonstrated in the ACUITY trial. Patients who presented with ACS were randomized to heparin plus a glycoprotein IIb/IIIa inhibitor, bivalarudin plus a glycoprotein IIb/IIIa inhibitor, or bivalarudin alone. As a whole, the data suggest that bivalarudin alone has similar ischemic outcomes with lower rates of bleeding when compared to heparin. [46]

In summary, the addition of antithrombotic medication is certainly beneficial in ACS. There are several choices, and each agent has distinct advantages and disadvantages that should be evaluated in each clinical situation.

Statins

While the HMG coA reductase inhibitors are commonly used for preventative therapy in patients with coronary artery disease, diabetes mellitus, and peripheral artery disease, statins also have a role in treating patients with acute coronary syndrome. In MIRACL, patients with ACS were randomized to high dose atorvastatin or placebo within 24-96 hours of admission. Patients who received upfront atorvastatin had a significant benefit in the prevention of recurrent ischemic events. [47] The PROVE-IT trial demonstrated that more intense statin therapy upfront in patients with ACS further reduced ischemic events by comparing atorvastatin to pravastatin. Those who received the higher statin dose had a significant benefit over patients who received the lower statin dose. [48] These findings suggest that in addition to lowering the LDL levels, statin therapy has an immediate pleiotropic effect that has a benefit if given to patients early in the course of acute coronary syndrome at a high dose.

Approach to Acute Coronary Syndrome

After diagnosing acute coronary syndrome, medical therapy should be instituted immediately. Next, management should be aimed towards a conservative or aggressive treatment plan. While it may seem intuitive that revascularization is better than a conservative approach, early studies suggested that there was no benefit of invasive cardiac procedures in patients with non-ST segment elevation myocardial infarction/unstable angina. [49,50] However, these trials were performed before newer medical agents and advanced equipment was developed. Therefore the data may not be applicable to contemporary practice.

Recent data suggests that there is a significant benefit when opting for an invasive approach in treating ACS. The Treat Angina with Aggrastat and Determine Cost of Therapy with an Invasive or Conservative Strategy (TACTIS-TIMI 18), The Randomized Intervention Trial of unstable Angina (RITA-3), and The Fragmin and Fast Revascularization during Instability in CAD (FRISC II) trials demonstrated that an early invasive approach provides a significant benefit over conservative therapy. [51, 52, 53] Specifically, it seems that the benefit of invasive and aggressive treatment is remarkably beneficial in patients who have a large burden of disease/high risk features. [54] That is, the larger the ischemic burden, the greater the benefit gained when treatment is invasive.

Conclusion

Thousands of patients present to the emergency room with the chief complaint of chest pain. After excluding other causes of non-cardiac chest pain, a work up to diagnosis acute coronary syndrome should incorporate the patient's history & physical, laboratory testing, and diagnostics including the surface 12 lead EKG. When ACS is diagnosed, and the 12 lead EKG is not consistent with ST elevation myocardial infarction, there is a plethora of medications that should be instituted, unless contraindications exist. While the medications between unstable angina/non-ST segment elevation myocardial infarction and ST segment myocardial infarction overlap, the latter diagnosis requires more aggressive immediate treatment upfront.

Anti-ischemic medications have a symptomatic and long term cardiovascular benefit. Every patient should be considered for dual antiplatelet therapy, which should include aspirin. The additional antiplatelet can range from glycoprotein IIb/IIIa inhibitors to clopidogrel, prasugrel, or ticagrelor. The decision to choose between these different agents is dictated by each clinical scenario. Similarly, an antithorombotic should be started, and the choice of a specific agent is individualized to the case. Finally, a high dose statin should be started upfront given the immediate and long term benefits of these agents in treating acute coronary syndrome.

After initiating medical therapy, patients with acute coronary syndrome and high risk features including elevated cardiac biomarkers, unstable hemodynamics, or deleterious dysrhythmias should be considered for an invasive strategy. The timing of intervention is dictated by the degree of disease. The larger the burden of disease, the greater the benefit gained the earlier the intervention is initiated.

The mode of revascularization is either percutaneous coronary intervention or coronary artery bypass surgery (CABG). Traditionally, CABG was performed for triple vessel disease or left main disease due to a benefit across all combined ischemic end points. However, newer stent design and antiplatelet therapy has decreased the gap between CABG and PCI. Regardless of the route chosen, medical therapy must be continued. Finally, risk factor modification is absolutely necessary. Cardiac rehabilitation is a class I recommendation after acute coronary syndrome. [55] The benefits of exercise should never be underestimated.

References

[1] Go, AS; Mozaffarian, D; Roger, VL; et al. Heart disease and stroke statistics--2013 update: a report from the American Heart Association. *Circulation.*, 2013 Jan 1, 127(1), e6-e245.

[2] Boersma, E; Pieper, KS; Steyerberg, EW; et al. Predictors of outcome in patients with acute coronary syndromes without persistent ST-segment elevation. Results from an international trial of 9461 patients. The PURSUIT Investigators. *Circulation.*, 2000 Jun 6, 101(22), 2557-67.

[3] Antman, EM; Cohen, M; Bernink, PJ; et al. The TIMI risk score for unstable angina/non-ST elevation MI: A method for prognostication and therapeutic decision making. *JAMA.*, 2000 Aug 16, 284(7), 835-42.

[4] Rawlings, C; Oglesby, K; Turner, J; et al. Comparison of two clinical scoring systems in risk stratification of non-ST elevation acute coronary syndrome patients in predicting 30-day outcomes. *Emerg Med J.*, 2012 Jan, 29(1), 40-2

[5] Pitts, SR; Niska, RW; Xu, J; et al. National Hospital Ambulatory Medical Care Survey: 2006 emergency department summary. *Natl Health Stat Report.*, 2008 Aug 6, (7), 1-38.

[6] Keller, T; Zeller, T; Ojeda, F; et al. Serial changes in highly sensitive troponin I assay and early diagnosis of myocardial infarction. *JAMA.*, 2011 Dec 28, 306(24), 2684-93.

[7] Zimmerman, J; Fromm, R; Meyer, D; et al. Diagnostic marker cooperative study for the diagnosis of myocardial infarction. *Circulation.*, 1999 Apr 6, 99(13), 1671-7.

[8] Holmvang, L; Lüscher, MS; Clemmensen, et al. Very early risk stratification using combined ECG and biochemical assessment in patients with unstable coronary artery disease (A thrombin inhibition in myocardial ischemia [TRIM] substudy). The TRIM Study Group. *Circulation*, 1998 Nov 10, 98(19), 2004-9.

[9] Goldman, L; Cook, EF; Johnson, PA; et al. Prediction of the need for intensive care in patients who come to the emergency departments with acute chest pain. *N Engl J Med.*, 1996 Jun 6, 334(23), 1498-504.

[10] Konstantinides, S; Geibel, A; Olschewski, et al. Importance of cardiac troponins I and T in risk stratification of patients with acute pulmonary embolism. *Circulation.*, 2002 Sep 3, 106(10), 1263-8

[11] Punukollu, G; Gowda, RM; Khan, IA; et al. Elevated serum cardiac troponin I in rhabdomyolysis. *Int J Cardiol.*, 2004 Jul, 96(1), 35-40.

[12] Punukollu, G; Khan, IA; Gowda, RM; et al. Cardiac troponin I release in acute pulmonary embolism in relation to the duration of symptoms. *Int J Cardiol.*, 2005 Mar 18, 99(2), 207-11.

[13] Agewall, S; Giannitsis, E; Jernberg, T; et al. Troponin elevation in coronary vs. non-coronary disease. *Eur Heart J.*, 2011 Feb, 32(4), 404-11

[14] Alhadi, HA; Fox, KA. Do we need additional markers of myocyte necrosis: the potential value of heart fatty-acid-binding protein. *QJM.*, 2004 Apr, 97(4), 187-98.

[15] Valle, HA; Riesgo, LG; Bel, MS; et al. Clinical assessment of heart-type fatty acid binding protein in early diagnosis of acute coronary syndrome. *Eur J Emerg Med.*, 2008 Jun, 15(3), 140-4

[16] McMahon, CG; Lamont, JV; Curtin, E; et al. Diagnostic accuracy of heart-type fatty acid-binding protein for the early diagnosis of acute myocardial infarction. *Am J Emerg Med.*, 2012 Feb, 30(2), 267-74

[17] Viswanathan, K; Kilcullen, N; Morrell, C; et al. Heart-type fatty acid-binding protein predicts long-term mortality and re-infarction in consecutive patients with suspected acute coronary syndrome who are troponin-negative. *J Am CollCardiol.*, 2010 Jun 8, 55(23), 2590-8

[18] Brennan, ML; Penn, MS; Van Lente, F; et al. Prognostic value of myeloperoxidase in patients with chest pain. *N Engl J Med.*, 2003 Oct 23, 349(17), 1595-604.

[19] Aukrust, P; Müller, F; Ueland, T; et al. Enhanced levels of soluble and membrane-bound CD40 ligand in patients with unstable angina.Possible reflection of T lymphocyte and platelet involvement in the pathogenesis of acute coronary syndromes. *Circulation.*, 1999 Aug 10, 100(6), 614-20.

[20] Keller, T; Tzikas, S; Zeller, T; et al. Copeptin improves early diagnosis of acute myocardial infarction. *J Am CollCardiol.*, 2010 May 11, 55(19), 2096-106

[21] Goldstein, S. Propranolol therapy in patients with acute myocardial infarction, the Beta-Blocker Heart Attack Trial. *Circulation.*, 1983 Jun, 67(6 Pt 2), I53-7.

[22] Metoprolol in acute myocardial infarction (MIAMI). A randomised placebo-controlled international trial.The MIAMI Trial Research Group. *Eur Heart J.*, 1985 Mar, 6(3), 199-226.

[23] Lewis, HD; Jr. Davis, JW; Archibald, DG; et al. Protective effects of aspirin against acute myocardial infarction and death in men with unstable angina. Results of a Veterans Administration Cooperative Study. *N Engl J Med.*, 1983 Aug 18, 309(7), 396-403

[24] Cairns, JA; Gent, M; Singer, J; et al. Aspirin, sulfinpyrazone, or both in unstable angina.Results of a Canadian multicenter trial. *N Engl J Med.*, 1985 Nov 28, 313(22), 1369-75.

[25] Serebruany, VL1; Steinhubl, SR; Berger, PB; et al. Analysis of risk of bleeding complications after different doses of aspirin in 192,036 patients enrolled in 31 randomized controlled trials. *Am J Cardiol.*, 2005 May 15, 95(10), 1218-22

[26] DiNicolantonio, JJ1; Norgard, NB; Meier, P; et al. Optimal aspirin dose in acute coronary syndromes: an emerging consensus. *Future Cardiol.* 2014 Mar, 10(2), 291-300.

[27] The Clopidogrel in Unstable Angina to Prevent Recurrent Events Trial Investigators. Effects of Clopidogrel in Addition to Aspirin in Patients with Acute Coronary Syndromes without ST-Segment Elevation. *N Engl J Med.*, 2001, 345, 494-502.

[28] Steinhubl, SR; Berger, PB; Brennan, DM; et al. Optimal timing for the initiation of pre-treatment with 300 mg clopidogrel before percutaneous coronary intervention. *J Am CollCardiol.*, 2006 Mar 7, 47(5), 939-43

[29] Sabatine, MS; Cannon, CP; Gibson, CM; et al. Effect of clopidogrel pretreatment before percutaneous coronary intervention in patients with ST-elevation myocardial infarction treated with fibrinolytics: the PCI-CLARITY study. *JAMA.*, 2005 Sep 14, 294(10), 1224-32

[30] Cuisset, T; Frere, C; Quilici, J; et al. Benefit of a 600-mg loading dose of clopidogrel on platelet reactivity and clinical outcomes in patients with non-ST-segment elevation acute coronary syndrome undergoing coronary stenting. *J Am CollCardiol.*, 2006 Oct 3, 48(7), 1339-45.

[31] Patti, G; Colonna, G; Pasceri, V; et al. Randomized trial of high loading dose of clopidogrel for reduction of periprocedural myocardial infarction in patients undergoing coronary intervention: results from the ARMYDA-2 (Antiplatelet therapy for Reduction of MYocardial Damage during Angioplasty) study. *Circulation.*, 2005 Apr 26, 111(16), 2099-106

[32] Wiviott, SD; Braunwald, E; McCabe, CH; et al. Prasugrel versus clopidogrel in patients with acute coronary syndromes. *N Engl J Med.*, 2007 Nov 15, 357(20), 2001-15.

[33] Wiviott, SD1; Antman, EM; Braunwald, E. Prasugrel. *Circulation.*, 2010 Jul 27, 122(4), 394-403

[34] Wallentin, L1; Becker, RC; Budaj, A; et al. Ticagrelor versus clopidogrel in patients with acute coronary syndromes. *N Engl J Med.*, 2009 Sep 10, 361(11), 1045-57

[35] A comparison of aspirin plus tirofiban with aspirin plus heparin for unstable angina.Platelet Receptor Inhibition in Ischemic Syndrome Management (PRISM) Study Investigators. *N Engl J Med.*, 1998 May 21, 338(21), 1498-505.

[36] Inhibition of platelet glycoprotein IIb/IIIa with eptifibatide in patients with acute coronary syndromes.The PURSUIT Trial Investigators. Platelet Glycoprotein IIb/IIIa in Unstable Angina: Receptor Suppression Using Integrilin Therapy. *N Engl J Med.*, 1998 Aug 13, 339(7), 436-43.

[37] Randomised placebo-controlled trial of abciximab before and during coronary intervention in refractory unstable angina: the CAPTURE Study. *Lancet.*, 1997 May 17, 349(9063), 1429-35.

[38] Stone, GW; Bertrand, ME; Moses, JW; et al. Routine upstream initiation vs deferred selective use of glycoprotein IIb/IIIa inhibitors in acute coronary syndromes: the ACUITY Timing trial. *JAMA.*, 2007 Feb 14, 297(6), 591-602

[39] Giugliano, RP; White, JA; Bode, C; et al. Early versus delayed, provisional eptifibatide in acute coronary syndromes. *N Engl J Med.*, 2009 May 21, 360(21), 2176-90

[40] Oler, A; Whooley, MA; Oler, J; et al. Adding heparin to aspirin reduces the incidence of myocardial infarction and death in patients with unstable angina. A meta-analysis. *JAMA.*, 1996 Sep 11, 276(10), 811-5.

[41] Théroux, P1; Ouimet, H; McCans, J; et al. Aspirin, heparin, or both to treat acute unstable angina. N Engl J Med., 1988 Oct 27, 319(17), 1105-11

[42] Cohen, M1; Demers, C; Gurfinkel, EP; et al. comparison of low-molecular-weight heparin with unfractionated heparin for unstable coronary artery disease. Efficacy and Safety of Subcutaneous Enoxaparin in Non-Q-Wave Coronary Events Study Group. *N Engl J Med.*, 1997 Aug 14, 337(7), 447-52.

[43] Antman, EM; McCabe, CH; Gurfinkel, EP; et al. Enoxaparin prevents death and cardiac ischemic events in unstable angina/non-Q-wave myocardial infarction. Results of the thrombolysis in myocardial infarction (TIMI) 11B trial. *Circulation.*, 1999 Oct 12, 100(15), 1593-601.

[44] Ferguson, JJ; Califf, RM; Antman, EM; et al. Enoxaparin vs unfractionated heparin in high-risk patients with non-ST-segment elevation acute coronary syndromes managed with an intended early invasive strategy: primary results of the SYNERGY randomized trial. *JAMA.*, 2004 Jul 7, 292(1), 45-54.

[45] Mehta, SR; Boden, WE; Eikelboom, et al. Antithrombotic therapy with fondaparinux in relation to interventional management strategy in patients with ST- and non-ST-segment elevation acute coronary syndromes: an individual patient-level combined analysis of the Fifth and Sixth Organization to Assess Strategies in Ischemic Syndromes (OASIS 5 and 6) randomized trials. *Circulation.*, 2008 Nov 11, 118(20), 2038-46.

[46] Stone, GW1; McLaurin, BT; Cox, DA; et al. Bivalirudin for patients with acute coronary syndromes. *N Engl J Med.*, 2006 Nov 23, 355(21), 2203-16.

[47] Schwartz, GG1; Olsson, AG; Ezekowitz, MD; et al. Effects of atorvastatin on early recurrent ischemic events in acute coronary syndromes: the MIRACL study: a randomized controlled trial. *JAMA.*, 2001 Apr 4, 285(13), 1711-8.

[48] Cannon, CP; Braunwald, E; McCabe, CH; et al. Intensive versus moderate lipid lowering with statins after acute coronary syndromes. *N Engl J Med.*, 2004 Apr 8, 350(15), 1495-504

[49] Boden, WE; O'Rourke, RA; Crawford, MH; et. Al. Outcomes in patients with acute non-Q-wave myocardial infarction randomly assigned to an invasive as compared with a conservative management strategy. Veterans Affairs Non-Q-Wave Infarction

Strategies in Hospital (VANQWISH) Trial Investigators. *N Engl J Med.*, 1998 Jun 18, 338(25), 1785-92.

[50] Yusuf, S; Flather M; Pogue J; et al. Variations between countries in invasive cardiac procedures and outcomes in patients with suspected unstable angina or myocardial infarction without initial ST elevation. OASIS (Organisation to Assess Strategies for Ischaemic Syndromes) Registry Investigators. *Lancet.*, 1998 Aug 15, 352(9127), 507-14.

[51] Cannon, CP; Weintraub, WS, Demopoulos, LA; et al. Comparison of early invasive and conservative strategies in patients with unstable coronary syndromes treated with the glycoprotein IIb/IIIa inhibitor tirofiban. *N Engl J Med.*, 2001 Jun 21, 344(25), 1879-87.

[52] Fox, KA; Poole-Wilson, PA; Henderson RA; et. al. Interventional versus conservative treatment for patients with unstable angina or non-ST-elevation myocardial infarction: the British Heart Foundation RITA 3 randomised trial. Randomized Intervention Trial of unstable Angina. *Lancet.*, 2002 Sep 7, 360(9335), 743-51.

[53] Wallentin, L; Lagerqvist, B; Husted S; et al. Outcome at 1 year after an invasive compared with a non-invasive strategy in unstable coronary-artery disease: the FRISC II invasive randomised trial. FRISC II Investigators. Fast Revascularisation during Instability in Coronary artery disease. *Lancet.*, 2000 Jul 1, 356(9223), 9-16.

[54] Mehta, SR; Granger, CB; Boden, WE; et al. Early versus delayed invasive intervention in acute coronary syndromes. *N Engl J Med.*, 2009 May 21, 360(21), 2165-75

[55] Anderson, JL; Adams, CD; Antman, EM; et al. ACC/AHA 2007 guidelines for the management of patients with unstable angina/non ST-elevation myocardial infarction: a report of the American College of Cardiology/American Heart Association Task Force on Practice Guidelines (Writing Committee to Revise the 2002 Guidelines for the Management of Patients With Unstable Angina/Non ST-Elevation Myocardial Infarction): developed in collaboration with the American College of Emergency Physicians, the Society for Cardiovascular Angiography and Interventions, and the Society of Thoracic Surgeons: endorsed by the American Association of Cardiovascular and Pulmonary Rehabilitation and the Society for Academic Emergency Medicine. *Circulation.*, 2007 Aug 14, 116(7), e148-304.

Index

B

C

D

E

F

G

H

I

J

K

L

M

Q

R

S

T

U

V

W

X

Y

Z